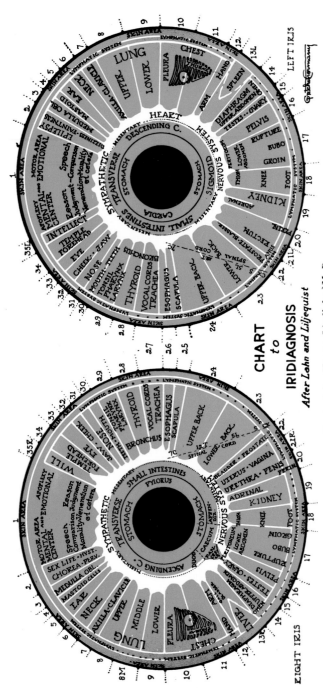

CHART
to
IRIDIAGNOSIS
After Lahn and Liljequist
Revised by Henry Lindlahr, M. D.

PHILOSOPHY

OF

NATURAL THERAPEUTICS

HENRY LINDLAHR M.D.

EDITED AND REVISED

By

JOCELYN C. P. PROBY, M.A., B.Litt (Oxon), D.O. (Kirksville, U.S.A.).

The C.W. Daniel Company Limited
Saffron Walden, Essex, England

First published in 1975 by
The Maidstone Osteopathic Clinic in Great Britain.

This edition published by
The C.W. Daniel Company Limited
1 Church Path, Saffron Walden, Essex, CB10 1JP, England

Revisions & Additions © Jocelyn Proby 1975

ISBN 0 85207 159 0

Reprinted 1987
Reprinted 1988
Reprinted 1993

Printed in Great Britain by
Hillman Printers (Frome) Ltd., Frome, Somerset.

CONTENTS

CONTENTS

"Ho, ye who suffer! Know ye suffer from yourselves. None else compels . . . no other holds ye
that ye live or die"

Siddartha

Evil is not an accident, not an arbitrary punishment, not always an "error
of mortal mind". It is the natural and inevitable result of violation of
nature's laws. It is instructive and corrective in purpose, and will remain
with us only so long as we need its salutary lessons.

ACKNOWLEDGEMENT

I wish to express my thanks to the many friends who have helped me in the preparation of this volume by giving advice and information and by typing and reading proofs. I would specially mention Mr. L. R. Ogden who went through the whole text with me in detail and made many useful criticisms and suggestions, and Mr. John Wernham who has undertaken the carrying out of printing and publication. It is my hope that I shall be able to prepare in the coming months two or three further volumes covering the other writings of Dr. Lindlahr.

J.P. Arklow, Ireland, 1975

EDITOR'S INTRODUCTION

Having decided that I should attempt to bring out a new edition of the works of the late Dr. Henry Lindlahr a few words of explanation are necessary. Ever since I became acquainted with these books some forty years ago I have become more and more convinced of their enormous importance and more and more astonished that they appear now to be neglected and almost unknown even among those who claim to be practising one of those techniques or forms of therapy which are said to be "natural".

The works of Lindlahr consist of four volumes, (1) The Philosophy of Natural Therapeutics, (2) Practice of Natural Therapeutics, (3) The Lindlahr Vegetarian Cook Book and A.B.C. of Natural Dietetics, (4) Iridiagnosis and other Diagnostic Methods. Lindlahr certainly intended to bring out one or two further volumes but, as far as I can discover, they did not reach the point of being published. One volume entitled "Nature Cure Eugenics, or Man-Building on the Physical, Mental and Moral Planes of Being" was certainly planned and would undoubtedly have been of great interest as carrying further his teaching and ideas on a number of matters which are only touched upon in the existing volumes.

The editing of these works of fifty years ago for the contemporary reader poses a number of problems and requires a knowledge of the development of orthodox medicine and scientific research in which I feel myself to be in many respects deficient. I have, however, tried to follow a certain plan and certain principles in carrying out the work. Though I have cut out sentences and paragraphs here and there where they appeared to be repetitive or no longer of interest or importance in these days, I have not altered Dr. Lindlahr's wording or the current of his arrangement and discourse except in a few instances where I have felt that his wording or phraseology is very dated or archaic or where for reasons of taste it grates upon the ear. For there is no doubt that he is on the whole a master of very clear, concise and expressive English prose and that he is also a person of such distinguished mind and such wide knowledge and experience that I have not felt justified in altering or censoring what he has to say even when I did not agree with it. Moreover, although he wrote so long ago, one is astonished by how little he can be said to be out of date and by how often he appears to be ahead of his age. There are, however, some places

1

in which I have felt notes to be required to draw attention to other points of view, to changes which have taken place in medical thought and practice and to advances in scientific knowledge which appear to have a bearing on his arguments or conclusions.

The importance of his work may be stated in the light of his own claim to be laying the foundations of a true Science of Medicine, and I verily believe that this he has in fact done. For if we think of it we must acknowledge that there is really no such thing as a Science of Medicine in the true sense of the term. We hear much indeed of Medicine being scientific and it is true that it makes much use of scientific terms and phraseology and uses many techniques and methods of a scientific nature. Also it is true that some of the subsidiary sciences which are useful and essential to the building of a Science of Medicine have reached a very considerable degree of advancement. Yet it cannot truthfully be said that a Science of Medicine really exists, though it may perhaps be struggling to be born. The basic idea of Science is, surely, that we live in an universe which is governed and proceeds according to law. It is recognised that if we can discover the laws governing any particular objects or phenomena and devise techniques for using those laws we shall be able to use and command Nature by first learning to obey. If, therefore, there is to be a true Science of Medicine it must be before all else a Science of Health and it must recognise that Health and Disease, like everything else, are subject to laws and are not matters of chance and beyond our control, as is now so very generally believed. A beginning must be made to discover at least some of the basic laws and principles which govern Health and the violation of which lead to Disease. This work has so far scarcely been begun either by mankind at large or by doctors and scientists of the orthodox school. This, it would seem, is because disease in general and particular diseases are studied far more than health, in the belief that it may be possible to find an explanation and a specific cure for every disease and that by so doing health will come to the world. Thus it is that most methods of treatment which are at present used are really empirical rather than scientific however much they may profess to be the latter. Empiricism is not necessarily a bad thing and may indeed sometimes come from an intuitive perception of what is the right thing to do in a particular situation, but it also has very great dangers, for it can very easily do harm rather than good in the long run if it in fact violates one or more of the great natural laws by which health and disease are governed.

What is important about Dr. Lindlahr's work is that he has studied and does lay down some at least of the basic laws on which Health depends. He shows very convincingly that disease is in fact the result of our individual or collective violation of those laws either through ignorance or wilfulness and that it is therefore in our power within a very reasonable time to rid ourselves of disease. This is a cheering and optimistic thought. What is less cheering is that he shows also very convincingly that much disease is not only self-made but doctor-made. In spite of very good progress in certain directions and in the technique of such things as surgery and obstetrics it is sometimes difficult not to feel that the negative and suppressive methods which are so widely employed are putting doctors in the unhappy position of creating more disease than they cure. For there is not much doubt that, if, for a variety of reasons of which perhaps improved hygiene is the most important, acute disease is less prevalent and less dangerous than it once was, the same cannot be said of chronic diseases. Nervous, mental, malignant and rheumatic diseases are certainly not on the decrease, and also there is an immeasurable quantity of non-health and sub-health, so that it is not very easy to find many people who can be described as perfectly healthy.

It will be noted by those reading and studying the Philosophy of Natural Therapeutics that it contains an amount of material which could be regarded or criticized as being philosophical or even religious rather than medical. Though some of this material may be controversial and unacceptable to some people, it appears to me that its inclusion is entirely justifiable and, indeed, necessary if a true and complete picture is to be obtained of the problems of health, disease and therapeutics in the contemporary world. While therapeutics is primarily concerned with the health of the physical body and the physical body is a physical and chemical entity which is subject to the laws of physics and chemistry, it is becoming more and more clear that the whole answer to the problems of disease and therapeutics is not to be found in the study of physics and chemistry and the material sciences allied thereto. This surely, is, because it is now very obvious that the physical body as we perceive it and know about it through our ordinary senses is not the whole man and perhaps not really the essential man at all. Lindlahr seems to make two points in this connection. The first is that the physical body should be looked upon as something which is part of a much larger whole and that it is linked to other bodies which act upon it and are acted upon by it. The second is that the physical body is subject to the influence of energies which are brought to bear on it and flow into it both from these other bodies and from outside. It follows from this that much disease which appears to be entirely physical is due to something being wrong in the mental, emotional or spiritual sphere of which the physical trouble is merely the reflexion. Conversely much mental and psychological trouble has for its origin a condition of the body which has so impaired the functioning of the brain and nervous system that they cease to be able to meet the demands made upon them. Thus it follows that the physician must learn to judge and to distinguish and to approach his cases in such a way as to bring the whole man into a harmonious and healthy state. In one case the physical approach will be the most important and may, indeed, be all that is required, but in another case it is more the mental, emotional or spiritual condition of the patient that requires to be changed and corrected and this will call for different and more subtle types of technique which have in the past been looked upon as being in the sphere of the psychologist, the priest or the spiritual healer rather than the doctor. Experience would seem to show that in actual fact most cases which we meet require both types of approach in different proportions.

In reading and editing Lindlahr's books I am aware that the expression "Nature Cure" constantly repeated is irritating and apt to conjure up a picture of loosely dressed people dancing in the dew. However, "Nature Cure" is the name which Dr. Lindlahr has chosen to give to the system of therapeutics which he sets forth and advocates and I have not felt justified in altering it to "Naturopathy" or "Natural Therapeutics" wherever it occurs. The point to be remembered is that in fact all genuine Cure is and must be "natural" in the sense that it must work in accordance with natural law. If it does not do so it is not scientific and not really Cure at all. Much that now passes for Cure is in fact not Cure but is at best a palliation and at worst an aggravation of a condition of non-health.

Another difficulty which an editor of an English version of an American publication has to face is the differences in spelling of medical and some other words in the two countries. While I have made an effort to be consistent I may not always have succeeded.

In conclusion, I must add that I did myself obtain some experience of Dr. Lindlahr's ideas and methods in action. I corresponded for some time with Daniel Mackinnon, a Scot who had been trained by Dr. Lindlahr and worked with him in his institution, and subsequently I worked with him (Mackinnon) for a period as his pupil and assistant in Windsor, Ontario. Mackinnon, who was himself the author of a book entitled "The Conquest of Pain" was undoubtedly the person upon whom the mantle of Lindlahr had fallen. I have made use of extracts from his writings in some of my notes and appendices.

J.P. 1975

ANNOUNCEMENT

The term Natural Therapeutics has been adopted to designate that system of natural living and healing which I have evolved and demonstrated in many years of institutional work. While the pioneers of Nature Cure inaugurated the great world wide movement for simpler and more rational ways of living and treating human ailments, their teachings and methods were very limited in scope as compared with our present comprehensive system of Natural Therapeutics which covers not only the original theories and practices but includes all that has been found good in up to date drugless and bloodless therapy.

As the term "Nature Cure" became more generally adopted by the public and the healing professions it did not stand for anything definite in the way of a school or scientific system. The time has come when order and unity must be evolved out of this chaos of theoretical teachings and practical methods.

TO THE PROGRESSIVE PHYSICIANS OF THE AGE

There are two principal methods of treating disease. One is the combative, the other the preventive. The trend of modern medical research and practice in our great colleges and endowed research institutes is almost entirely along combative lines, while the individual, progressive physician learns to work more and more along preventive lines. The slogan of modern medical science is, "Kill the germ and cure the disease." The usual procedure is to wait until acute or chronic diseases have fully developed, and then, if possible, to subdue them by the use of drugs, surgical operations, and by means of the morbid products of disease, in the form of serums, antitoxins, vaccines, etc. The combative method fights disease with disease, poison with poison, and germs with germs and germ products. In the language of the Bible, it is "Beelzebub against the Devil."

The preventive method does not wait until disease has fully developed and gained ascendancy in the body, but concentrates its best endeavours on preventing, by hygienic living and by natural methods of treatment, the development of disease. Thus it endeavours to put the human body in such a normal, healthy condition that it is practically proof against infection or contagion by disease taints and miasms, and against the inroads of bacteria and parasites.

The question is, which method is the more practical, the more successful and more popular? Which will stand the test of "the survival of the fittest" in the great struggle for existence?

The medical profession has good reason to be alarmed by the inroads made in its work by irregular, unorthodox systems, schools and cults of treating human ailments; but instead of raging at the audacious presumption of these interlopers, would it not be better to inquire if there is not some reason for the astonishing spread and popularity of these therapeutic innovations? Their success is undoubtedly based on the fact that they concentrate their best efforts on preventive instead of combative methods of treating disease. People are beginning to realise that it is cheaper and more advantageous to prevent disease than to cure it. To create and maintain continuous, buoyant good health means greater efficiency for mental and physical work; greater capacity for the true enjoyment of life, and the best insurance against failure and poverty. Therefore, he who builds health is of greater value to humanity than he who allows people to drift into disease through ignorance of nature's laws, and then attempts to cure them by doubtful and uncertain combative methods. It is said that in China the physician is hired and paid by the year; that he receives a certain stipend as long as the members of the family are in good health, but that the salary is suspended as long as one of his charges is ill. If some similar method of engaging and paying for medical services were in vogue in this country the trend of medical research and practice would soon undergo a radical change.[1]

The diet expert, the hydrotherapist, the physical culturist, the adjuster of the spine, the mental healer and Christian Scientist, pay little attention to the pathological conditions or the symptoms of disease. Each of these, in accordance with his theory of disease and cure, regulates the diet and

---

[1]
The inauguration in recent times of public health services and the consequent payment of many doctors on some kind of salary basis has undoubtedly led to a change of thinking among some sections of the medical profession. As doctors no longer have the same vested interest in disease as they did formerly and are often very overworked, some of them have begun to ask themselves the reason for the enormous amount of disease with which they have to deal rather than to be contented with treating in some way the cases which come to them.

habits of living on a natural basis, promotes elimination, teaches correct breathing and wholesome exercises, corrects the mechanical lesions of the framework of the body, or establishes the right mental and emotional attitude, and, in so far as he succeeds in doing this, builds health and so diminishes the possibility of disease. The successful doctor of the future will have to fall in line with the procession and do more teaching than prescribing.(1)

I realize that many of the statements and claims made in this volume will seem radical and irrational to my colleagues of the allopathic school of medicine. They will say that most of my teachings are contrary to the firmly established theories of medical science. All I ask of them is to judge not too hastily; to observe, to think and to test, and I am certain that they will find verified in actual experience many of the teachings of the Nature Cure philosophy. Medical science has been forced to abandon innumerable theories and practices which were at one time as firmly established as some of the pet theories of today. By none of the statements made in this book do I mean to deny the necessity of combative methods under certain circumstances. What I wish to emphasize is that the allopathic school of medicine is spending too much of its effort along combative lines and not enough along preventive lines. It would be foolish to deny the necessity of surgery in traumatism and in abnormal conditions which require mechanical means of adjustment or treatment. Such necessity, for instance, will exist in certain obstetrical cases as long as women have not learned to live, or are not willing to live, in such a way as to make surgical intervention at childbirth unnecessary. It is also true that so long as people persist in violating the laws of their being, thereby making their bodies prolific breeding grounds for disease taints, germs and parasites which are bound to provoke inflammatory, feverish processes (nature's cleansing and healing efforts), combative measures will have to be resorted to by the physician, and precautionary measures against infection will have to be observed. These, however, should be in harmony with nature's endeavours, not contrary and suppressive; they should tend to conserve and not to destroy. Natural dietetics, fasting, hydrotherapy, osteopathy, chiropractic, naprapathy, and mental therapeutics, are combative as well as preventive, but if properly applied they do not in any way injure the organism or interfere with nature's intent and nature's methods. This cannot be said for much of the surgical and medical treatment of the old school of medicine. We criticize and condemn only those methods which

(1)
It is not perhaps a matter of chance that the old word "doctor" in its origin denotes one who teaches. This is ideally his true role though he must, of course, also be an expert in the special techniques required in dealing with disease when it has arisen.

are suppressive and destructive rather than curative.

In many instances the warnings and teachings of Nature Cure philosophy have already been verified, and have had to be heeded and accepted by medical science. The exponents of Nature Cure protested against the barbarous practice of witholding water from patients burning in fever heat, and against the exclusion of fresh air from the sick room by order of the doctor. The cold water and no drug treatment of typhoid fever, the water treatment for other acute diseases, as well as the open air treatment for tuberculosis, were forced upon the medical profession by the advocates of Nature Cure. For more than half a century the latter have been curing all inflammatory, feverish diseases, from simple colds to scarlet fever, diphtheria, cerebro-spinal meningitis, smallpox, appendicitis etc., etc., by hydrotherapy, fasting and other natural methods, without resorting in any case to the use of poisonous drugs, antitoxins or surgical operations.

For many years before the terrible after effects of X-Ray treatment and of extirpation of the ovaries, of the womb and of other vital organs, became so patent that the physicians of the regular school could no longer ignore them, Nature Cure physicians had strongly warned against these unnatural practices, and called attention to their destructive after effects.

As long as seventeen years ago, when the X-Rays were in high favour for the treatment of cancer, lupus, and other diseases, I warned against the use of these rays, claiming that their vibratory velocity was too high and powerful, and that they were therefore destructive to the tissues of the human body. Since the failure of the X-Rays and the discovery of Radioactivity, the rays and emanations of radium and other radio-active substances are widely advertised and exploited as therapeutic agents, but these rays also are far beyond the vibratory ranges of the physical body in velocity and power. Therefore, it remains to be seen whether their injurious after effects do not in the long run outweigh any beneficial effects. The destructive action of these high power rays, as well as that of inorganic minerals, is very slow and insidious, manifesting only in the course of many years. This new field of therapeutics, therefore, has not yet passed the stage of dangerous experimentation. Inorganic minerals also prove injurious and destructive to the tissues of the human body because they are too slow in vibratory velocity, and too coarse in molecular structure.

It is the intent and purpose of this volume to warn against the exploitation of destructive combative methods to the neglect of preventive constructive and conservative methods. If these teachings contribute something towards this end they will have fulfilled their mission.

CHAPTER I

MISSING LINKS

The fundamental principles of Nature Cure philosophy, which radically differ from allopathic theory and practice, and which are destined to revolutionize the chaotic teachings of the old schools and to establish in their place an exact science of medicine, are the following:

Every acute disease is the result of a purifying, healing effort of nature. The inflammatory processes back of all acute and sub-acute diseases are identical in nature and purpose and in the way they run their courses through the five stages of inflammation. The bacteria found associated with acute, sub-acute and chronic diseases are not the *primary* causes and instigators of these abnormal processes, but rather the product of pathogenic conditions and the agents through which nature breaks down complex, disease-producing (pathogenic) substances into simpler compounds suitable for neutralization by alkaline elements and for elimination through the organs of depuration. The primary cause of germ activity is the morbid soil in which bacteria breed and multiply. Basing our practice on these fundamental propositions, we do not endeavour to "kill the germs" with poisonous drugs, vaccines, serums and antitoxins, but instead we endeavour through natural ways of living and natural methods of treatment to purify the organism of the systemic waste, morbid encumbrances and disease taints which furnish the soil for the development and multiplication of disease germs.

Many who have carefully studied my previous writings over the years were probably not entirely satisfied with the evidence presented in proof of these fundamental laws and principles. When I described the processes of inflammation solely from the viewpoint of the teachings of Pasteur and Metchnikoff, they may have wondered why the white blood cells should destroy the disease germs if the latter were scavengers of morbid matter and disease taints. Also many enquiries have come to me from readers and from students running somewhat as follows: "You say that scabies (itch), lice, crab lice and many other so-called contagious diseases develop in the form of "healing crises" under circumstances where infection or contagion is improbable or impossible. If this be true, where do the germs or para-

9

sites come from? In the case of scabies, lice, crab lice, etc., do you believe in spontaneous generation?" In my former writings I anticipated and answered these questions by saying: "If our bodies contain the morbid soil, we need not worry about the microbes of disease; they will come from somewhere, because the spores of germs are present everywhere. Our bodies are alive with them." At that time, however, I could not have answered the question: "What are these spores of disease germs, these seed germs of bacteria? Where do they come from?"

Lately the solution of this problem also has come to me in an unexpected manner. Until a few weeks ago I was not aware of the fact that a French scientist, Antoine Béchamp, as far back as the middle of the last century, had given a rational, scientific explanation of the origin, growth and life activities of germs and of the normal living cells of vegetable, animal and human bodies. This information came to me first in a pamphlet entitled "Life's Primal Architects", by E. Douglas Hume. Thus was I led to my investigation of Béchamp's work at first hand. Especially have I made a careful study of his last work, entitled "The Blood", in which he summarizes the microzymian theory of cell life. He demonstrated in his lectures at the University of Montpelier and at the Sorbonne, as early as 1864, that cells and germs are not the smallest individual living organisms, as taught by Pasteur and his followers, but that they are in turn made up of infinitely smaller living beings which he named "microzymes". This term means in English "minute ferment bodies". According to Béchamp, then, cells and germs are associations of microzymes. The physical characteristics and vital activities of cells and germs depend upon the soil in which their microzymes feed, grow and multiply. Thus microzymes, growing in the soil of procreative germ plasm, develop into normal, permanent, specialized cells of the living vegetable, animal or human organism. The same microzymes feeding on morbid materials and systemic poisons in these living bodies develop into bacteria.

I shall cite here only one of the many experiments made by Professor Béchamp and his collaborators, which go to prove the correctness of his deductions. Beer yeast becomes active and multiplies normally only in a sugar solution. While feeding on sugar and digesting it, it decomposes the sugar into alcohol, carbonic acid and small amounts of acetic acid. When Béchamp added creosote or other antiseptic substances to the fermenting fluid the normal activity of the yeast germs gradually subsided. They deteriorated and decomposed, their detritus gradually changing into bacteria, which appeared although the experiment was conducted under conditions which made invasion of bacteria from without impossible. The bacteria in their turn, when they had consumed the decaying materials on which they had subsisted, disintegrated until there was nothing left but the original microzymes. Thus he showed that microzymes are at the beginning and at the end of all organized beings, He found the chalk of Sens and other calcareous rocks alive with microzymes, which started processes of fermentation in blood, milk and other fermentable substances. When we consider that these geological microzymes are the remains of fossil organisms which lived in remote prehistoric ages we must come to the conclusion that these primal architects of life are practically indestructible and must be endowed with life in its most primitive form.

The researches and teachings of Béchamp and the discovery of microzymes confirm in a wonderful way the claims of Nature Cure philosophy, according to which bacteria and parasites cannot cause and instigate inflammation and other disease processes unless they find their own peculiar morbid soil in which to feed, grow and multiply.

Béchamp's profound revelations were soon superseded by the plausible theories of Pasteur and Metchnikoff, which fully justified the suppressive poison treatment of the allopathic school. Pasteur compared the human body to a barrel of beer and pronounced it, like beer, to be at the mercy of extraneous organisms. As these produce good or bad beer — a liquid diseased, as it were, or healthy — so on entering animal bodies microorganisms create disease, each after its own order. It only needed Professor Metchnikoff's theory of phagocytosis and the alleged discovery of "opsonins" or natural antitoxins in the blood, by Sir Almroth Wright and Dr. Bulloch, to furnish the medical profession with a delightfully simple theory as to the origin of disease comprehensible to the least intelligent. Upon this basis rests the entire structure of modern medical theory and practice.

The microzyme evidently is one of the missing links in the chain of evidence in proof of the Nature Cure philosophy of health, disease and cure. The other one was discovered by Dr. Thomas Powell of Los Angeles. As far as I know he was the first to advance the claim that the so-called white corpuscles or "phagocytes" instead of being valiant germ fighters and germ eaters are in reality particles of morbid, pathogenic matter; that instead of destroying the disease germs they are, in the inflammatory processes, destroyed by the germs. It is interesting to note that Béchamp already ridiculed the idea of "phagocytosis". In his book "The Blood" he says — "although their master (Pasteur) had declared that the cellules (leucocytes) were not living, his disciples imagined that the leucocytes (under the name of phagocytes) were living like amoebae and able to perform movements called amoeboid. And it was believed that these phagocytes formed themselves into troops to pursue and devour the microbes. There was thus a phagocytosis, which was trumpeted forth as providential. The precise knowledge of the blood reduces to its just value this latest form of the struggle against the microzymian theory". Later on I shall explain more fully Béchamp's reasons for opposing the idea of phagocytosis.

Dr. Powell's discovery of the true nature of the so-called leucocyte together with our knowledge of the activity of the microzymes furnishes for the first time in medical history a rational and consistent explanation of the process of inflammation. Inflammation always starts with obstruction of the capillary circulation, caused by "white blood corpuscles" and other colloid or pathogenic matter. The obstruction causes the white blood corpuscles in the blood stream to be forced out into the neighbouring tissues ("emigration of the leucocytes"). Stagnation causes them to disorganize and putrefy. This morbid soil develops the microzymes of the normal cells into various kinds of "disease germs" or bacteria. According to this theory, then, the microzymes are the spores or the seeds of disease germs which grow and thrive in morbid matter only. Thus the chain of evidence which proves the "disease germ" as constructive and the white blood corpuscle (or phagocyte) as pathogenic material, is complete, and Nature Cure philosophy throughout stands justified in theory and practice. Dr. Thomas Powell's theory of the pathogenic nature of the leucocytes is also absolutely verified by the clinical records of our patients. This conclusive evidence of the true character of the "phagocyte" and the correctness of natural treatment is given in Chapter IX.[1]

An interesting confirmation of the truth of Nature Cure philosophy

---

[1]
Lindlahr here and elsewhere in his writings has firmly based his ideas of acute disease and infection on the writings and researches of Béchamp and Powell. Since his death there has been much research in the fields of micro-biology, virology, bacteriology, haematology, etc. Some at least of this research would certainly seem to point to conclusions somewhat in line with those of Béchamp, but the basic Pasteurian concept of the parasitic nature of acute disease would still appear to hold sway in scientific and medical circles as a whole. In contra-distinction to this Béchamp's contention, as I understand it, is that "pathogenic" bacteria are not so much the cause of disease as its result and accompaniment. In some circumstances they may spread or communicate disease and they may condition it and modify it in various ways, but they are not in any real sense the cause of it, which is to be found rather in a changed and abnormal condition of the blood and tissues. He also holds that "microzymes" of the body which are, rather than the cells, the ultimate units of life, are capable of themselves evolving or changing into various kinds of bacteria both in disease and in death. We are therefore capable of creating our own bacteria in addition to, or apart from, any which may enter our bodies from outside. Moreover, Béchamp very definitely implies that bacterial action in the body is a constructive and natural process which may sometimes require to be guided or restrained but should not be violently prevented or interfered with, as is so frequently done today. At the moment the work of Béchamp and Powell is almost unknown in the scientific world and their books are practically unobtainable, but there has been of recent years some revival of interest in Béchamp in France, England and the United States. It would appear highly desirable that more scientists should read his works with care, perhaps repeat some of his key experiments with more modern technique, separate what is sound from what is not, restate his conclusions in more modern language and correlate his work to that of other recent investigators.

and practice comes from the battle fields of Europe. Ever since I began to teach and practice Nature Cure I have advocated the exposure of wounds to air and light with no antiseptic treatment whatever. We have cured during the last seventeen years, the worst kind of wounds, many of which under antiseptic treatment had entered upon advanced stages of necrosis. The treatment in all such cases consisted in exposing the wounds freely to air and light, and in keeping them clean and fresh by frequent washing with diluted lemon juice. For many years I have been denounced as a dangerous ignoramus and quack for this and other deviations from orthodox theory and practice. During the last few years, however, reports have come from the battle fields of Europe, according to which the wounds of soldiers, who were left exposed out of doors and did not receive hospital care and antiseptic treatment, healed much quicker and more perfectly than those who received the ordinary surgical treatment. Of late medical men have frequently lectured on this wonderful discovery in several Chicago colleges. This, of course, upsets completely the allopathic theory of the danger of germ invasion and of the necessity of antiseptic treatment, and it confirms absolutely the truth of the Nature Cure teachings as to the true character of germ activity. The natural treatment of wounds will be discussed more fully in Volume II of this Series.

What the Electron is to the Atom, the Microzyme is to the Cell

What a remarkable correspondence this theory of the origin of cell life bears to the latest scientific opinions concerning the constitution of the atom. As all elements of matter and their atoms are made up of electrons vibrating in the primordial ether, so all cells and germs are made up of microzymes. As the electrons, according to their numbers in the atom and their modes of vibration, produce upon our sensory organs the effects of various elements of matter, so the microzymes, according to the medium or soil in which they live, develop into various cells and germs, exhibiting distinctive structure and vital activities.

New Light on Heredity

Modern biology teaches us that all permanent, specialized cells present in the complicated adult body are actually contained in the original procreative cell which results from the union of the male spermatazoon and the female ovum. Science, however, has failed to explain this seeming miracle — how is it possible that all the permanent cells of the large adult body can be present from the beginning in the minute procreative cell and in the rudimentary body of the foetus. Béchamp's theory of microzymes brings a rational and scientific explanation. If these microzymes are as minute in comparison to the cell as the electrons are in comparison to the atom, and the atom in comparison to the visible particles of matter, then the mystery of the genesis of the complex human body from the pro-creative cell, as well as the mysteries of heredity in its various phases, are amenable to explanation. If the microzymes are the spores, or seeds, of cells, it is possible to conceive that these infinitesimal, minute living organisms may bear the impress of the species and of radical and family characteristics and tendencies, finally to reappear in the cells, organs and nervous system of the adult body.

CHAPTER II

WHAT IS NATURE CURE?

Nature cure is vastly more than a system of curing aches and pains; it is in truth, a complete revolution in the art and science of living. It is the practical realization and application of all that is good in natural science, philosophy and religion. About seventy years ago this greatest and most beneficient of reformatory movements was inaugurated by Priessnitz, in Grafenberg, a small village in the Silesian mountains. He was a simple farmer, but he had a natural genius for the art of healing. His pharmacopeia consisted not in poisonous pills and potions, but in plenty of exercise, fresh mountain air, water treatments in the cool, sparkling brooks, and simple, wholesome country fare, consisting largely of black bread, vegetables, and milk fresh from cows fed on nutritious mountain grasses.

The results accomplished by these simple means were wonderful. Before he died, a large sanitarium, filled with patients from all over the world and from all stations of life, had grown up around his forest home. Among those who made the pilgrimage to Grafenberg to become patients and students of this genial healer, the simple-minded farmer-physician, were wealthy merchants, princes and doctors from all parts of the world. Rapidly the idea of drugless healing spread over the civilized world. Hahn the apothecary, Kuhne the weaver, Rikli the manufacturer, Father Kneipp the priest, Lahmann the doctor, Adolph Just the teacher, and Turnvater Jahn, the founder of physical culture, became enthusiastic pupils and followers of Priessnitz. Each one of these men enlarged and enriched some special field of the great realm of natural healing. Some elaborated the water cure and natural dietetics, others invented various systems of manipulative treatment, earth, air, and light cures, magnetic healing, mental therapeutics, curative gymnastics, etc. etc. Von Peckzely added the Diagnosis from the Iris of the Eye, which reveals not only the innermost secrets of the human organism, but also nature's ways and means of cure, and the changes for better or for worse continually occurring in the body.

In this country, Dr. Trall of New York, Dr. Jackson of Danville, Dr. Kellogg of Battle Creek, and others caught the infection and crossed the ocean to become students of Priessnitz. Quimby, the itinerant spiritualist and healer, became successful and renowned by the application of the natural methods of cure. At first his favourite methods were water, massage and mental treatment. Gradually he concentrated his efforts on metaphysical methods of cure, and before he died he evolved a complete system of magnetic and mental therapeutics. Quimby's methods and teachings were adopted by Mrs. Eddy, his most enthusiastic pupil, and by her elaborated into Christian Science, the latest and most successful of the modern mental healing cults. Dr. Still, of Kirksville, Missouri, made a valuable addition to natural healing methods by the development of osteopathy, a system of scientific manipulation of the framework of the body. Later developments of manipulative treatment are chiropractic, originated by Dr. D. D. Palmer of Davenport, Iowa; neurotherapy, evolved by Drs. Arnold and Walter of Philadelphia, Pennsylvania; naprapathy, founded by Dr. Oakley Smith of Chicago, Illinois; and spondylotherapy, developed by Dr. Albert Abrams of Los Angeles, California.[1]

Thus the simple pioneers of Nature Cure laid the foundation for the world wide modern health culture movement. They refused to be blinded or confused by the conflicting theories of books and authorities, or by the action of a thousand different drugs on a legion of different symptoms, but rather applied common sense reasoning to the solution of the problems of health, disease and cure. They went for inspiration to field and forest rather than to the murkier atmosphere of the dissection and vivisection rooms. They studied the whole and not only the parts; causes as well as effects and symptoms. Realizing that man had lost his natural instinct and strayed far away from nature's ways, they studied and imitated the natural habits of the animal creation rather than the confusing doctrines of the schools. Thus they proclaimed the "return to nature" and the "new gospel of health" which they looked upon as destined to free humanity from the destructive influences of alcoholism, meat eating, the dope and tobacco habit, of drug poisoning, vaccination, surgical mutilation, vivisection, and many other abuses practised in the name of science.

These thoughts were not and are not the mere dreams of visionaries. When we see the wonderful changes which can be wrought in a human being by a few months or years of rational living and treatment, it seems not impossible that these ideals could be reached within a few generations.

[1]
In view of Dr. Lindlahr's very severe criticisms of Christian Science which appear later in his works it is somewhat surprising that he includes it here among the methods contributing to the armamentarium of Nature Cure. The kind of mental treatment which he did believe in and recommend differs very much from Christian Science.

Moreover, when parents learn how to beget children in accord with natural law, how to mould their bodies and their characters into harmony and beauty before the new life sees the light of day, when they learn to rear their offspring in health of body and soundness of mind, then we shall have true types of beautiful manhood and womanhood, and children will not so often be a curse and a burden to themselves, to those who bring them into the world or to society at large. Children so born and reared in harmony with the laws of their being could well be the future masters of the earth, a true and noble aristocracy of health.

CHAPTER III

CATECHISM OF NATURE CURE

The philosophy of Nature Cure is based on sciences dealing with newly discovered and rediscovered natural laws and principles, and with their application to the phenomena of life and death, health, disease and cure. Every new science embodying new modes of thought requires exact modes of expression and new definitions of words and phrases already in common use. Therefore I have endeavoured to define, as precisely as possible, certain words and phrases which convey meanings and ideas peculiar to the teachings of Nature Cure. The student of Nature Cure and kindred subjects will do well to study closely these definitions and formulated principles, as they contain the pith and marrow of our philosophy and greatly facilitate its understanding.

(1)　What is Nature Cure?
Nature Cure is a system of man-building in harmony with the constructive principle in nature of the physical, mental and moral planes of being.

(2)　What is the Constructive Principle in Nature?
The constructive principle in nature is that principle which builds up, improves, and repairs, which always makes for the perfect type, whose activity in nature is designated as evolutionary, and which is opposed to the destructive principle in nature.

(3)　What is the Destructive Principle in Nature?
The destructive principle in nature is that principle which disintegrates and destroys existing forms and types, and whose activity in nature is designated as devolutionary.

(4)　What is Normal or Natural?
That is normal or natural which is in harmonic relation with the life purposes of the individual.

(5) What is Health?
Health is normal and harmonious vibration of the elements and forces composing the human entity on the physical, mental and moral planes of being, in conformity with the constructive principle in nature applied to individual life.

(6) What is Disease?
Disease is abnormal or inharmonious vibration of the elements and forces composing the human entity on one or more planes of being, in conformity with the destructive principle in nature applied to individual life.

(7) What is the Primary Cause of Disease?
The primary cause of disease, barring accidental or surgical injury to the human organism and surroundings hostile to human life, is violation of nature's laws.

(8) What are the Effects of Violation of Nature's Laws on the Physical Human Organism?
The effects of the violation of nature's laws on the physical human organism are: 1. Lowered vitality.
2. Abnormal composition of blood and lymph.
3. Accumulation of waste matter, morbid materials and poisons.

These conditions are identical with disease, because they tend to lower, hinder or inhibit normal function (harmonious vibration), and because they engender and promote destruction of living tissues.

(9) What is Acute Disease?
What is commonly called "acute" disease is in reality the result of nature's efforts to eliminate from the organism waste material, foreign matter and poisons, and to repair injury to living tissues. In other words every so-called acute disease is the result of a cleansing and healing effort of nature.

(10) What is Chronic Disease?
(a) Chronic disease is a condition of the organism in which lowered vibration (lowered vitality), due to the accumulation of waste material and poisons, with the consequent destruction of vital parts and organs, has progressed to such an extent that nature's constructive and healing forces are no longer able to react against the disease conditions by acute corrective efforts (healing crises).

(b) Chronic disease is a condition of the organism in which morbid encumbrances, having gained the ascendancy, prevent acute reaction (healing crises) on the part of the constructive forces of nature.

(c) Chronic disease is the natural consequence of the inability of the organism to react by acute efforts, or "healing crises", against conditions inimical to health.

(11) What is a "Healing Crisis"?

A healing crisis is an acute reaction, resulting from the ascendancy of nature's healing forces over disease conditions. Its tendency is towards recovery, and it is, therefore, in conformity with nature's constructive principle.

(12) Are all Acute Reactions Healing Crises?

No; there are healing crises and disease crises.

(13) What is a Disease Crisis?

A disease crisis is an acute reaction resulting from the ascendancy of disease conditions over the healing forces of the organism. Its tendency is, therefore, toward fatal termination.[1]

(14) What is Cure?

Cure is the readjustment of the human organism from abnormal to normal conditions and functioning.

(15) What Methods of Treatment are in Conformity with the Constructive Principle in Nature?

Those methods which:
1. Establish normal surroundings and natural habits of life in accord with nature's laws;
2. Economize vital force;
3. Build up the blood on a natural basis; that is, supply the blood with its natural constituents in right proportions;
4. Promote the elimination of waste material and poisons without in any way injuring the human body;
5. Correct mechanical lesions;

---

[1] It would appear that in practice many crises which would under this definition be described as "disease crises" may, by wise treatment, be turned into "healing crises". Conversely it may lead to very serious consequences if a "healing crisis" is treated by suppressive measures.

6. Arouse the individual in the highest possible degree to the consciousness of personal responsibility and to the necessity of intelligent personal effort and self-help.

(16) Are Medicines in Conformity with the Constructive Principle in Nature?

Medicines are in conformity with the constructive principle in nature in so far as they, in themselves, are not injurious or destructive to the human organism and in so far as they act as tissue foods and promote the neutralization and elimination of morbid matters and poisons.

(17) Are Poisonous Drugs and Promiscuous Surgical Operations in Conformity with the Constructive Principle in Nature?

Poisonous drugs and promiscuous operations are not in conformity with the constructive principle in nature because:

1. They suppress acute diseases or reactions (crises), the cleansing and healing efforts of nature;

2. They are in themselves harmful and destructive to human life;

3. Such treatment fosters the belief that drugs and surgical operations can be substituted for obedience to nature's laws and for personal effort and self-help.

(18) Is Metaphysical Healing in Conformity with the Constructive Principle in Nature?

Metaphysical systems of healings are in conformity with the constructive principle in nature in so far as:

1. They do not interfere with or suppress nature's healing efforts;

2. They awaken hope and confidence (therapeutic faith), and thereby increase the inflow of vital force into the organism;

3. They teach the law of cause and effect and thus awaken and strengthen the consciousness of personal responsibility.

They are *not* in conformity with the constructive principle in nature in so far as:

1. They fail to assist nature's healing efforts, but ignore, obscure and deny the laws of nature and defy the dictates of reason and common sense;

2. They substitute in the treatment of disease a blind, dogmatic belief in the wonder-working power of metaphysical formulae and prayer, for intelligent co-operation with nature's constructive forces and for personal effort and self-help;

3. They weaken the consciousness of personal responsibility.

(19) Is Nature Cure in Conformity with the Constructive Principle in Nature?

Nature Cure is in conformity with the constructive principle in nature that:

1. It teaches that the primary cause of weakness and disease is disobedience to the laws of nature;

2. It arouses the individual to the study of natural laws and demonstrates the necessity of strict compliance with these laws;

3. It strengthens the consciousness of personal responsibility of the individual for his own status of health and for the hereditary conditions, traits and tendencies of his offspring;

4. It encourages personal effort and self-help;

5. It adapts surroundings and habits of life to natural laws;

6. It assists nature's cleansing and healing efforts by simple natural means and methods of treatment which are in no wise harmful or destructive to health and life, and which are within the reach of everyone.

(20) What are the Natural Methods of Living and of Treatment?

1. Return to nature by the regulation of eating, drinking, breathing, bathing, dressing, working, resting, thinking, the moral life, sexual and social activities, etc., establishing them on a normal and natural basis.

2. Elementary remedies such as water, air, light, earth cures, magnetism electricity, etc.

3. Chemical remedies such as scientific food selection and combination, homoeopathic medicines, simple herb extracts, and vitochemical remedies.

4. Mechanical remedies, such as corrective gymnastics, massage, magnetic treatment, structural adjustment and, in cases of accident, surgery.

5. Mental and spiritual remedies, such as scientific relaxation, normal suggestion, constructive thought, the prayer of faith, etc.

CHAPTER IV

WHAT IS LIFE?

In our study of the cause and character of disease we must endeavour to begin at the beginning, and that is LIFE itself; for the processes of health, disease and cure are manifestations of that which we call life, vitality, life elements. While endeavouring to fathom the mystery of life we soon realize that we are dealing with an ultimate which no human mind is capable of solving or explaining. We can study and understand life only in its manifestations, not in its origin and real essence.

There are two prevalent but widely differing conceptions of the nature of life or vital force — the *material* and the *vital*. The former looks upon life or vital force with all its physical, mental and psychical phenomena as manifestations of the electric, magnetic and physiochemical activities of the physical material elements composing the human organism. From this viewpoint, life is a sort of "spontaneous combustion" or, as one scientist expresses it, a "succession of fermentations" or chemical changes. The vitalistic conception of life, on the other hand, regards vital force as the primary force of all forces, coming from the great central source of all life. This force, which permeates, heats and animates the entire created universe, is an expression of divine intelligence and will, the "logos" the "word" of the great Creative Intelligence. It is the divine energy which sets in motion the whirls in the ether, the electric corpuscles that make up the atoms and elements of matter.

These electrons are positive and negative forms of electricity. Electricity is a form of energy. It is intelligent energy; otherwise it could not act with that same wonderful precision in the electrons of the atoms as in the suns and planets of the sidereal universe. This intelligent energy can have but one source: the will and intelligence of the Creator — or as Swedenborg expresses it, of "the great Central Sun of the Universe". If this supreme Intelligence should withdraw its creative energy, the electric charges (forms of energy) and with it the atoms, elements, and the entire material universe, would disappear in the flash of a moment. From this it appears that crude matter, instead of being the source of all life and of all its complicated mental and spiritual phenomena (which assumption on the face of it, is absurd), is but an expression of the Life Force, itself a manifestation of the great Creative Intelligence which some call God, others Nature, the Oversoul, Brahma, Prana, The Great Spirit, etc., each according to his best understanding.

It is this supreme intelligence and Power acting in and through every atom, molecule and cell in the human body, which is the true healer, the 'vis medicatrix naturae" which always endeavours to repair, to heal and to restore the perfect type. All that the physician can do is to remove obstructions and to establish normal conditions within and around the patient, so that "the healer within" can do his work to the best advantage.

Here the Christian Scientist will say: "That is exactly what we claim. All is God! All is Mind! There is no matter! Our attitutde to disease is based on these facts". But suppose that, in the final analysis, matter is nothing but vibration, an expression of Divine Mind and Will; that, surely, does not justify me in denying and ignoring its reality. Because I have an "all mind" body, is it advisable for me to place myself in the way of an "all mind" train moving at the rate of sixty miles an hour?

The question is not what matter is in the final analysis, but how matter affects us. We have to take it and treat it as we find it. We must be as obedient to the laws of matter as to those of the higher planes of being.

Life is Vibratory

All things in nature, from a fleeting thought or emotion to the hardest piece of diamond or platinum, are modes of motion or vibration. Until a few years ago physical science assumed that an atom was the smallest imaginable part of a given element of matter; that although infinitesimally small, it still represented solid matter. Now, in the light of more recent evidence, we have good reason to believe that there is no such thing as solid matter; that every atom is made up of charges of negative and positive electricity acting in and upon an omnipresent ether; that the difference between an atom of iron and one of hydrogen, or any other element, depends solely upon the number of electrons it contains and upon the velocity with which these vibrate around one another in the ether. Thus, the atom, which was thought to be the ultimate particle of solid matter, is found to be a little universe in itself in which electrons revolve around one another like the sun and planets in the sidereal universe. This explains what we mean when we say that life and matter are vibratory. Over two thousand years ago Pythagoras taught that all matter was made up of three elements, viz., a primordial substance, motion, and number. It is interesting to note how up-to-date modern science appears to verify the teachings of this ancient philosopher. In the language of modern science the primordial substance is the all-pervading ether, motion is electricity, and number is the number of electrons vibrating in the atom.

As early as 1863 John Newlands discovered that when he arranged the elements of matter in the order of their atomic weight, they displayed the same relation to one another as do the tones in the musical scale. Thus modern chemistry appears to demonstrate the verity of the "music of the spheres" and how the entire sidereal universe is built on the laws of harmony. That which is orderly, lawful, good, beautiful, natural, healthy, vibrates in unison with the harmonics of this great "Diapason of Nature": in other words it is in alignment with the constructive principle in nature. That which is disorderly, abnormal, ugly, unnatural, unhealthy vibrates in discord with nature's harmonies. It is in alignment with the destructive principle in nature. What we call "inanimate nature" is beautiful and orderly because it plays in tune with the score of the symphony of life. Man only can play out of tune. This is his privilege, if he chooses, by reason of his freedom of choice and action.

We can now better understand the definitions of Health and Disease given in the Catechism of Nature Cure (Chapter III); namely, that Health is normal and harmonious vibration and Disease abnormal and inharmonious vibration. If there is to be health the vibratory conditions of the organism must be in harmony with nature's established harmonic relations in the physical, mental and psychical realms of human life and action.

What is an "Established Harmonic Relation"?

A simple illustration may help to make this clear. If a watch is in good condition, "in harmonious vibration", its movement is so adjusted that it coincides exactly in point of time, with the rotations of our earth around its axis. The established, regular movement of the earth forms the basis of the established harmonic relationship between the vibrations of a normal "healthy" timepiece and the revolutions of our planet. The watch has to vibrate in unison with the harmonics of the planetary universe in order to be normal, or "in harmony". In like manner, everything that is to be normal, natural, healthy, good, beautiful, must vibrate in unison with its correlated harmonics in nature.

Obedience the Only Salvation

Orthodox medical science attributes disease largely to accidental causes: to chance infection by disease taints, germs or parasites, or to draughts, chills, wet feet, etc. The religiously inclined frequently attribute disease and other tribulations to the arbitrary rulings of an inscrutable

Providence. Christian Scientists tell us that sin, suffering, disease and all kinds of evil are only "errors of mortal mind", or the products of diseased imagination (though this in itself admits the existence of something abnormal and diseased).

Nature Cure philosophy, on the other hand, presents a more rational concept of evil, its cause and purpose, namely: that it is brought on by violation of nature's laws; that it is corrective in its purpose; that it can be overcome only by compliance with the law. There is no suffering, disease nor evil of any kind anywhere unless the law has been transgressed somewhere by someone. These transgressions of the law may be due to ignorance or to wilfulness and viciousness. The effects will always be commensurate with the causes. This places the responsibility for disease and evil in general where it belongs — on ourselves. "We are not punished for our sins but by our sins." The great all-wise and all-loving Father-Mother principle does not impose or enforce suffering on its children. We create it in ourselves through ignorant or wilful violation of the laws of our being. There is no accident, no ill luck nor misfortune, — there is nothing but cause and effect.

The science of natural living and healing shows clearly that what we call disease is primarily nature's effort to eliminate morbid matter and to restore the normal functions of the body; that the processes of disease are just as orderly in their way as everything else in nature; that we must not check or suppress them, but co-operate with them. Thus we learn slowly and laboriously the all-important lesson that obedience to natural law is the only means of prevention of disease and the only cure. The fundamental law of cure, the law of action and reaction and the law of crisis, as revealed by Nature Cure philosophy, impress upon us the truth that there is nothing accidental nor arbitrary in the processes of health, disease and cure; that every changing condition is either in harmony or in discord with the laws of our being; that only by complete surrender and obedience to these laws can we attain and maintain perfect physical health.

Selfcontrol the Master Key

Thus Nature Cure brings home to us constantly and forcibly the inexorable operation of natural law and the necessity of compliance with the law. Herein lies its great educational value to the individual and to the race. The man who has learned to master his habits and his appetites so as to conform to nature's laws on the physical plane, and who has thereby regained his bodily health, realizes that personal effort and selfcontrol are the master key to all further development on the mental and spiritual planes of being as well; that selfmastery and unremitting and unselfish personal effort are the only means of self completion, of individual and social salvation.

The naturist, who has regained health and strength through obedience to the laws of his being, enjoys a measure of selfcontent, gladness of soul and enthusiasm which cannot be explained by the mere possession of physical health. These highest and purest attainments of the human soul are not the results of mere physical well-being, but of the peace and harmony which come only through obedience to natural law. Such is the peace which passeth understanding.

CHAPTER V

THE PRIMARY CAUSE OF DISEASE AND ITS MANIFESTATIONS

We have learned in the previous chapter that, barring trauma (injury) and surroundings uncongenial to human life, the primary cause of all disease is violation of nature's laws. Violation of nature's laws in thinking, breathing, eating, drinking, working, resting, as well as in moral, sexual and social conduct, results in certain primary and secondary manifestations of disease.

The three primary manifestations of disease coincide with the three primary life requirements of the cell. Biology teaches us that these are innervation, nutrition and drainage. By innervation is meant a copious influx of life force and an adequate nerve supply from headquarters in the brain and spinal cord. Anything, therefore, which obstructs the nerve connection of the cell with the sympathetic and central nervous systems lowers the vitality of the cells, tissues and organs and of the organism as a whole, and interferes with the transmission of afferent and efferent nerve impulses. Nutrition, the second requirement of the cell, necessitates normal composition of blood, lymph and other fluids of the body; therefore, abnormal composition of vital fluids constitutes the second of the primary manifestations of disease. The third requirement is perfect drainage. Accumulations of waste and morbid matter interfere with drainage as well as with the nutrition of the cell by obstruction of venous and lymphatic circulation and so constitute the third of the primary manifestations of disease.

To go more into detail, we have primarily: (1) Lowered vitality due to such things as over-work, night work, weakening habits, excesses, over-indulgence, over-stimulation, poisonous drugs, ill-advised surgical operations, mechanical factors, and to wrong thinking and feeling. (2) Abnormal composition of blood and lymph due to improper selection and combination of food and especially to lack of mineral salts in organic form. (3) Accumulation of waste material, morbid matter and poisons (pathogen). These accumulations are caused by lowered vitality, faulty diet, over-eating, use of alcoholic and narcotic stimulants, drugs, vaccines, antitoxins, and by suppression of acute disease, by poisonous drugs, ice and surgical operations. There are also secondary stages and manifestations of disease. These include: (1) More deep-seated hereditary and acquired taints of sycosis, scrofula, psora, syphilis, mercurialism, cinchonism, iodism and many other forms of systematic and drug poisoning. (2) Disease germs, parasites, etc. (3) Fevers, inflammation, skin eruptions, catarrhal discharges, ulcers, abscesses, haemorrhages, etc. — processes which indicate the oxidation and elimination of morbid or pathogenic material.

The Unity of Disease and Treatment

There is, or should be, a unity or correspondence between disease and the methods of treatment to be used, and Nature Cure methods do correspond with the three primary manifestations of disease. Everything is done to improve and economize vital force, to build up the body fluids on the right basis and to promote elimination of waste and poisons. In the following chapters I intend to show how all the different forms, phases and phenomena of disease arising within the human organism, apart from those caused by accident or by external conditions unfavourable to human life, grow out of one or more of the three primary manifestations of disease. If this is true and all disease originates from a few simple causes, it will not seem strange and improbable that all disease can be treated successfully by a few simple, natural methods of living and treatment, thereby establishing the right of Nature Cure to be classed among the exact sciences.

We must now consider more in detail these three primary stages of manifestations of disease.

(1).   Lowered Vitality. Health Positive. Disease Negative.

The freer the inflow of life force into the organism, the greater the vitality the more there is of strength, of positive resisting and recuperative power.

At the very foundation of the manifestation of life lies the principle of polarity which expresses itself in the duality of positive and negative affinity. The swaying to and fro of the positive and the negative, the effort to balance incomplete polarity, constitutes the very ebb and flow of life. Disease is disturbed polarity or unbalanced chemical equilibrium. Exaggerated positive or negative conditions, whether physical, mental or psychical, tend to disease on the respective planes of being. Foods, medicines, suggestions and all other methods of treatment exert on the individual subjected to them either a positive or a negative influence. It is, therefore, of the greatest importance that the physician and every one who wishes to live and work in harmony with nature's laws should understand this all important question of magnetic polarity.

Lowered vitality means lowered, slower and coarser vibration, which results in weakened resistance to the accumulation of morbid matter, poisons, disease taints, germs and parasites. This is what we designate ordinarily as the "negative" condition. Let us explain this more fully by an homely illustration. Many of my readers have probably seen in operation in amusement parks the "human roulette". This contrivance consists of a large wheel, board covered, somewhat raised in the centre and sloping towards the circumference. The wheel rotates horizontally, parallel with the ground and competitors throw themselves down on the wheel and try to cling to it while it rotates with increasing swiftness. While the wheel moves slowly it is easy enough to cling to it; but the faster it revolves, the more strongly the centrifugal force tends to throw off the human "flies" trying to hold fast. The accelerated repelling power of the revolving wheel may serve as an illustration of what we call vigorous vibration, good vitality, natural immunity or recuperative power. This is the positive condition.

The more intense the action of the life force, the more rapid and vigorous are the vibratory activities of the atoms and molecules in the cells, and of the cells in the organs and tissues of the body. The more rapid and vigorous the vibratory activity the more powerful is the repulsion and expulsion of morbid matter and poisons which encumber the organism and tend to its destruction. This explains why, with advancing age, waste and morbid matter accumulate more readily in the body. Lowered vitality means lowered vibration and this means lowered resistance to the accumulation of waste and morbid materials. This in turn further obstructs the inflow and distribution of vital energy. In many ways the primary manifestations of disease tend to act on and aggravate one another.

Health or disease, in the final analysis, is resident in the cell. Though a minute, microscopic organism, the cell is an individual living being, which eats, drinks, grows, throws off waste matter, multiplies, ages and declines, just like man, the large conglomerate cell. If the individual cell embodies health, man, the complex cell is well also, and vice versa. From this it becomes apparent that in all our considerations of the processes of health, disease and cure, we have to deal primarily with the individual cell. The vibratory activity of the cell may be lowered through the decline of vitality brought about in a natural way by advancing age, or in an artificial way, through wrong thinking and feeling, wrong habits of living, overwork, unnatural stimulation and excesses of various kinds. On the other hand, the inflow of vital force into the cells may be obstructed and their vibratory activity lowered by the accumulation of waste and morbid matter in the tissues of the body. Such clogging interferes with the inflow of life force and with the free and harmonious vibration of the cells and organs of the body as surely as dust in a watch interferes with the normal action and vibration of its wheels and balances.

I would here call attention to the fact that many people are under the impression that fasting, vegetarian diet or raw food diet and certain eliminative methods of treatment necessarily result in the creation of negative conditions and that negative patients must be kept on a heavy meat diet. Though there may be a few cases in which I would recommend the inclusion of some meat in the diet of some patients, as will be explained in a later chapter, it must be emphasized that the "positive nourishing" diet consisting largely of meat, eggs, fats and gluten, clogs the system heavily with pathogenic waste and morbid materials, thereby obstructing the inflow and distribution of the life elements, which is equivalent to lowered vitality or a negative condition. On the other hand, it is clear that in all cases where negative conditions are caused by clogging with waste and morbid matter, the Nature Cure methods of eliminative treatment, such as pure food diet, hydrotherapy, etc., must be invaluable means of removing obstructions and promoting the inflow and free circulation of positive electromagnetic and vitochemical energies.

(2) Abnormal Composition of Blood and Lymph

As the second of the primary manifestations of disease, we cited abnormal composition of blood and lymph. The human organism is made up of a certain number of elements in well defined proportions. Chemistry has discovered, so far, about eighteen of these in appreciable quantities and has ascertained, to a certain extent, their functions in the economy of the body. These elements must be present in the right proportions in order to insure normal texture and functioning of the component parts and organs of the body.

The cells and organs receive their nourishment from the blood and lymph streams. Therefore they must contain all the elements needed by the organism in the right proportions, and this, of course, depends upon the character and combination of food elements. Every disease arising in the organism from internal causes is accompanied by a deficiency in blood and tissues of certain important mineral elements (organic salts) and this in turn is caused by an unbalanced diet. Improper food combinations create an over-abundance of waste and morbid matter in the system, while failing to supply the positive mineral elements or organic salts on which depends the elimination of waste materials and systemic poisons. The great problem of natural dietetics is, therefore, how to restore and maintain the positivity of the blood and of the organism as a whole through providing in food, drink and medicine an abundant supply of the positive mineral salts in organic form.

(3) Accumulation of Morbid Matter and Poisons

This is the third of the primary manifestations of disease. We have learned how lowered vitality and the abnormal composition of the vital fluids favour the retention of waste and systemic poisons in the body. If, in addition to this, food and drink contain too much of the waste-producing proteins, carbohydrates and hydrocarbons, and not enough of the eliminating positive mineral salts, then waste and morbid materials are bound to accumulate in the system and this results in the clogging of the tissues with pathogenic materials. Such accumulation in blood and tissues creates a great variety of diseases arising within the human organism, as will be explained more fully in subsequent chapters. More harmful and dangerous and more difficult to eliminate than systemic poisons which have arisen within the body, are drug poisons, especially when they are administered in the inorganic mineral form.

As already pointed out the three primary causes of disease tend to reinforce one another. Health is dependent upon an abundant supply of life force, upon the unobstructed, normal circulation of the vital fluids and upon perfect oxygenation and elimination of waste. Anything which interferes with these essentials causes disease; anything which promotes them establishes health. Nothing so interferes with the inflow of life force, with free and normal circulation of blood and lymph and with the combustion of food materials and systemic waste as the accumulation of foreign matter and poisons in the tissues of the body.

Mental and Emotional Influences

In conclusion, something must be said about how health and disease are affected by mental and emotional factors, for our mental and emotional states exert a most powerful influence upon the inflow and distribution of vital force. Fear, worry, anxiety and all kindred emotions create in the system conditions similar to those of freezing. These destructive vibrations congeal the tissues, contract the minute channels of life and thereby paralyze the vital activities. Emotional conditions of impatience, irritability, anger, fury, wrath, etc. have a heating, corroding effect upon brain and nerve substance and consume it like burning fire. Self-pity has been called the consumption of the soul, or psychic phthisis. In like manner, all other destructive emotional vibrations obstruct the inflow and normal distribution of the life forces through the organism, while the constructive emotions of faith, hope, cheerfulness, happiness, love and altruism exert a relaxing, harmonizing and vitalizing influence upon the tissues of the body, thus opening wide the floodgates of the vital energies and raising the discords of weakness, disease and discontent to the harmonics of buoyant health and happiness.

I shall be dealing more in detail with the mental, emotional and psychic causes of disease and their treatment in Volume II of this series, but let us now observe a little how mind controls matter and how it acts on the changing conditions of the physical body. Life manifests through vibration. It acts on the mass by acting through its minutest particles. Changes in the physical body are wrought by vibratory changes in atoms, molecules, microzymes and cells. Health is "satisfied polarity"; that is, the balancing of the positive and negative elements, forces and energies in harmonious vibration. Anything which interferes with the free, vigorous and harmonious vibration of the minute parts and particles composing the human organism tends to disturb and unbalance polarity and natural affinity, thus causing discord or disease. When we fully realize these things we shall not stand so much in awe of our physical bodies. In the past we thought of the body as a solid and imponderable mass difficult to control and to change. This conception left us in a condition of utter helplessness in the presence of weakness and disease. We now think of the body as composed of minute electrons rotating around one another within the atom at relatively immense distances, We know that in similar manner the atoms vibrate in the molecule, the molecules in the microzyme, and these in the cell, the cells in the organ, and the organs in the body — the whole capable of being changed by a change in the vibrations of its particles. Thus the erstwhile solid physical mass appears plastic and fluid, readily swayed and changed by the vibratory harmonies and discords of thoughts and emotions as well as by foods, medicines and treatment.

Under the old concept the mind fell readily under the control of the body and became the abject slave of its physical conditions, swayed by fear and apprehension under every sensation of physical weakness, discomfort or pain. The servants lorded it with high hand over the master of the house and the result was chaos. Under the new concept, control is placed where it belongs. Dictatorship is assumed by the real master of the house, the soul man, while the servants, the physical members of the body, remain obedient to his bidding. This is the new man, the ideal progeny of new thinking and high philosophy. Understanding the structure of the body, the laws of its being and the operation of the life elements within it, this man retains poise and confidence under the most trying circumstances. Animated by faith in the supremacy of the healing forces within him and sustained by the power of his will, he governs his body as the artist controls his violin, and attunes its vibrations to nature's harmonies of health and happiness.

CHAPTER VI

THE UNITY OF ACUTE DISEASE

In the previous chapter I have been concerned mostly with explaining the three primary manifestations of disease, namely: (1) Lowered Vitality, (2) Abnormal Composition of Blood and Lymph, (3) Accumulation of Waste, Morbid Matter and Poisons in the System. We now come to the consideration of some of the secondary manifestations, the first of which is "Hereditary and Acquired Taints". On first impression, it might be thought that heredity is a primary cause of disease; but on further consideration it seems right to regard it as an effect rather than a primary cause. If the parents possess good vitality and pure, normal blood and tissues and if they apply in the prenatal and postnatal treatment of the child the necessary insight and foresight, there cannot be any inherited disease. In order to create abnormal hereditary tendencies, the parents, or earlier ancestors, must have ignorantly or wantonly violated nature's laws, such violation resulting in lowered vitality and in deterioration of blood and tissues.

The female and male germinal cells unite and form the primitive reproductive cell — the prototype of marriage. The human body with its millions of cells and cell colonies is developed by the multiplication, with gradual differentiation, of the germ plasm of the reproductive cell, or rather of its microzymes. Herein lies the simple explanation of heredity which is proved to be an actual fact, not only by common experience and scientific observation but also in a more definite way by nature's records in the iris of the eye. The iris of the new born child reveals in its diagnostic details, not only in a general way hereditary taints, lowered resistance and deterioration of vital fluids, but frequently special weakness and deterioration in those organs which were weak or diseased in the parents. Under the conventional (unnatural) care of the infant, which is now so common, these hereditary and congenital tendencies and their corresponding signs in the iris become more and more pronounced, proceeding through the various stages of infantile diseases, through chronic conditions to the final destructive stages. In the face of the well established facts of disease inheritance we have, however, this consolation: if the child be treated in accordance with the teachings of Nature Cure philosophy, the abnormal hereditary encumbrances and tendencies can be overcome and eliminated within a few years. If the infant organism be brought under the right conditions of living and treatment, in harmony with the laws of its being, the life principle within will approach ever nearer to the establishment of the perfect type. Many living proofs of this are to be seen.

Natural Immunity

Next among the "Secondary Manifestations of Disease" are germs, parasites, inflammations, fevers, skin eruptions, catarrhal discharges, ulcers, etc. Modern medical science is built upon the germ theory of disease and treatment. Since the microscope has revealed the presence and seemingly entirely pernicious activity of certain micro-organisms in connection with certain diseases, it has been assumed that bacteria are the direct, primary causes of most diseases, and that they represent definite species of living beings whose natural habitat is the air, earth and water. According to this theory human beings are at the mercy of these invaders; — health and disease, life and death, are largely matters of accident over which we have no control. Basing their prophylaxis and treatment on this idea, the slogan is "kill the bacteria (by poisonous antiseptics, serums, antitoxins, etc.) and you will cure the disease".

Nature Cure philosophy takes an entirely different view of the problem. Bacteria develop from microzymes, the primal units of living organisms, but this occurs only under morbid, pathogenic conditions. These microzymes may be the remains of decomposing bacteria entering the system from without, or the microzymes of normal cells may develop into bacteria under pathogenic conditions within the body. According to this conception the cycle of germ life works out as follows: The microzymes of the normal healthy cells under morbid, pathogenic conditions may develop into bacteria (as would appear from the experiments of Béchamp which are discussed in a later chapter). These bacteria feed on and decompose the morbid matter which brought them into being. Thus nature, with the evil, provides the remedy. When the morbid food supply has been exhausted the microzymes devour the protoplasm of their own bacteria until there is nothing left but themselves, and they seem to be practically indestructible under ordinary conditions, as is shown by the finding of living microzymes in calcarous rocks of ancient geological formation. It is undoubtedly true that these morbid microzymes may again develop into disease germs if they enter a living body and find morbid soil on which to feed, but otherwise they are not harmful.

At first glance it may seem that this does not differ materially from the germ theory of the old school of medicine. On closer consideration, however, it will be found that there is a vast difference between the two concepts which leads to entirely different methods of treatment. According to orthodox belief, disease germs are special creations which of their own accord create disease. If this were true then "killing the germs" would be good practice. On the other hand, if our concept is the right one, then we must prevent the development of morbid conditions and, if such exist, our treatment must be directed to their removal. Killing the germs will not remove the morbid soil and therefore will leave the way open for the development of bacteria from the microzymes present in all living matter. Thus the microzymian theory of disease positively confirms the claims of Nature Cure philosophy that bacteria and parasites are scavengers of pathogenic materials, that inflammation is a purifying, healing process and that therefore acute, febrile diseases are as normal and orderly as anything else in nature.

Thus it would appear to be demonstrated that micro-organisms are only secondary manifestations of disease, that bacteria and parasites live, thrive and multiply to the danger point only in a weakened and diseased organism. If this were not so the human family would be extinct within a few months' time. The fear instilled by the germ theory of disease is frequently more destructive than the micro-organisms themselves. We have had under observation and treatment a number of insane patients whose peculiar delusion or monomania was an exaggerated fear of germs, a genuine "bacteriophobia".

The Nature Cure philosophy is the antithesis of all this. It recognizes that bacteria or their microzymes are practically omnipresent, that we absorb them in food and drink and inhale them in the air we breathe, and that our bodies are alive with them; but that it is not possible for us to be affected by disease taints and germs from without if our bodies are in a clean and vigorous state. The proper thing to do, therefore, is not to try to kill the germs, but to remove the morbid matter and disease taints on which they subsist and which they are capable of reducing to simpler forms suitable for elimination through the organs of depuration. Everything is good Nature Cure treatment which invigorates the system, builds up the blood and lymph on a normal basis, and purifies the tissues from their morbid encumbrances in such a way as to make germ activity unnecessary. To seek to kill germs without purifying and invigorating the organism would be like trying to keep a house free from fungi and vermin by sprinkling it daily with carbolic acid and other germ killers, instead of flooding it with fresh air and sunshine and washing it out thoroughly. The antiseptic would only add to the filth.

Bacteriologists are unanimous in declaring that the various disease germs are found not only in diseased bodies, but also in the bodies of seemingly healthy persons. A celebrated French bacteriologist reports that in the mouth of a healthy infant, two months old, he found almost all the disease germs known to medical science. A celebrated physician in the same country who had been appointed by the government to investigate the causes of tuberculosis declared before an International Tuberculosis Congress that he had found tubercle bacilli in 95 per cent of all the children he had examined. Dr. Osler, one of the greatest living medical authorities, mentions repeatedly that the bacilli of diphtheria, pneumonia and of many other virulent diseases are found in the bodies of healthy persons.

The inability of bacteria, by themselves, to create disease is further confirmed by the well known facts of natural immunity to specific infection or contagion. All mankind is more or less affected by hereditary or acquired disease taints, morbid encumbrances and drug poisoning, resulting from age-long violation of nature's laws and from the suppression of acute diseases; but even under the almost universal conditions of lowered vitality, morbid heredity and physical and mental degeneration, it is found that under identical conditions of exposure to draughts or infection, only a certain percentage of individuals will "take cold" or "catch disease". The fact of natural immunity is repeatedly corroborated by common experience as well as in the clinics and laboratories of our medical schools and research institutes. Also of a specific number of mice or rabbits inoculated with cancer, only a small percentage develop the malignant growth and succumb to its ravages. The development of infectious and contagious diseases necessitates a certain predisposition, or, as medical science calls it, "Disease Diathesis". This predisposition to infection and contagion consists in and is explained by the unity of disease as demonstrated in the previous pages.

Why Epidemics?

When giving these explanations in lectures I am frequently asked the question: "If what you say is true — if disease arises within the body organism rather than through invasion from without, — how do you explain epidemics in which many people become affected at the same time by similar kinds of disease germs?" The answer to this is: That it is common for the majority of people in a certain locality or area to be addicted to the same bad habits of living and of treating their ailments, thus producing in them the same kind of morbid soil, and this favours the development of normal or diseased microzymes into similar forms of bacteria and of the corresponding inflammatory processes. Also certain atmospheric and cosmic influences and conditions which we do not fully understand have much to do with the periodic appearance of epidemic or endemic diseases.(1)

Bacteria: Secondary not Primary Manifestations of Disease

We have already seen how lowered vitality weakens the resistance of the system to the attacks and inroads of disease germs and poisons. The development of microzymes into bacteria depends furthermore upon a congenial morbid soil. Just as the ordinary yeast germ multiplies in a sugar solution only, so the various micro-organisms of disease thrive and multiply, each in its own peculiar and congenial kind of morbid matter. Thus, the typhoid bacillus develops and thrives in a certain kind of effete matter which accumulates in the intestines; the pneumonia germs flourish best in the morbid excretions of the lungs; and meningitis germs in the diseased meninges of the brain and spinal cord.

Dr. Pettenkofer, a celebrated physician and professor of the University of Vienna, also reached the conclusion that bacteria by themselves cannot create disease, and for years he defended his opinion on the lecture platform and in his writings against the solid opposition of the medical profession. On one occasion he supported his theory by picking up a glass containing millions of live cholera bacilli and swallowing its contents before the eyes of his astonished students. The seemingly dangerous experiment resulted only in a slight nausea. Numerous cases are on record of persons in this country who subjected themselves in similar manner to infection, inoculation and contagion with the most virulent kinds of bacteria and disease taints, without developing the corresponding diseases. A few years ago Dr. Rodermund, a physician in the state of Wisconsin, created a sensation by smearing his body with the exudate of smallpox sores in order to demonstrate to his medical colleagues that a healthy body could not be infected with the disease. He was arrested and quarantined in jail, but not before he had come in contact with many people. Not a single case of smallpox developed through this "exposure".

During the many years I have been connected with sanitarium work, my workers and myself, in administering the various forms of manipulative treatment, have handled intimately thousands of cases of contagious diseases, and I do not remember a single instance where any one of us was the least affected by such contact. Ordinary cleanliness, good vitality,

(1)
   The full explanation of epidemics, particularly those of a very destructive kind, which from time to time sweep across large areas of the world causing very high mortality especially among people living in primitive conditions, is not easy to find. This matter is further discussed in an appendix at the end of this volume. (See Appendix I).

clean blood and tissues, the organs of elimination in good, active condition and a positive, fearless attitude of mind, will practically establish natural immunity to excessive and destructive activity of bacteria and disease taints. If infection takes place the organism reacts to it through inflammatory processes and by means of these endeavours to overcome it and so to eliminate micro-organisms and poisons from the system.

In this connection it is of interest to learn that the danger to life from bites and stings of poisonous reptiles and insects has been greatly exaggerated. According to popular opinion, anyone bitten by a poisonous insect or reptile, as the rattlesnake, Gila monster or tarantula, is doomed to die, while as a matter of fact statistics show that only from two to seven per cent of such cases prove fatal. I am often asked: "What is the right thing to do in case of snake bite? Would you not give plenty of whiskey to save the victim's life?" It is my belief that of the "seven per cent" who die after being bitten by rattlesnakes and other poisonous reptiles, a goodly proportion do so because of the effects of enormous doses of strong whiskey poured into them under the mistaken idea that it is an efficient antidote to the poison. People do not know that the death rate from snake bite is so very low, and therefore they attribute the recoveries to the whiskey, just as recoveries from other diseases under medical or metaphysical treatment are attributed to the virtues of the particular medicine or method of treatment applied, instead of to the real healer, the "vis medicatrix naturae", which in most cases eliminates the rattlesnake venom without injury to the organism.(1)

To recapitulate: Just as yeast cells are not only the cause but also the product of sugar fermentation, so disease germs are not only a cause (secondary) but also a product of morbid fermentation (inflammation) in the system. Furthermore, just as the yeast germs devour and decompose sugar, so the disease germs consume and decompose morbid matter and systemic poisons. In a way, therefore, micro-organisms are just as much the product as the cause of disease and act as scavengers or eliminators of morbid matter (see Chapter X). In order to hold in check the destructive activity of bacteria and to prevent their multiplication beyond what is safe, nature manufactures her own "antitoxins". We have an apt illustration of this in the activity of yeast germs. While digesting sugar they change it

(1)
     There is no doubt that very grave emergencies can arise from the bites and stings of animals and from puncturing wounds which can carry poison or infection into the actual tissues and blood stream. Tetanus and rabies as well as snake and insect bites are conditions which come to mind in this connection. Apart from the washing out or sucking out of wounds as far as possible, hydrotherapy and particularly the use of the whole sheet pack is the treatment above all others which, according to the Nature Cure view, should be applied in these cases.

into alcohol and carbonic acid. As the alcohol accumulates in the fermenting fluid it gradually checks and finally stops the activity of the yeast germs. Thus nature holds in check the activity of germs by their own waste products. To this it may be answered, if that is so, then the administration of antitoxin must be good and natural treatment. There is a difference, however. Nature does not check or suppress the activity of bacteria until they have decomposed the disease matter (pathogen) on which they live. The powerful and highly poisonous doses of medical serums and antitoxins check and suppress the inflammatory process before it has run its natural course, and thus, if the patient survives, leaves the system in a condition of chronic encumbrance. This will be more fully explained later.

Whatever tends to build up the blood on a natural basis, to promote elimination of morbid matter and thereby make unnecessary the activity of bacteria and parasites without injuring the body or depressing its vital functions, is good Nature Cure practice. The first consideration, therefore, in the treatment of inflammation must be not to interfere with its natural course. Secondly, the natural method of treatment must keep the inflammatory activities below the danger point and within constructive limits. This the physician must accomplish by careful regulation of diet, or by fasting, by hydropathic, manipulative and homeopathic treatment as described in Vol. II of this series.

By the various statements and claims made in this chapter, I do not wish to convey the idea that I am opposed to scrupulous cleanliness and to surgical asepsis. These are matters of common sense. But I do affirm that the danger from infectious disease lies as much, or more so, in internal filth as in external uncleanness. Cleanliness and asepsis must go hand in hand with the purification of the inner man in order to insure "natural immunity". It should be noted that the argument of this chapter is corroborated by Béchamp's microzymian theory and by Dr. Powell's interpretation of the phenomenon of "leucocytosis". These matters will be more fully discussed later.

CHAPTER VII

THE LAWS OF CURE

This brings us to the consideration of acute inflammatory and feverish diseases. From what has been said, it follows that inflammation and fever are not primary, but secondary manifestations of disease. No form of inflammatory disease can arise in the system unless there is present some handicap to health which nature is endeavouring to overcome and to get rid of. On this fact in nature is based what I claim to be the fundamental law of cure. "Give me fever and I can cure every disease". Thus Hippocrates, the "Father of Medicine", formulated the fundamental Law of Cure over two thousand years ago. I have expressed this law in the following statement: Every acute disease is the result of a cleansing and healing effort of nature. This law, thoroughly understood and applied in the treatment of diseases, will eventually do for medical science what the discovery of other natural laws has done for physics, astronomy, chemistry and other exact sciences. It will, by demonstrating the unity of disease and treatment, transform the medical empiricism and confusion of the past and present into an exact science.

Making a general application of the law, we deduce that all acute diseases, from a simple cold to measles, scarlet fever, diphtheria, smallpox, pneumonia, etc., represent nature's efforts to remove from the system some form of morbid matter, virus or poison dangerous to health and life. In other words, acute disease cannot develop in a perfectly normal, healthy body living under conditions favourable to human life. The question may be asked: "If acute diseases represent nature's healing efforts, why is it that people die as a result of them?" The answer to this is: that the vitality may be too low, the injury or morbid encumbrance too great, or the treatment may be inadequate or harmful, so that nature loses the fight; still, acute disease represents an effort of nature to remove the causes of disease and thus to re-establish normal, healthy conditions.

It is a curious fact that this fundamental principle of Nature Cure and law of nature has been acknowledged and corroborated by medical science. The most advanced works on pathology admit the constructive and beneficial character of inflammation. However, when it comes to the treatment of acute diseases, physicians seem to forget entirely this basic principle of pathology and treat inflammation and fever as though they were, in themselves, inimical and destructive to health and life. From this inconsistency in theory and practice arise all the errors of allopathic medical treatment. Failure to understand this fundamental law of cure accounts for the confusion on the part of exponents of the different schools of healing science, and for the greater part of human suffering. Nature Cure philosophy never loses sight of the fundamental law of cure. While allopathy regards acute disease conditions as in themselves harmful and hostile to health and life, as something to be "cured" (we say "suppressed") by drug, ice or knife, the Nature Cure school regards these forcible house cleanings as beneficial and necessary — necessary so long as human beings continue to disregard nature's laws. While, through its simple, natural methods of treatment, Nature Cure easily modifies the course of inflammatory and feverish processes and keeps them within safe limits, it never checks nor suppresses acute reactions by poisonous drugs, ice, serums, antiseptics, surgical operations, suggestion or any other suppressive treatment. Skin eruptions, boils, ulcers, catarrh, diarrhoea, and all other forms of inflammatory febrile disease processes are indications that there is something hostile to life and health in the organism, which nature is trying to remove and overcome by these so-called "acute" diseases. What then, is to be gained by suppressing them with poisonous drugs and surgical operations? Such practice does not allow nature to carry on her work of cleansing and repair and to attain her ends. The morbid matter which she is endeavouring to eliminate by acute reaction is thrown back into the system. Worse than that, drug poisons are added to disease poisons. Is it any wonder that fatal complications arise, or that the acute process is changed to chronic disease?

Why does the Greater Part of Allopathic Materia Medica consist of Virulent Poisons?

The statements made in the preceding pages are a severe indictment of so-called "regular" medical science, but they point out the difference in the basic principles of the old school of healing and those of Nature Cure philosophy. The fundamental Law of Cure explains why allopathic medical science is in error, not in a few but in most things. The foundation — the orthodox conception of disease — being wrong, it follows that everything built thereon must be wrong also. The fundamental law of cure explains also why the great majority of allopathic prescriptions contain virulent poisons in some form or other, and why surgical operations are in high favour with the disciples of the old school. The answer of allopathy to the question, "Why do you give poisons?" usually is, "Our materia medica contains poisons because drug poison kills and eliminates disease poison". We, however, claim that drug poison merely serves to paralyse vital force, whereby the deceptive results of allopathic treatment are obtained.

The following will explain this more fully. If acute diseases are nature's cleansing and healing efforts, all acute reactions represent increased activity of vital force, resulting in feverish and inflammatory conditions, accompanied by pain, redness, swelling, high temperature, rapid pulse, catarrhal discharges, skin eruptions, boils, ulcers, etc. Allopathy regards these violent activities of vital force as detrimental and harmful in themselves. Anything which will inhibit the action of vital force will, in allopathic parlance, "cure" acute disease. As a matter of fact, nothing more effectively paralyzes vital force and impairs vital organs than poisonous drugs, ice and the surgeon's knife. These, therefore, must necessarily constitute the favourite means of "cure" of the old school of medicine. But this school is in reality mistaking effect for cause. It fails to see that the local inflammation arising within the organism is not the disease, but merely marks the locality and the method through which nature is trying her best to discharge the morbid encumbrances; — that the acute reaction may be local, but that its causes or "feeders" are always constitutional and must be treated constitutionally. When under the influence of rational, natural treatment, the poisonous irritants are eliminated from blood and tissues, the local symptoms take care of themselves; it does not matter whether they manifest as pimple or cancer, as a simple cold or as consumption.

The Law of Dual Effect

Everywhere in nature rules the great Law of Action and Reaction. In the realms of physical nature, giving and receiving, action and reaction, balance each other mechanically and automatically. This makes it possible for the mechanic, the scientist and the astronomer to predict with mathematical precision for ages in advance the results of certain activities in nature. This great law of dual effect also forms the foundation of healing science. It is related to and governs every phenomenon of health, disease and cure. When I formulated the fundamental law of cure in the words: "Every acute disease is the result of a healing effort of nature", this was but another expression of the great law of action and reaction. What we commonly call crisis, acute reaction or acute disease, is in reality nature's attempt to establish health. Applied to the physical activity of the body, the Law of Compensation may be expressed as follows: Every agent

44

affecting the human organism produces two effects: a first, temporary effect, and a second, lasting effect. The second, lasting effect is always contrary to the first, transient effect. For instance, the first temporary effect of cold water applied to the skin consists in sending the blood to the interior; but in order to compensate for the local depletion, nature responds by sending greater quantities back to the surface, which results in increased warmth and better surface circulation. Conversely, the first effect of a hot bath is to draw the blood to the surface; but the second effect sends the blood back to the interior, leaving the surface bloodless and chilled. Stimulants, as we shall presently see, produce their deceptive effects by consuming the reserve stores of vital energy in the organism. This is inevitably followed by weakness and exhaustion in exact proportion to the previous excitation. The first effect of relaxation and sleep is weakness, numbness and death-like stupor; the second effect, however, is an increase of vitality.

The law of Dual Effect governs all drug action. The first, temporary, violent effect of poisonous drugs, is usually due to nature's efforts to overcome and eliminate these substances. The second, lasting effect is due to the retention of the drug poisons in the system and their destructive action on the organism. In theory and in practice, allopathy considers the first effect only and ignores the lasting after effects of drugs and surgical operations. It administers remedies whose first effect is contrary to the disease condition. Therefore, in accordance with the law of action and reaction, the second, lasting effect of such remedies must be similar to the disease condition. Common, everyday experience should teach us that this is true, for laxatives and cathartics always tend to produce chronic constipation. The second effect of stimulants and tonics of any kind is increased weakness. Their continued use often results in complete exhaustion and paralysis of mental and physical powers. Headache powders, pain killers, opiates, sedatives and hypnotics may paralyze brain and nerves into temporary insensibility; but, if due to constitutional causes, the pain, nervousness and insomnia will always return with redoubled force. If taken habitually these agents invariably tend to create heart disease and paralysis and ultimately develop addiction. Cold and catarrh "cures" such as quinine, coal tar products, etc., suppress nature's efforts to eliminate waste and morbid matter through the mucous linings of the respiratory tract, causing retention of disease matter, thus breeding pneumonia, chronic catarrhs, asthma and consumption. Mercury, iodin, salvarsan and other alteratives, by suppression of external elimination, and even more so by their own destructive effects, create internal chronic diseases of the most dreadful types, such as locomotor ataxia, paresis, paralysis agitans, etc. So the recital might be continued through all the orthodox materia medica. Each drug breeds new disease symptoms which are in their turn "cured" by other poisons, until the insane asylum or merciful death brings down the curtain on the tragedy of a ruined life.

The teaching and practice of homoeopathy, on the other hand, is fully in harmony with the law of action and reaction. Proceeding upon its basic principle — "Similia similibus curantur", or "like cures like" — it administers remedies whose first, temporary effect is similar to the disease condition. In accordance, then, with the law of dual effect, the second effect of the remedies must be contrary to the disease condition, that is, truly curative.

CHAPTER VIII

SUPPRESSION VERSUS ELIMINATION

My claim that the conventional treatment of acute diseases is suppressive and not curative will probably be denied by my medical colleagues. They will maintain that their methods also are calculated to eliminate morbid matter from the system. But what are the facts in actual practice? Is it not true that preparations of mercury, lead, zinc, silver and other powerful poisons are constantly used to suppress skin eruptions, boils, abscesses, etc., instead of allowing nature to rid the system through these "skin diseases" of scrofulous, venereal and psoric taints? Some time ago Dr. Wiley, former Government Chemist, published a list of the ingredients of a number of popular remedies for colds, coughs and catarrhs. Every one of them contained some powerful opiate or astringent. These poisonous drugs relieve the cough and catarrhal conditions by paralyzing the eliminative activity of the membranous linings of the nasal passages, bronchi and lungs, the digestive and genito-urinary organs; but in doing so they throw back into the system morbid matter which nature is trying to get rid of, and add drug poisons to disease poisons.

Equally harmful is suppression by means of the surgeon's knife. It may be a quicker and apparently more effective process to remove the inflamed appendix or diseased tonsils than to cure them by building up the blood and inducing elimination of systemic poisons by natural methods. But operative treatment is not eliminative. It does not remove from the system the original cause of inflammation or deterioration of tissues and organs, but it does remove the outlet which nature had established for the escape of morbid material. These morbid encumbrances, forcibly retained in the body, weaken and destroy other parts and organs or affect the general health of the patient. My own observations during nearly eighteen years of practical experience prove positively that the average length of life after a "major" operation, performed on important, vital parts and organs, is less than ten years, and after such an operation the general health of the patient is, in the great majority of cases, not as good as before. This is confirmed by many other conscientious observers of many different schools.

Some common instances of suppression and the usual chronic after effects which it produces may be mentioned. Diarrhoea is often suppressed with laudanum and other opiates which paralyze the peristaltic action of the bowels and, if repeated, soon produce chronic constipation. Gonorrhoeal discharges and syphilitic ulcers are checked and suppressed by local injections, cautery and by prescriptions containing mercury, iodine, arsenic (salvarsan) and other poisonous alteratives which effectually prevent nature's efforts to eliminate the venereal poisons from the system. All feverish diseases are more or less interfered with or suppressed by antiseptics, antipyretics, serum and antitoxins. Professors in colleges and the best books on Materia Medica teach that these remedies lower the fever because they are "protoplasmic poisons"; because they paralyze the red and white blood corpuscles, benumb heart action and respiration and depress all vital functions. Nervousness, sleeplessness, and pain are suppressed by sedatives, opiates and hypnotics. Every one of the drugs used for such purposes is a powerful poison which benumbs brain and nerve action, in that way interfering with nature's healing efforts and frequently preventing the consummation of beneficial healing crises. Epileptic attacks and other forms of convulsions are suppressed, but never cured, by bromides which benumb and paralyze brain and nerve centres. All that these "sedatives" accomplish is to produce in course of time idiocy and different forms of paralysis and premature senility. However, is he not considered the best doctor who can most promptly bring about these and similar deceptive results through artificial inhibition or stimulation by means of the most virulent poisons found on earth?

It is not realised that dandruff and falling hair are connected with the elimination of systemic poisons through the scalp. The thing to do, therefore, is not to suppress this elimination and thereby cause accumulation of poisons in the brain area, but to stop the manufacture of poison in the body and to promote its removal through natural channels. Dandruff "cures" and hair tonics contain glycerin, poisonous antiseptics and stimulants which are absorbed by scalp and brain, causing dizziness, headaches, loss of memory, neurasthenia, deafness, weakness of sight, etc. Head lice and similar parasites peculiar to other parts of the body live on scrofulous and psoric taints. When these are consumed, the lice depart as they came. The microzymian theory furnishes an explanation of this and similar phenomena, and this is confirmed by the fact that these noxious pests do not remain with all people who have been infected with them, but only with those whose external or internal conditions furnish them with the means of subsistence. In a number of cases we have seen healing crises take the form of lice. At that time the patients were living in the most cleanly surroundings, taking various forms of water treatment every day, so that infection was practically impossible. In each of these cases the patient recalled having been infested with parasites at some previous time, and remembered that sulphur and molasses, mercurial salves or other means of suppression had been applied. We prescribe for the removal of lice only cold water and the comb. Even antiseptic soaps should be avoided.

The foregoing statements, more than any other portion of this volume, have brought down upon it violent criticism and condemnation. However, many of our patients who have developed, under natural treatment, such parasitic crises will testify to their reality. Indeed, as I am writing this, one of our guests is just recovering from one of these parasitic crises. Before this woman came to us she had lived for many years in her luxurious home and since she has been with us during the last four months she has not left our institution. She has occupied a room alone and has received several water treatments, including head bath, every day, so that infection was impossible. Yet, four weeks ago, the attendant who gave her treatment discovered her scalp covered with nits which a few days later developed into swarms of lice. She was much alarmed and shed tears of mortification, until she better understood the nature of the phenomenon. I showed her the passage in this volume dealing with psora and parasitic diseases; also her original examination report which, in the section devoted to diagnosis from the iris, had the entry "psora positive, several itch spots", indicating suppression of itchy parasitic skin eruptions. When told that the psora taints on which these parasites live is the soil of tuberculosis and cancer, she endured her crisis with great equanimity. The visitors remained with her for about three weeks and then suddenly disappeared as they had come. Nothing was used to combat the parasites except fresh cold water and the comb. Lice, crab lice, scabies (itch parasites), belong to the same psoric family. They live on psoric taints, just as bacteria live on other disease taints and systemic poisons. This patient is now fully convinced of the reality of parasitic crises. This subject is more fully treated in Volume II of this series.

The Results of Suppression of Children's Diseases

Sycotic eruptions on the heads and bodies of infants, also called "milk scurf", if suppressed by salves, cream, unsalted butter, or even by warm bathing, are often followed by chorea (St. Vitus's dance), epilepsy, a scrofulous constitution, and, in later life, by tuberculosis. Measles, scarlet fever, diphtheria, cerebro-spinal meningitis, and other febrile diseases of childhood, if properly treated by natural methods, are curative or at least corrective in their effects on the system, and represent well defined, orderly, natural processes for the elimination of inherited or acquired disease taints, drug poisons, etc. But if arrested or suppressed before they have run their natural course, or before nature has had time to re-establish normal conditions, then the abnormal conditions become fixed and permanent (chronic). In addition to this, the poisons, serums and antitoxins employed to arrest the disease process very often affect vital parts and organs permanently, causing the gradual deterioration of cells and tissues, and paving the way for cancer, tuberculosis, chronic affection of the kidneys, etc. in later years.

These simple facts, which can be verified by any unprejudiced observer, account for the "mysterious sequelae" of drug and serum treated acute diseases. These never occur where natural methods of healing have been correctly employed. Among these chronic after effects are deafness, blindness, heart and kidney diseases, nervous affections, idiocy, infantile paralysis, tuberculosis, cancer etc.

Further Consideration of Suppression as the Cause of Chronic Disease

A few years ago Dr. Nicholas Senn, a celebrated Chicago surgeon, after a long trip to Africa and other parts of the world, expressed views very much in conformity with Nature Cure doctrine, at least in part. He maintained that cancer and many other chronic diseases were practically unknown among primitive peoples living simply and naturally, and that such diseases are the result of "civilization" with its accompaniments of "over-feeding and over-living". This is undoubtedly true, and the majority of disease would gradually disappear if men and women lived more naturally. "Civilization has become almost synonymous with artificiality of life and unnatural habits. We hope and believe that a higher civilization, yet to come, will combine the most exquisite culture of mind and soul with true simplicity and naturalness of living. Meanwhile excessive meat eating, strong spices and condiments, alcohol, coffee, tea, over-work, night work, fear, worry, sensuality, corsets, high heels, foul air, improper breathing, lack of exercise, loveless marriages, race suicide, — all of these and many other evils of "hyper-civilization" have contributed their share to the universal degeneracy of civilized nations commented upon by Dr. Senn. Dr. Senn, however, seems to have failed to recognize a most important cause of the rapid increase of destructive chronic diseases; namely, the suppression of acute diseases by poisonous drugs and surgical operations. When the unnatural habits of life alluded to have so lowered the vitality and favoured the accumulation of waste matter and poisons that the sluggish bowels, kidneys, skin and other organs of elimination are unable to keep a clean house, nature is forced to resort to other, more radical means of purification or we would choke in our own impurities. These forcible house-cleanings of nature are colds, catarrhs, skin eruptions, diarrhoeas, boils, ulcers, abnormal perspiration, haemorrhages, and many other forms of inflammatory and febrile diseases. Sulphur and mercury may drive back the skin eruptions, antipyretics and antiseptics may suppress fever and catarrh; the patient and the doctor may congratulate themselves on a speedy cure; but what is the true state of affairs? Nature has been thwarted in her work of healing and cleansing. She has to give up the fight against disease matter in order to combat the more potent poisons of mercury, quinine, iodine, strychnine, etc. The disease matter is still in the system, plus the drug poison. Proof positive of the retention of drug poisons in the organism is furnished by the diagnosis from the iris of the eye, which is explained more fully in a later volume of this series.

When vitality has been sufficiently restored, nature may make another attempt at purification, this time, possibly, in another direction; but again her well meant efforts are defeated. This process of suppression is repeated over and over again until blood and tissues become so loaded with waste matter and poisons that the healing forces of the organism can no longer react against them by acute diseases. Then results the "chronic condition" which in the vocabulary of the old school of medicine is only another name for "incurable". The more skilled the allopathic school becomes in the suppression and prevention of acute diseases by drugs, knife, X-rays, serums, vaccination virus, antitoxin, etc., the greater will be the increase of chronic dyspepsia, nervous prostration, insanity, locomotor ataxia, paresis, cancer, secondary and tertiary syphilis, tuberculosis and many other so-called incurable diseases.

Suppression of acute diseases, by drug and knife, is the all important factor in the creation of malignant diseases which Dr. Senn overlooked in his discourse on the causes of chronic destructive ailments. If he had analysed his experiences more deeply he would have found that the great scourges of chronic disease exist only in those parts of the earth where drug stores flourish. These statements may seem exaggerated; but I would like to cite a few typical cases of suppression and its effects from the records of our institutional practice. Paresis, locomotor ataxia and paralysis agitans are not, as is usually assumed, due to secondary and tertiary syphilis but to mercury and other alteratives administered for the cure of luetic and other diseases. In less than six months' time we cure the so-called specific diseases by our natural methods, provided they have not been suppressed and complicated by mercury, iodine or other poisonous drugs. We never interfere with the original lesion, but assist nature to discharge the poison through the channels established for this purpose. By the natural methods of treatment we moderate the inflammatory processes and keep them within constructive limits. A bonfire is useful to burn up the rubbish on the premises but it must be watched and tended so that it will not destroy the buildings. Under rational treatment, discharges and ulcers act as fontanels to the system. Not only the specific poison, but much of hereditary and acquired disease matter also is eliminated in the process. After such a cure, blood and tissues are purer than before the infection. On the other hand, we claim that the dreadful sufferings of the "secondary" and "tertiary" stages are brought on by suppressive drug treatment by means of mercury, the iodides, "606" etc. These drugs suppress the initial lesions and diffuse the disease poison through the system. Nature takes up the work of elimination by means of skin eruptions and ulcers in various parts of the body, but these also are promptly suppressed with mercurial ointments and other alteratives. This process of suppression is continued for months and years, until the organism is so thoroughly saturated with alterative poisons that vital force can no longer arouse the body to acute reactions against the original syphilitic taint. This condition of vital paralysis is called "cure". However, many of the medical teachers know better and instruct their students somewhat as follows: "When, after two or three years of mercurial treatment, syphilitic symptoms cease to appear, you may permit the patient to marry — but never guarantee a cure." This is because it is well known that the children of such a marriage may be born with "hereditary" symptoms, and because the patient may himself at any time confront the doctor with a hole in his palate, ulcers on his body, caries in his bones, or other second and tertiary symptoms. Mercury will work its way into the nerve matter of the brain and spinal cord, causing inflammation, excruciating headaches, nervous symptoms, girdle pains, etc. These stages of acute and subacute inflammation are followed in a few years by sclerosis (hardening) of nerve matter and blood vessels, resulting in paresis, locomotor ataxia, or paralysis agitans. Neither is it necessary to contract specific diseases in order to fall a victim to these dreadful conditions; mercury, iodine, salvarsan and other destructive alteratives are given in a hundred different forms for a multitude of other ailments.

A few years ago we had under our care a patient in the last stages of locomotor ataxia, who for years had been suffering the tortures of the damned. There had never been a taint of specific disease in her system, but four different times she had been salivated by calomel. This dreadful poison had been administered in large doses for the cure of liver trouble and constipation. She was only fourteen years old when, on account of this, she first suffered from acute mercurial poisoning (salivation). Another patient who, after fifteen years of "slow and torturous dying by inches", succumbed to the same disease, had absorbed the mercurial poison in his boyhood while attending a boarding school. He was twice salivated by mercurial ointments applied to cure the itch (scabies), a disease which was epidemic at times among the boys. He likewise never had a syphilitic infection. A young man, insane at the age of thirty, absorbed the poison when four years of age. He had at the time a psoric skin eruption. The family physician, suspecting syphilitic infection from the nurse girl, kept the child under mercury for six months. That this diagnosis was false was confirmed by the iris of the eye which revealed psora as the cause of the suspicious eruption which reappeared several times later in life, and because the servant girl was afterwards absolutely exonerated by competent physicians.

The subject of venereal diseases, their natural and unnatural treatment, will be treated more fully later in this work.

Proofs by the Diagnosis from the Eye

We have treated many hundreds of cases of so-called chronic neuralgia, neuritis, rheumatism, neurasthenia, epilepsy, tuberculosis, cancer and idiocy, due to the pernicious effects ofquinine, iodine, arsenic, strychnine, coal tar products and other virulent poisons taken under the guise of "medicine".

We know that this is so for the following reasons:

(a). Because the diagnosis from the iris of the eye plainly reveals the presence of these poisons in the system.

(b). Because the drug signs in the iris are accompanied by the symptoms of these poisons in the system.

(c). Because the history revealed the fact that the patient had at some time taken the poison revealed in his iris.

(d). Because, under natural living and treatment, diseases long ago suppressed by drugs or knife reappear as healing crises.

(e). Because in these healing crises, drugs indicated in the iris are frequently eliminated, each under its own peculiar symptoms.

(f). Because, to the extent that a drug is eliminated from the system by a healing crisis, its sign will disappear from the iris.

As an illustration:

(a). The diagnosis from the iris reveals quinine poisoning in the region of the brain.

(b). This enables us to say to the patient, without questioning him, that he suffers from severe frontal headaches and ringing in the ears, that he is very irritable, and so on through the various symptoms of quinine poisoning, or, as the medical men call it, "chronic cinchonism".

(c). The history of the patient reveals the fact that he has taken large amounts of quinine for colds, grippe, or malaria.

(d). Under our methods of natural living and treatment, the patient improves; the organism becomes more vigorous, and the organs of elimination act more freely; the latent poisons are stirred up in their hiding places; healing crises make their appearance. The processes of elimination thus inaugurated develop various symptoms of acute quinine poisoning.

(e). The eliminating crises are accompanied by headaches, ringing in the ears, nasal catarrh, bone pains, neuritis, strong taste of quinine in the mouth, etc.

(f). Every healing crisis, if naturally treated, diminishes the signs of disease and drug poisons in the eye.

CHAPTER IX

INFLAMMATION

From what has already been said it will have become apparent that the inflammatory and feverish diseases are just as natural, orderly and lawful as anything else in nature; that, therefore, after they have once started, they must not be checked or suppressed by drugs, ice, surgery or any other agent. Inflammatory processes can be kept within safe limits, and they must be assisted in their constructive tendencies by the natural methods of treatment. To check and suppress acute diseases before they have run their natural course means to suppress nature's purifying and healing efforts, to bring about fatal complications, and to change acute, constructive reactions into chronic disease conditions. Those who have followed the preceding chapters will remember that their general trend has been to prove one of the fundamental principles of Nature Cure philosophy namely, the Unity of Disease and Cure. We claim that all acute diseases are uniform in their causes, their purpose, and, where conditions are favourable, uniform also in their progressive development. In former chapters I have endeavoured to prove and to elucidate the unity of acute diseases in regard to their causes and their purpose, the latter not being destructive, but constructive and beneficial. I have pointed out that the micro-organisms associated with disease are not the terrible menace they are commonly thought to be, but that, like everything else in nature, they serve a useful purpose. I have shown that it depends upon ourselves whether their activity is harmful and destructive, or beneficial; that is upon our manner of living and of treating acute elimination. Let us now trace the unity of acute diseases in regard to their general course by a brief examination of the processes of inflammation and their development through five well-defined stages. I shall base our studies on recognized works on pathology and bacteriology.

A. The Story of Inflammation according to the Orthodox Interpretation

Before inflammation can arise, there must exist an exciting cause in the form of some obstruction or of some agent inimical to health and life.

Such excitants may be systemic poisons, dead cells, blood clots, fragments of bone, and other effete matter produced in the system itself, or they may be drug poisons, or foreign bodies such as particles of dust, soot, stone, iron, or other metals, slivers of wood, etc.; again they may be micro-organisms or parasites.

When one or more of these exciting agents of inflammation are present in the tissues in sufficient strength to call forth the reaction and opposition of the healing forces, the microscope always reveals the following phenomena, slightly varying under different conditions. The circulation in the affected parts or organ seems to be obstructed. Owing to the increased blood pressure, the minute arteries and veins in the immediate neighbourhood become dilated. The distension of the blood vessels stretches and thereby weakens their walls. Through these the white blood corpuscles squeeze their mobile bodies and work their way into the neighbouring tissues. In some mysterious way they seem to sense the exact location of the danger point, and hurry towards it in large numbers like soldiers summoned to meet an invading army. The faculty of the white blood corpuscles to apprehend the presence and exact location of the enemy (bacteria) has been ascribed to chemical attraction and is called chemotaxis. The "army of defence" is made up of white blood corpuscles or leucocytes. These wandering cells possess the faculty of absorbing and digesting microbes. They contain certain proteolytic or protein-splitting ferments, by means of which they decompose and "digest" poisons and hostile micro-organisms. On account of their activity as germ destroyers, these cells have been called germ killers or phagocytes. In their movements and actions these valiant little warriors act very much like intelligent beings, animated by the qualities of patience, perseverance, courage, foresight and self-sacrifice. The phagocytes absorb morbid matter, poisons, or micro-organisms by enveloping them with their own bodies. It is a hand-to-hand fight, and many of the brave little soldiers are destroyed by the poisons and bacteria which they attack. What we call "pus" is made up of the bodies of live and dead phagocytes, disease taints and germs, blood serum, broken-down cells, in short, the "debris of the battlefield". We can now understand how the processes just described produce the well-known "cardinal symptoms" of inflammation and fever; the redness, heat and swelling due to increased blood pressure, congestion and accumulation of exudates; the pain due to irritation and to pressure on nerves. We can also comprehend how impaired nutrition, obstruction and destruction in the affected parts and organs interfere with and inhibit functional activity. The organism has still other means of defending itself. At the time of bacterial infection, certain germ-killing substances are developed in the blood serum. Science has named these defensive proteids opsonins and alexins. It is also claimed that the phagocytes and tissue cells in the neighbourhood of the area of irritation produce antibodies or natural antitoxins which neutralize the bacterial poisons and kill the micro-organisms of disease.

It must further be seen that the growth and development of bacteria and parasites is inhibited and finally arrested by their own waste products. We have an example of this in the yeast germ, which thrives and multiplies in the presence of sugar in solution. Living on and "digesting" the sugar, it decomposes the sugar molecules into alcohol and carbonic acid. As the alcohol increases during the process of fermentation, it gradually arrests the development and activity of disease germs and parasites. They produce certain waste products which gradually inhibit their own growth and multiplication. The vaccines, serums and antitoxins of medical science are prepared from these bacterial excrements and from extracts made of the bodies of bacteria. In the serum and antitoxin treatments, therefore, the allopathic school is imitating nature's procedure in checking the growth of micro-organisms, but with this difference: nature does not suppress the growth and multiplication until the morbid matter on which they subsist has been decomposed and consumed, and until the inflammatory processes have run their natural course through the five stages of inflammation; while serums and antitoxins given in powerful doses at the different stages of any disease may check and suppress germ activity and the processes of inflammation before the latter have run their natural course and before the morbid matter has been eliminated. Besides that, these powerful poisons cause permanent injury to the cells, tissues and organs of the body, which frequently results in serious chronic after effects, the "mysterious sequelae" of medical science. There is no excuse for resorting to these doubtful and dangerous agents in the treatment of inflammatory processes when Nature Cure methods will produce satisfactory results in a simple natural way.

What has been said in former chapters confirms our claim that all acute diseases are uniform in their causes and in their purpose. From the foregoing description of inflammation it will have become clear that they are also uniform in their pathological development. The uniformity of acute inflammatory processes becomes still more apparent when we follow them through their five successive stages, viz: Incubation, Aggravation, Destruction, Abatement and Reconstruction, as illustrated in the following diagram:

Destruction

Aggravation   **Abatement**

Incubation   **Reconstruction**

1. **Incubation.** The period of incubation is the time between the exposure to an infectious disease and its development. This period may last from a few moments to several days, weeks, months or even years. During this stage morbid matter, poisons, micro-organisms and other excitants of inflammation congregate in certain parts and organs of the body. When they have accumulated to such an extent as to interfere with the normal functions or to endanger the health and life of the organism, the life forces begin to react to the obstruction or threatening danger by means of the inflammatory processes before described. (From the foregoing it appears that allopathy figures the period in incubation from the time of germ invasion, while according to our conception, incubation is co-existent with the three primary manifestations of disease. (Chapter V.))

2. **Aggravation.** During the period of Aggravation the battle between the phagocytes and nature's antitoxins on the one hand, and the poisons and micro-organisms of disease on the other hand, gradually progresses, accompanied by a corresponding increase in fever and inflammation, until it reaches a climax, marked by the greatest intensity of feverish symptoms.

3. **Destruction.** The battle between the forces of disease and the healing forces is accompanied by the disintegration of tissues due to the accumulation of exudates, to pus formation, the development of abscesses, boils, fistulae, open sores, etc. and to other morbid changes. It involves the destruction of phagocytes, bacteria, blood vessels and tissues just as a battle between contending human armies results in loss of life and property. The stage of destruction ends in crisis, which may be either fatal or beneficial.

4. **Abatement or Absorption.** If the healing forces of the organism are in the ascendant, and if they are supported by right treatment which tends to build up the blood, increase the vitality, and promote elimination, then the poisons and the micro-organisms of disease will gradually be overcome, absorbed or eliminated, and by degrees the tissues will be cleared of the "debris of the battlefield". This is accompanied by the gradual lowering of the temperature, pulse rate and other symptoms of fever and inflammation.

5. **Reconstruction.** When the period of abatement has run its course and the affected areas have been cleared of the morbid accumulations and obstructions, then, during the fifth stage of inflammation, the work of rebuilding begins. The struggle having been more or less destructive to the cells, tissues, blood vessels and organs of the areas involved, these must

now be reconstructed, and this last stage of the inflammatory process is, therefore, in a way the most important. On the thoroughness of regeneration of the injured parts depends the final effect of the acute disease upon the organism.

B. The story of Inflammation according to the Pathogenic Theory

The theory of inflammation according to Metchnikoff and the pathology of the allopathic school of medicine is certainly a most interesting and romantic story. The campaigns and battles of the tiny heroic defenders of the body, the phagocytes or "germ-eaters" against the micro-organisms of disease and infectious taints and poisons read very much like the accounts of skirmishes, battles, captures and killings in human warfare between the armies of defence of a country and the invading enemy. It looks, however, as though we may have to relegate this romance of pathology to the realm of fairy tales. There is one phase of this allopathic conception of inflammation, first advanced by Professor Metchnikoff, which does not fully agree with the Nature Cure idea of the activities of bacteria and parasites, and their effect upon the processes of disease and cure. Nature Cure philosophy teaches that these micro-organisms are scavengers which live, thrive, and multiply on disease matter only. According to the Metchnikoff theory, the bacteria are the enemies of the body, the creators of disease, which have to be killed and eliminated from the system by the brave little phagocytes and by antibodies and antitoxins secreted by certain cells and glandular structures.

Dr. Thomas Powell of Los Angeles has advanced another theory of the pathology of inflammation which is more in line with the Nature Cure conception of acute disease and of the origin and functions of bacteria and parasites in the economy of nature. For the last three years we have examined in our clinical and laboratory work the two theories from all possible viewpoints and closely observed the action of leucocytes and bacteria under varying conditions of health and disease. Our studies along these lines of research have convinced us that the phagocytic theory of inflammation is incorrect and that Dr. Powell's interpretation is the true one. Everyone interested in the subject should study Dr. Powell's work, "Fundamentals and Requirements of Health and Disease". A careful perusal of his book will show that all his teachings as to the fundamental causes of disease, lowered vitality, degeneration of the vital fluids, accumulation of waste and morbid matter (his "pathogen"), are straight Nature Cure philosophy. The only, and certainly very valuable, addition which he has made to Nature Cure theory is his version of the nature and activities of the leucocytes.

Dr. Powell agrees with Nature Cure when he attributes all disease arising in the human body to the accumulation in the system of certain morbid materials, the end and by products of digestion and of the metabolic changes in the cells and tissues of the body. I have, in the past, referred to these as "acids, ptomaines, xanthins, and poisonous alkaloids" and collectively as "colloids", and to the resulting conditions and symptom of disease as "collemia". Uric acid and other morbid materials mixed with it form in the system a sticky, mucoid substance which obstructs the capillary circulation, irritates the nervous system, forms deposits, and in that way causes all kinds of symptoms and disease conditions. I chose these names because "colloid" means glue-like and "collemia" signifies a glue-like condition of the blood. Dr. Powell has made a happy selection of the word "pathogen" (which means "disease-creating") for these accumulations of morbid materials. Therefore, I shall in future discussions employ this word.

Briefly stated, Dr. Powell's theory of inflammation works out as follows: After the period of "incubation" during which "pathogen" is accumulating in the system the period of aggravation is explained thus: The congestion of blood in the area of inflammation is caused by the accumulation of pathogen in the circulation which obstructs the tiny capillaries in the affected parts. This accumulation, aside from the great viscosity of the blood, is due to lowered vitality, lowered resistance, or to some kind of irritation or obstruction. As the result of this obstruction in the capillary circulation the blood cannot pass, it surges back and bulges or distends the capillaries and gradually the larger blood vessels. This explains the congestion, which is always the first symptom of inflammation. The capillaries expand in such a way that the leucocytes are forced out into the neighbouring tissues. This throws new light on the migration of the leucocytes, for according to Dr. Powell's theory, these are particles of pathogenic matter which have been condensed into globular bodies resembling cells. This condensation of pathogen takes place in the trabeculae of the spleen, and in the lymph glands of lymph nodes. This explains why in many diseases characterized by accumulations of morbid matter in the system, the lymphatic glands and the spleen become considerably enlarged. In such cases the allopathic surgeon not infrequently cuts out the glands. I have always claimed this is an irrational and destructive practice. From the Nature Cure viewpoint the functions of the lymphatic glands and of the spleen are to condense morbid material (pathogen) from the circulation. Enlargement and the ensuing suppuration of these structures, therefore, means that they are overcharged or engorged with pathogenic matter. A perfect analogy of this is found in inflammation and suppuration of the tonsils and adenoid tissue, which are also important parts of the drainage system of the body. The extirpation of these useful eliminating organs is just as senseless and destructive as the cutting out of lymphatic glands or any other useful organ of the body. We might as well remove the sewers from a house because they are clogged with refuse.

We have left the leucocytes after they had "migrated" or as we now believe, after they had been forced out through the distended capillaries into the surrounding tissues. Next we see them engaged in a life and death struggle with the bacteria. This coincides with the stage of destruction. According to the old version, the leucocytes were devouring and digesting the bacteria, but now the story can be read in another way. The leucocytes or rather the condensed particles of pathogen, disintegrate into pus under the proteolytic action of bacteria. Thus the pathogenic conception of inflammation reverses the old theory from beginning to end. The leucocytes, instead of being the intelligent and heroic defenders of the body, are its deadliest enemies. Instead of pursuing the disease germs and destroying them, the leucocytes or particles of pathogen, forced into the tissues, decompose and form the morbid soil for the development of microzymes into bacteria, which in turn cause the oxidation and disintegration of these morbid products of faulty metabolism.

Many questions will naturally be asked by critical people asked to accept this new interpretation. For instance: "If leucocytes are particles of pathogen, why have they nuclei and amoeboid motion — why do they resemble so closely the living cells of the body?" Now, while it is true that these particles do in a general way resemble genuine cells in their appearance and activities, this resemblance may easily be explained by the new theory of pathogenesis. We have been convinced that the more or less cellular form of the particles is due to the forcing of the pathogen through the trabeculae of the spleen and the lymph glands, which condenses it into compact particles.([1]) Another question which may be asked is: "Why is it necessary that the spleen and the lymph nodes condense the albuminous pathogenic material of the blood into the so-called white blood corpuscles?" In order to explain this we must briefly consider the processes of nutrition and elimination as they take place in the tissues of the body. The elements of nutrition in the forms of oxygen and carbohydrates and protein substances are carried in the salty blood serum through the walls of the capillaries into the intercellular spaces to be absorbed by the cells. This passage from the tiny blood vessels into the neighbouring tissues is

([1])
It should perhaps be noted that it has recently been claimed by certain scientists that they have succeeded in propagating leucocytes on culture media. If this is so it would seem to point to their being in some sense cells.

called osmosis. By this word osmosis is meant the passage of a salty fluid through an animal membrane. To illustrate: If a bladder filled with pure water be suspended in a larger vessel also full of pure water, and if salt then be added to the water in the vessel, the salt will penetrate through the membrane of the bladder into the water which it contains. On the other hand, the carbonic acid and other waste materials effected by the cells are collected by the capillary vessels of the venous and lymphatic systems and through these are carried to the organs of elimination. This passage of the "fæces of the cells" from the intercellular spaces into the venous and lymphatic vessels also takes place by means of osmosis.

From the foregoing it becomes apparent that the freer from pathogenic materials the blood serum and the lymph fluid, the more rapidly will they pass and repass through the walls of the blood and lymph vessels into and out of the intercellular spaces. If, on the other hand, the blood is in a mucoid, viscous, sticky condition with excessive amounts of colloid or pathogenic matter in diffuse form, then the passage of the blood serum through the walls of the capillary vessels and the cells will be greatly impeded and may become impossible. This gives rise to obstruction, stagnation, congestion, colloid degeneration or inflammation. It is to prevent this mucoid or colloid condition of the blood serum and lymph fluid that the lymph nodules and the spleen condense the pathogenic materials into the comparatively compact leucocytes. It is also reasonable to assume that pathogen in the compact form of leucocytes offers a better soil for the action of microzymes than in the diffuse colloid form.

According to Dr. Béchamp's theory the microzymes in the decomposing leucocytes create the bacteria. This does away with the idea that the leucocytes in a mysterious way (chemotaxis) hunt up disease germs in the tissues and then destroy them. May this not explain why in the worst chronic destructive diseases, as in the advanced stages of tuberculosis, we find the leucocytes diminished in number. If phagocytosis were a fact in nature we would expect the opposite condition. That is, in the more advanced stages of the disease the phagocytes should be present in larger numbers. We find, however, that the opposite is the case and that the lymph nodes are engorged and enlarged with leucocytes and other colloid materials. This condition is easily explained by the new version of leucocytosis. Excessive amounts of pathogenic materials in the circulation cause obstruction in the lung tissues, giving rise to the inflammatory tuberculous processes. Finally, the accumulations of pathogen in the circulation becomes so great that the spleen and lymph nodes, being no longer able to cope with them, become engorged. Thus the number of leucocytes in the circulation diminishes but at the same time the vital fluids become more viscous and pathogenic. This explains the enlargement of the spleen and the swelling and degeneration of the lymphatic glands in such diseases as tuberculosis, typhoid, malaria, etc. These facts, instead of contradicting it, are strong evidence in support of the pathogenic theory of leucocytosis.

Another question which can be asked is: "If the white blood corpuscle is not a living cell, why has it a nucleus and amoeboid motion?" Dr. Powell's work gives an explanation of the granulated and nucleated appearance of the leucocytes. He says: "When first formed the leucocytes are neither granular nor nucleated and are known as 'young cells' or 'round cells'. In time they begin to decay in one of several ways; Sometimes they succumb to the external assaults of Pasteur's 'Microbe generateur du pus', masquerade for a while as pus corpuscles and finally fall to pieces and disappear as such; sometimes they yield to the internal assaults of other micro-organisms with which they have come in contact. As this form of decay progresses a 'nucleus' appears; to this other nuclei are soon added. As time advances these foci increase in size as well as number, the constituents thereof becoming susceptible first to one dye and then to another i.e. at one stage eosin, at another methyl and so on. Sometimes they undergo fatty degeneration, in which they are called myelocytes. The myelocyte is simply a leucocyte in process of hydrocarbonization, the dangerous leucocyte being thus changed into a less dangerous thing — namely fat. There is no lack of evidence that the white blood corpuscle is adead thing, that its destiny is dissolution and that in its downward course it carries disease and destruction to its host, the living organism. Those distortions on which the migratory or amoeboid movement of the leucocyte depend and which have seemed to indicate that it is endowed with life, are chiefly attributable to the action of the carbon dioxide gas which is generated within it as it passes into decay. Thus it is the expansion of this gas which gives rise to those protrusions of the leucocyte which are called pseudopodia, while the escape of the gas into the aqueous element of the blood permits it to resume its former shape. . . . In short, the leucocyte, or so-called white blood corpuscle, is not what it appears to be. It has impressed the world that it is a living organism — a living cell — while the fact is, it is not a living cell, but a mortuus corpusculum, or lifeless corpuscle, owing its motility to the forces not of life, but of death — to adhesion, gaseous expansion and chemotaxis. I do not hesitate to affirm that every nucleus or nucleolus which we see in a leucocyte is simply a collection of residual matter (the earthy remains of that arch destroyer, pathogen) and is to be regarded, therefore, as a focus of decay; that the segmentation of the leucocyte is not a matter of 'vital duplication' as has been supposed, but of progressive disintegration; that the increase of its size is due not to growth, but to accretion of the adherence of particles of kindred material which are floating on the blood stream. The fact that the leucocyte becomes less active in consequence of the lowering of its temperature, is attributable to the consequent increase of the disintegrating process; the fact that it is 'killed' as biologists have declared, by iodin, arsenic and other poisons, is due, not to the destruction of its life, but to the preservative action of these drugs. The leucocytes are not the 'vigilant policemen as we have been led by their performances to believe, but owe their so-called 'phagocytic' powers to their viscidity, or extreme adhesiveness. The leucocytes gather the bacteria by sticking to and flowing round them. This is followed by the destruction, not of the bacteria, but of the leucocytes. The leucocyte is not the destroyer but the thing destroyed."

As is explained more fully in the next chapter, we should understand that the microzymes develop into bacteria while feeding on the decaying materials of the leucocytes. The amoeboid motions of the latter are caused by the expansive action of the carbonic acid which is formed in the oxidation and disintegration of their morbid materials, somewhat as dough is "raised" by the carbon dioxide gas which is a product of fermentation.

The foregoing description of osmotic nutrition and lymphatic elimination throws additional light on the importance and modus operandi of massage treatment. The lymph stream has not behind it the powerful pressure of the heart pump. Both the venous and lymphatic circulations become sluggish through pathogenic obstruction of the capillary vessels and intra-cellular lymph spaces. It is readily seen how deep manipulation of the fleshy tissues and systematic kneading and stroking from circumference to centre will stir up and accelerate the movement of the venous blood and lymph fluids toward the heart and toward the outlet into the subclavian vein.

This way of looking at things is supported by practical experience. The examination of the records of patients in our Institution discloses the fact that in ninety per cent of all the cases which improved under our care and treatment, the white blood corpuscles decreased by from 1000 to 4000 or more in number; while the red blood corpuscles showed a proportionate increase. Practically all these patients were of the stubborn chronic type. The few cases that went into a decline and ended fatally showed an increase in leucocytes, except in tuberculosis, which in the last stages usually shows a decrease. This is because the lymphatic glands and the spleen are so completely engorged and obstructed with leucocytes and colloid material that they can no longer condense the pathogen into white corpuscles. Some cases which at the commencement of treatment showed an exceedingly low number of leucocytes, ranging from 2000 to 3000, increased up to 4000 under natural living and treatment. In these the low number at the beginning of treatment was due to the fact that the lymphatic system and spleen were in a diseased condition and unable to condense the pathogen. As these organs improved, the number of leucocytes increased. The average number of the white corpuscles, after six months of natural living and treatment, seems to be about 4000. This is 3500 lower than the average adopted as normal by the allopathic school. Their standard in this case is too high for the same reason that their standard acidity of the urine is too high; namely, because they accept the average as the normal, leaving out of consideration that the average individual is abnormal. People following the conventional habits of living suffer from hyperacidity as well as from excessive amounts of colloid or pathogenic materials because the ordinary diet is too rich in pathogen-producing proteins, starches and fats, and deficient in the acid-neutralizing alkaline mineral elements. According to allopathic standards, the ratio of the white to the red corpuscles is as 1 to 666. In animals the proportion is considerably lower than in the human. I firmly believe that with proper prenatal care, natural management after birth, and rational habits of living throughout life, the average number of leucocytes can be reduced far below 4000.

It may be said, if the foregoing theories are correct, it would be good policy to increase as much as possible the number of bacteria and parasites in the body, and if this be desirable then it would be good practice to expose one's self to infectious diseases. The answer to this is, there is no need of artificially introducing the micro-organisms of disease or infectious disease taints, because the presence of pathogenic matter in the system will bring about germ activity, whenever that becomes necessary for the protection of health and life. Pathogenic matter breeds its own destroyers the same as any decaying putrefying material generates the fungi, parasites or bacterial micro-organisms which decompose and destroy it. Proof of this we see in the putrefying cadaver and in the uncleaned house full of filthy rubbish. The rational way is to keep the system, through right living, free from pathogenic matter, then there will be no need for bacterial scavengers. They cannot live and cause trouble in a clean body endowed with good vitality and governed by a positive mind. The question, where do the micro-organisms come from, I have answered as follows: The spores and seeds of disease germs and parasites are practically omnipresent; they are at the same time the product of disease and the disintegrators of morbid matter. This is briefly explained in the following chapter which deals with Professor Béchamp's teachings.

CHAPTER X

THE DISCOVERY OF MICROZYMES

It may be interesting at this point to enter more fully into the researches and deductions of the great French scientist whose discoveries are destined one day to revolutionize Biology. Antoine Béchamp who was a contemporary of Louis Pasteur and of Professor Metchnikoff was, among other things, a Professor of the Department of Medicine at the University of Montpelier and later in the Free University of Lille. Impartial investigators now claim that Pasteur appropriated from Béchamp many of the ideas and discoveries which made him world famous. When these men lived and worked in their respective fields, a battle royal was raging in the scientific world as to whether substances such as flesh, blood, milk and saccharinaceous (sweet) fluids remained intact when preserved from all contact with the atmosphere. Pasteur claimed that they did; that organisms in the air were needed to cause in such fluids processes of putrefaction or fermentation. He compared the human body to a barrel of beer and pronounced it, like that beverage, to be at the mercy of extraneous organisms. Just as these produce good or bad beer — a liquid diseased, as it were, or healthy — so on entering animal bodies micro-organisms create disease, each after its own order. Pasteur looked upon atmospheric germs as individual entities, endowed with specific, well defined functions; it was a special germ ferment that soured milk, a special ferment that turned grape juice to wine and wine to vinegar, etc. At that time definite organisms had been noticed in sick animals, particularly tiny rod-like bodies in cattle suffering from anthrax. Pasteur assumed that these were caught from the atmosphere and on this he established the doctrine of specific malignant germs, each dealing out its specific malady. It only needed Professor Metchnikoff's theory of phagocytosis and the discovery of "obsonins" or natural antitoxins in the blood, by Sir Almroth Wright and Dr. Bulloch, to furnish the medical profession with a delightfully simple theory as to the origin of disease, comprehensible to the least intelligent. Upon this flimsy basis rests the entire structure of medical theory and practice.

Unfortunately, the world "and all that therein is" is the reverse of simple and these crude explanations of disease leave many questions unanswered.

Firstly, the origin of malignant, microscopic entities is left an unexplained problem. If plagues be caused by bacilli which pass into man through the flea from the rat, whence did the rat catch them? Secondly, if a specific organism produces a specific disease, why should its effects differ in different species? Why, for instance, should the organism associated with anthrax cause splenic fever in cattle and pustules on the skin of humans? Thirdly, the laboratory-made sicknesses of experimental work are not produced by organisms caught from the air, but result from the inoculation of substances taken from diseased bodies. Fourthly, the postulates of Koch, which formulate rules for the recognition of disease germs, have been disproved by the latter's contradictory behaviour. It has to be admitted that all these postulates are rarely, if ever, complied with.

Let us now examine the teachings of Professor Béchamp concerning these problems. During the course of his researches he observed fermentative effects in all parts of living bodies. His work on yeasts had taught him that fermentation was nothing more than the chemical changes produced by living organisms in their environment through feeding and eliminative processes. For this reason he had always combated Pasteur's idea of a specific role being attached to a specific ferment and maintained that under changed circumstances the achievement of the ferment might be different. The fermentative effects he noticed in living bodies were frequently quite dissociated from the presence of bacteria. This gave him cause for reflection, being to him clear proof that all organisms were formed of infinitely minute living bodies, all largely occupied, like ourselves, in the business of feeding. He understood why believers in spontaneous generation had never been satisfied that the intrusion of air borne organisms was the one explanation for various phenomena.

There was life everywhere. Bodies of plants and animals alike were made up of living particles. This explained the necessity for the application of great heat, as well as the exclusion of atmospheric germs, in order to prevent putrefactive changes in living protoplasm. It was essential to kill the internal life, as well as to guard against external. Pasteur himself, in one of his experiments, described a piece of meat kept air proof, as yet having become odorous. This in itself should have shown him that either his method had been faulty, or else that alteration can take place apart from air borne organisms. What was Béchamp's explanation? What did he teach at a time when there was more or less complete acceptance of Virchow's view of the cell as the structural unit of life, or, so to speak, as the primary living thing? Béchamp taught that the cell or germ was no more than a transitory object, built up by the true entities found within it. To these he gave the name of microzymes, or minute ferment bodies. These are the same particles now known as microsomes. Of these primary units of life Edmund B. Wilson says in his text book "The Cell in Development and Inheritance": "Their behaviour is in some cases such as to have led to the hypothesis long since suggested by Henle (1841) and at a later period developed by Béchamp and Estor, and especially by Altmann, that microsomes are actually units or bioblasts, capable of assimilation, growth and division, and hence to be regarded as elementary units of structure, standing between the ultimate molecules of living matter and the cell".

The microzymes of Béchamp are the minute granules that mark the honeycomb structure of the cell and the cell nucleus, and have been distinguished as chromatin granules, owing to the deep shade they take when stained for observation under the microscope. Before the division of the cell nucleus takes place, the chromatin granules assume the appearance of a thread which breaks into pieces known as chromosomes. These subdivide lengthwise during cell cleavage, thus providing each derivative cell with an equal number of what are supposed to be the prime factors of new life and the transmitters of heredity.

Altmann inquired, "How can a granulum (microzyme) arise without its cell?" Béchamp answered, "Every living cell and therefore every living being is reducible to the microzyme." It was Béchamp's contention that processes of putrefaction are wrought by microzymes which, upon the corruption of the body that formed their habitat, are freed to the soil‘ water and air, and are themselves, either in their infinitesimal forms or else in larger shapes as bacteria, the ferments which play so great a role in life and for which the orthodox school of bacteriology provides no explanation. All the micro-organisms which teem in the air, the ground, the rocks, are, according to Béchamp, the remains of animal and vegetable matter. This seems to be proved by the fact that bacteria abound wherever decaying plant or animal life is found, and that they are equally scarce wherever such life is wanting, whether on the bleak post of a high mountain range or on the sterile tracts of the arid desert. The following statements epitomize Béchamp's important discovery: The birth of bacteria, as well as of normal cells of living bodies, is from within. These minute beings are nothing more nor less than the products of life's primal architects, the indwelling microzymes or microsomes of cells and germs. "The cell", he wrote, "is a collection of an infinite number of little beings which have an independent life, a special natural history. The microzymes of animal cells, (when living in morbid matter), associate two by two or in larger numbers and extend themselves into bacteria." These microzymes are those spores or seed germs of bacteria whose existence I presumed and postulated in my philosophy of the unity of disease and cure.

The fermentation of eggs is a puzzle which the germ theorists endeavour to solve by declaring that the shell is not impenetrable to external bacteria. When impenetrability is absolutely assured by artificial means, and yet change, though in a much lesser degree, takes place, they are driven to fall back on Pasteur's explanation that probably germs of putrefaction originally penetrated into the hen's oviduct. Béchamp, on the contrary, showed that the same causes which under normal conditions produce the chicken, give rise under abnormal conditions to fermentation and eventually to putrefaction. According to his demonstrations, the causes of the normal as well as the abnormal processes are the microsomes or, as he named them, the microzymes.

In this connection I may be permitted to quote from a later chapter in this volume in connection with an attack of smallpox from which my son suffered. "As far as I could learn, there was not another case of smallpox in Chicago or its vicinity at the time of the boy's illness. If the contagion theory be true, from whom did he 'catch' the disease, and why did not one of the many persons living in the same house become infected? My answer is, this acute eliminative process was nature's way of purifying the young body of inherited scrofulous and other disease taints."

The microzymes explain the possibility of contagion and infection from without as well as spontaneous generation of bacteria from morbid soil within the system. While bacteria entering the body from without may instigate disease processes, such germs must have originated in morbid soil somewhere and upon entering the body they cannot live and multiply to the danger point unless they find the morbid materials necessary to their existence. If all germs could suddenly be wiped out of existence the conditions which make them necessary would create them anew. In 1869 Béchamp said, "In typhoid fever, in gangrene, in anthrax, the existence has been proved of bacteria in the tissues and in the blood and this has been looked upon as a case of ordinary parasitism. It is evident, however, after what we have said, that the diseases were not caused by the introduction of foreign germs, but that we have to do here only with a deviation of function of microzymes, a deviation indicated also by the change that has taken place in their form. In cases where bacteria have been noted in the blood, it is not a case of ordinary parasitism, but rather of abnormal development of primitive normal organisms. The bacteria, far from being the cause, are on the contrary the effect of the malady."

The microzyme is a microcosm, the cell its macrocosm, just as man is the macrocosm of the cell, and as the sidereal universe is the macrocosm of man, its microcosm. As the well being of man depends upon normal nutrition and wholesome surroundings, so also the health of the cell and of the microzymes depends upon proper nutrition, drainage and innervation. Thus provided with its essential life requirements, the primary unit of life will develop into the normal cells of the vegetable, animal or human body, not into disease germs or parasites. This theory of the origin of bacteria would explain such problems as are voiced in the "Lancet" (Mar. 20th 1909). "When a casual organism is injected into an animal often it happens that it gives rise to a disease bearing no clinical resemblance to the original malady". This discrepancy, besides betraying the unreliability of experiments on animals, points to the conclusion that conditions in the body are the deciding factors, rather than parasitic invaders which, in any case, have not been taken from the air, but from a diseased subject. As Béchamp observes, "the inoculation of anthrax produces splenic fever in cattle and pustules (on the skin) in human beings, thus demonstrating the control factors of diseased conditions to be inborn, not extraneous". "Disease is born of us and in us" wrote Béchamp, "and that is as it should be, because the life of man, and of every other creature, is no more delivered over to chance than the course of the stars". "Life would be delivered over to chance if it depended upon primitive microbic germs created for destructive purposes" (Les Microzymes).

What an interesting confirmation this is of the fundamental postulate of Nature Cure philosophy, according to which disease is not an accident, nor an arbitrary infliction, but the inevitable result of the violation of nature's laws. If it is true that disease is bred in us and of us, health undoubtedly arises in the same way and can be maintained by attention to the well being of the infinitesimal entities which build up our bodies and which we may justly call "life's primal architects". The well being of these minute builders and workers depends upon right living; that is, our habits of thinking, feeling, breathing, eating, drinking, exercising, bathing, clothing, as well as our sexual and social activities, must be in harmonious relation with the laws of our being.(1)

In commenting upon Professor Béchamp's teachings, Douglas Hume says: "When all is said and done, could Professor Béchamp's microscope, or the most powerful lens of the present day, ever hope to pry into the primal entity of life, the first individual unit of organized existence? Far beyond all searching in its minuteness must such an element be, and well does August Weissmann in his 'Germplasm: a Theory of Heredity', write: "We are thus reminded afresh that we have to deal not only with the infinitely great, but also with the infinitely small; the idea of size is a

---

(1)
It is doubtful whether it could now be claimed that the microzyme is the ultimate unit of life, though it may be in the ordinary way the "primal architect" of the cell. It would perhaps be hard to say where life begins or to be sure that the bridge between organic and inorganic is not still being crossed as it must have been at some stage in the evolution of the planet.

purely relative one and on either hand extends infinity". Hume continues in his pamphlet: "Since from such infinitesimal beginnings the brain of a Newton, the music of a Beethoven, the beauty of a Lady Hamilton are evolved, we find ourselves reconsidering the Platonic theory of Ideation." The final reality is the idea in the mind of the creator. Thought forms are the souls of things and matter convolutes to these soul patterns. So the relation of thought and feeling to health and disease appears to be not without scientific basis — the physical reverts to the metaphysical. The ancient Vedic teaching is proved afresh — "The whole of the universe is evolved through Sankalpa (thought ideation) alone; it is only through Sankalpa that the universe retains its appearance". (The Varaha Upanishads of Krishna-Yajur Veda.) And so "the eternal thought in the eternal mind" (Bhagavad-Gita) precludes the disseverence of the thought from the thinker. If, on the one hand, man, in deep humility, realizes himself a pigmy in an incomprehensible universe, on the other hand, his consciousness of his oneness with the stupendous whole leaves him appalled by his dignity and the possibilities of his amazing destiny. Thus, in the mystery of life's primal architects (microzymes), there may be dimly discerned that unity of Creator and created which, in the oldest philosophic teachings in the world found voice in that triumphant cry of faith of the Vedic utterance: "That supreme Brahman, the self of all, the great abode of the universe, subtler than the subtle, the Eternal, That is thyself, and thou art That". (Kaivalya Upanishad.)

I leave it to the reader to decide for himself which theory of inflammation is the more rational, the old or the new. The new version removes the last doubt as to the beneficent character and constructive activity of the tiny organisms which so far have been looked upon as the greatest enemies of mankind. It makes the Nature Cure philosophy of health, disease and cure consistent and rational in all its principles and deductions.

CHAPTER XI

RESULTS OF SUPPRESSION

If the inflammation be allowed to run its course through the different stages of acute activity and the final stage of reconstruction, then every acute disease, whatever its name and description, will prove beneficial to the organism, because pathogen and poisons have been eliminated from the system; abnormal and diseased tissues have been broken down and built up again to a purer and more normal condition. The acute disease has, as it were, acted upon the organism like a thunder storm on the sultry, vitiated summer air. It has cleared the system of impurities and obstructions and re-established wholesome normal condition. Therefore, acute diseases, when treated in harmony with nature's intent, always prove beneficial. If, however, through neglect or wrong treatment, the inflammatory processes are not allowed to run their natural course, if they are checked or suppressed by drugs, ice bags, or surgical operations, or if the disease conditions in the system are so far in the ascendancy that the healing forces cannot react properly, then the constructive forces may lose the battle and the disease may take a fatal course or develop into chronic ailments. Whether we accept the old or the new interpretation of inflammation, the foregoing deductions are true. In either case the inflammatory process is constructive in nature and purpose.

Suppression during the First Two Stages of Inflammation

It may be argued that suppression during the stages of incubation and aggravation need not have fatal consequences if followed by natural living and eliminative treatment. To this I would reply: "Such procedure always involves the danger of concentrating the disease poisons in vital parts and organs, thus laying the foundation for chronic destructive diseases". Furthermore, it is not at all necessary to suppress inflammatory processes by poisonous drugs and other means, because we can easily and surely control them and keep them from becoming dangerous by our natural methods of treatment. I shall now support with proof and illustrations the foregoing theoretical expositions by following the development of various diseases through the five stages of inflammation.

Catching a Cold

To consider first the commonest of all diseases, the "cold": according to popular opinion, the catching of colds is responsible for the greater part of human ailments. Very frequently I hear from patients who come for consultation: "All my troubles date back to a cold I took at such and such a time", etc. Then I have to explain that colds are not contracted suddenly and from without but come from within; that their "period of incubation" may have extended over months or years or over several successive life-times; that a clean healthy body possessed of abundant vitality cannot "take cold" under the ordinary thermal conditions congenial to human life, no matter how sudden the change in temperature. At first this may seem to be contrary to common experience as well as to the theory and practice of medical science. But Nature Cure philosophy will throw light on the development of a cold from start to finish and on the question of whether it can be "caught", or whether it develops slowly within the organism by means of an incubation extending over a period of time.

"Taking cold" may be caused by chilling the surface of the body or part of the body. In the chilled portions of the skin the pores close, the blood recedes into the interior, and as a result the elimination of poisonous gases and exudates is locally suppressed. This "catching cold" through being exposed to a cold draught through wet clothing, etc. is not necessarily followed by more serious consequences. If the system is not too much encumbered with morbid matter and if kidneys and intestines are in fairly good working order, these organs will assist the temporarily inactive skin to take care of the extra amount of waste and morbid materials and eliminate them without difficulty. The greater the vitality and the more normal the composition of the blood, the more effectively the system as a whole will react in such an emergency and throw off the morbid materials which were not eliminated through the skin. If, however, the organism is already overloaded with waste and morbid materials; if the bowels and kidneys are already weakened or atrophied through continued overwork and over-stimulation; if, in addition, the vitality has been lowered through excesses or over-exertion, and the vital fluids are in an abnormal condition, then the morbid matter thrown into the circulation cannot find an outlet and endeavours to escape by way of the mucous linings of the nasal passages, the throat, bronchi, stomach, bowels, or genito-urinary organs. The waste materials and poisonous exudates which are being eliminated through these internal membranes cause irritation and pathogenic congestion, and thus produce the well known symptoms of inflammation and catarrhal elimination — sneezing (coryza), cough, expectoration, mucous discharges, diarrhoea, leucorrhoea, etc. We may safely assume that these forcible house-cleanings do not occur until it becomes necessary for the system to eliminate excessive accumulations of pathogen. In other words, the chilling of the surface is merely the spark which explodes the combustibles stored within.

Why is it necessary that such elimination must take the form of inflammation? Why cannot it proceed in the ordinary way without causing violent acute reaction? The reason is that the organs of depuration are so constructed that they eliminate only waste materials of comparatively simple chemical composition. Thus, the skin eliminates carbonic acid and salts which are neutralized acids. The kidneys eliminate normally urea and salts; in abnormal conditions, they also eliminate uric acid, indican and a few other kinds of acids and ptomaines. The intestines eliminate little but undigested food waste. Pathogen, however, is made up of chemically highly complex substances which cannot be eliminated through the organs of depuration. Pathogenic substances must first be broken down into simple compounds chemically adapted for elimination through these organs, and this decomposition is accomplished through inflammation and germ activity.

We now understand that these so-called "colds" are nothing more nor less than forms of vicarious elimination. The membranous linings of the internal organs are doing the work for the inactive, sluggish and atrophied skin, kidneys and intestines. The greater the accumulation of morbid matter in the system, the lower the vitality, and the more abnormal the composition of the blood and lymph, the greater the liability to the "catching" of colds. What is to be gained by suppressing the different forms of acute catarrhal elimination with cough and catarrh "cures" containing opiates, astringents, antiseptics and antipyretics? Is it not obvious that such procedures interfere with nature's purifying efforts, that they hinder and suppress the inflammatory processes and the accompanying elimination of morbid matter from the system? Such a course can have but one result — converting nature's cleansing and healing efforts into chronic disease.

From the foregoing it will have become clear how it is that the cause of a cold lies not so much in the cold draught, or the wet feet, as in the primary causes of all diseases: lowered vitality, deterioration of vital fluids, and the accumulation of morbid matter and poisons in the system, conditions which may have built up over many years.

What, then, is the natural cure for colds? There can be but one remedy; increased elimination through the proper channels. This is accomplished by judicious dieting and fasting, and through restoring the natural activity of the skin, kidneys and bowels by means of wet packs, cold sprays and ablutions, sitzbaths, massage, neurotherapy, homoeopathic remedies, exercise, sun and air baths and all other methods of natural treatment which save vitality, build up the blood on a normal basis and promote elimination without injuring the organism.

Suppression during the Third Stage of Inflammation

Should the inflammatory processes be suppressed during the stage of destruction, the results would be still more serious and far-reaching. We have learned that during this stage the affected parts and organs are involved more or less in a process of disintegration. They become filled with morbid exudates, pus, etc., which interfere with and make impossible normal nutrition and functioning. If suppression takes place during this stage, it is obvious that the affected areas will be left permanently in a condition of destruction. The following may serve as an illustration: Suppose changes and repairs have been found necessary in a building. Workmen have torn down the partitions, hangings, wallpaper, etc. At this stage of the proceedings the owner discharges the workmen, and the building is left in a condition of chaos. Surely this would be most irrational. It would leave the house unfit for habitation. But such a procedure exactly corresponds to the suppression of inflammatory diseases during the stage of destruction. Such suppression leaves the affected organs in an abnormal, diseased condition and accounts for the "mysterious sequelae" or chronic after effects which so often follow drug or ice-treated acute diseases. Numerous cases of chronic affections of the lungs and kidneys, of infantile paralysis, and of many other chronic ailments are directly traceable to such suppression.

The following case came under our care and treatment a few years ago. Several gentlemen of Greek nationality called on me with the request that I should visit a friend of theirs who had been confined to bed for about two months in one of our great hospitals. On investigation I found that the patient had entered the hospital while suffering from a mild attack of pneumonia. The doctors of the institution had ordered ice packs. Rubber sheets filled with ice were applied to the chest and other parts of the body. This had been continued for several days until the fever had subsided. As a matter of fact, ice is more suppressive than anti-fever medicines. Continued icy cold applications chill the parts of the body to which they are applied, depress the vital functions and effectually suppress the inflammatory processes. The result in this case was that the inflammation in the lungs had been arrested and suppressed during the stage of destruction, while the air cells and tissues were filled with exudates, blood serum, pus, live and dead blood cells, morbid microzymes, bacteria, etc., leaving the affected areas of the lungs in a consolidated condition. As a consequence of suppression the pneumonia had been changed from the acute to the sub-acute and chronic stages and the doctors had informed his friends that he was now suffering from "miliary tuberculosis", and would probably die within a week or two. Discouraged by this information, the friends of the patient asked me to take charge of the case. The man was transferred to our institution and we began at once to apply the natural methods of treatment. For ice packs we substituted cold water packs — strips of linen wrung out of water of ordinary temperature wrapped around the body and covered with several layers of flannel bandages. The wetpacks became warm on the body in a few minutes. They relaxed the pores and drew the blood to the surface, thus promoting heat radiation and the elimination of morbid matter through the skin. They did not suppress the fever, but kept it below the danger point. Under this treatment, accompanied by fasting and judicious manipulation, the inflammatory and feverish processes which had been suppressed by the ice packs soon revived, became once more active and were made to run their natural course through the stages of destruction, absorption (abatement) and reconstruction. The result of this Nature Cure treatment was that about two months after the patient entered our institution, his friends were able to send him on a holiday to Greece and he made a complete recovery.

I have observed a number of similar cases suffering from solidification of the lungs and the resulting asthmatic or tubercular conditions, which have been "doctored" into these chronic ailments by means of antipyretics and of ice. Frequently such treatment leads to the accumulation of fluids in the pleura and lung tissues. Then the allopathic physician resorts to "tapping", but the withdrawal of the fluids only results in quicker accumulation. Under natural treatment these morbid excretions absorb gradually through the lymphatic drains. Equally dangerous is the ice bag or pack if applied to the inflamed brain or to the spinal column. Only too often it results in paralysis or in death. In many instances, acute cerebro-spinal meningitis is changed in this way by drug and serum treatment or by the use of ice bags into the chronic, so-called incurable infantile paralysis. I say "so-called incurable" advisedly, because we have treated and cured such cases in all stages of development from acute inflammatory meningitis to chronic paralysis of long standing.

In our treatment of acute diseases we never use ice or icy water for packs, compresses, baths or ablutions, but always water of ordinary temperature as it comes from the well or tap. The water compress or pack warms up quickly and thus brings about a natural reaction within a few minutes, while the ice bag or pack continually chills and practically freezes the affected parts and organs. This does not permit the skin to relax; it prevents a warm reaction, the radiation of body heat and the elimination of morbid matter through the skin.(1)

Suppression During the Fourth and Fifth Stages of Inflammation

Let us see what happens when acute diseases are suppressed during the stages of absorption and reconstruction. If the healing forces of the body gain a victory over the pathogenic conditions which are threatening the health and life of the organism, then the symptoms of inflammation, swelling, redness, heat, pain and the accelerated heart action which accompanies them, gradually subside. The "debris of the battle field" is carried away through the venous and lymphatic circulation — the drainage system of the body. When in this way all morbid materials have been completely eliminated, in other words when conditions have become normal, then the microzymes will regenerate and reconstruct the injured and destroyed cells and tissues. If, however, these processes of elimination and reconstruction be interfered with or interrupted before they are completed, the microzymes will continue to create germs of putrefaction and the affected parts and organs will not have a chance to become entirely well or strong. They will remain in an abnormal, diseased condition, and their functional activity will be seriously handicapped.

The After Effects of Drug or Ice Treatment of Typhoid Fever

In many instances I have told patients after a glance into their eyes that they suffered from chronic indigestion, malassimilation and malnutrition caused by drug treated typhoid fever; and in every case these records in the eyes were confirmed by the history of the case. In such cases the outer rim of the iris shows a wreath of whitish or drug coloured specks or flakes. I have named this the typhoid or lymphatic rosary. It corresponds to the lymphatic glands and other absorbent vessels in the intestines. It appears in the iris of the eye when these structures have been injured or are engorged with pathogenic matter as a result of drug, ice or surgical treatment. Wherever this has happened, the venous and lymphatic vessels in the intestines do not absorb the food materials and these pass through the digestive tract and out of the body without having been properly digested and assimilated. During the destructive stages of typhoid fever, the intestines become denuded by the sloughing of their membranous linings.

(¹)
It does appear that there is a way in which an ice pack can be used which promotes elimination and is not suppressive. A compress with six to ten ice cubes is placed over the solar plexus and lower abdomen and the patient put to rest in bed for two or three hours. This method is described in "The Grape Cure" by Basil Shackleton, page 84. (Thorsons Ltd.).

These sloughed membranes give the stools of the typhoid fever patient their peculiar "pea-soup" appearance. In a similar manner the lymphatic, venous and glandular structures which constitute the absorbent vessels of the intestines atrophy and slough away. If the inflammatory processes are allowed to run their normal course under natural treatment through the stages of destruction, absorption, and reconstruction, the microzymes will rebuild the membranous and glandular structures of the intestinal canal perfectly; convalescence will be rapid; and the patient will enjoy better health than before the disease was contracted. If, however, through injudicious feeding, the application of ice or the administration of quinine, mercury, purging salts, opiates, or other destructive agents, nature's processes are interfered with, prematurely checked and suppressed, then the sloughed membranes and absorbent vessels are not reconstructed, and the intestinal tract is left in a denuded and atrophied condition. Such a patient may arise from bed thinking he is cured but, unless he is afterwards treated by natural methods, he will never make a full recovery. It will take him, perhaps, months or years to die a gradual, miserable death through malassimilation and malnutrition which frequently result in some form of wasting disease, such as pernicious anaemia or tuberculosis. If he does not actually die from the effects of the wrongly treated typhoid fever, he will be troubled for the rest of his life with intestinal indigestion, constipation, malassimilation and accompanying nervous disorders.

I am, however, glad to say that in the treatment of typhoid fever advanced medical science is now adopting the Nature Cure treatment as practised and taught by the pioneers of Nature Cure more than fifty years ago — that is, straight cold water and fasting, and no drugs. This treatment would prove equally efficacious in all other acute diseases if the allopaths would only condescend to try it. It is a strange and curious fact that, so far, they have never found it worth while to do so. Nature Cure physicians know from daily experience that the simple water treatment and fasting is sufficient to cure all other forms of acute disease just as easily and effectively as typhoid fever. By this is proved the unity of treatment in all acute diseases. For both typhoid fever and tuberculosis, progressive medical men have now abandoned the germ killing method of treatment. They have found it futile to hunt for drugs and serums to kill the typhoid and tuberculosis bacilli in these, the two most destructive diseases afflicting the human family. They have been forced to admit that the simple remedies of the Nature Cure school, cold water and fasting in typhoid fever and fresh air treatment in tuberculosis, are the only worth while methods of fighting these formidable enemies. If they could be induced to continue their researches and experiments along these natural lines, they would attain infinitely more satisfactory results than through their complicated germ hunting and germ killing theories and practices.(1)

The natural treatment of all acute diseases is fully described in Volume II of this series.

---

(1)
Whatever may have been the case when Dr. Lindlahr wrote it can now hardly be said that the treatment of either typhoid or tuberculosis is on Nature Cure lines. Vaccines, antitoxins, drugs and antibiotics are freely used for prophylaxis and treatment in both these diseases. It seems clear that tuberculosis, especially of the pulmonary variety, is on the decline. It is claimed that this decline is largely due to the methods of treatment being used. It would on the whole seem more likely that it is due to more healthy habits and living conditions in certain respects. It may also not be without significance that lung cancer appears to be on the increase while pulmonary tuberculosis is declining. Lung trouble of all other kinds is very widespread and damaging and much of it is no doubt attributable to smoking and other forms of pollution.

CHAPTER XII

SURGERY

The discoverers of anaesthetics are classed among the greatest bene-factors of humanity because it is believed that ether, chloroform, cocaine and similar nerve paralyzing agents have greatly lessened the sum of human suffering. I doubt, however, that this is true. Anaesthetics have made surgery technically easy and have done away with the pain caused directly by the incisions; but, on the other hand, these marvellous effects of pain killing drugs have encouraged indiscriminate and unnecessary op-erations to such an extent that at least nine tenths of all surgical operations performed today are uncalled for. In most instances these ill-advised mutilations are followed by lifelong weakness and suffering, which far outweigh the temporary pains formerly endured when unavoidable operations were performed without the use of anaesthetics. I do not wish to be understood as condemning unqualifiedly all surgical interventions in the treatment of human ailments. An operation may occasionally be absolutely necessary as a means of saving life. Surgery is also indicated in cases of injury, such as wounds or fractured bones, in certain obstetrical complications and in other affections of a purely mechanical nature. In all such cases anaesthetics prevent much suffering which cannot be avoided in any other way. But anyone who has had an opportunity to watch the prolonged misery of the victim of uncalled for operations will not doubt that anaesthesia has been a two edged sword which has inflicted many more wounds than it has healed. Many physicians have recognized more or less distinctly the uselessness and harmfulness of old school medical treatment. Dissatisfied and disgusted with old fashioned drugging, they turn to surgery convinced that in it they possess an exact scientific method of curing ailments. They seem to think that the surest way to cure a diseased organ is to remove it with the knife. I, for one, cannot understand how an organ can be cured when, having been extirpated and preserved in alcohol, it adorns the specimen cabinet of the surgeon.([1])

Surgeons are apt to say that they do not remove organs from the body unless they have become useless, or to declare that, since we do not know what this or that organ is good for, it might as well be removed and will never be missed. What opinion would you form of a watchmaker who put a spring, a wheel or a balance into a watch unnecessarily? Do we not know that every minute part is of importance and cannot be removed without throwing the whole out of equilibrium? Can we believe that the various parts of the wonderful mechanism of the human body are any less important for the perfect working of the whole?

Not long ago surgeons claimed that the thyroid gland could be removed without bad effects. They did not then know what functions it performed and therefore thought is could not be of much importance. It was found. however, that persons thus operated on died shortly afterwards. We read in the papers of daring and successful removals of spleens, stomachs, kidneys and parts of the brain, etc., but the subsequent sufferings and miserable and premature endings of the victims are never reported.

The inflamed part or organ is, in fact, usually but a symptom of the disease. The irritants which cause the inflammation, growth or tumour are contained in every drop of blood. They may belong to the scrofulous, psoric, gonnorrheal, syphilitic, tuberculous or pathogenic poisons which are present, or it may be some destructive drug poison which occasions the disturbance. Suppressing morbid discharges or cutting out inflamed parts does not eliminate the causes at the back of local symptoms. Nature usually seeks the easiest possible outlet. If you block this, the chances are that subsequent conditions will be worse than the first. The procedure is as futile as trying to stop running water by means of a dam. You may for a time arrest the flow but soon it will rise to the level of your obstruction, then you will be obliged to raise the dam. This will happen again and again until the rising flood will invade and damage the neighbouring fields and finally break through the artificial barrier, sweeping everything before it.

Everyday experience proves that the foregoing is not mere theorising, not slandering a noble profession. The claims of the surgeons are not borne out by actual facts. During the past seventeen years there have come under

(1)
It should be noted that very considerable developments have taken place since Dr. Lindlahr's time both in the technique and scope of surgery and in the use of various kinds of anaesthetics. Many of these developments may be traced to the experience gained by surgeons in two world wars and much real progress has been made in many fields, though one may have reservations about some new forms of surgery and of anaesthesia which are now in vogue. It may well be that in the field of anaesthesia we are about to see something of a revolution which will greatly reduce the use of drugs and gases in this connection. We hear of operations being performed with the patient fully conscious but relieved of pain by some form of nerve blocking by acupuncture or some similar procedure. We also hear of operations being performed with the patient being put into a kind of sleep and relieved of pain by techniques of deep relaxation akin to hypnosis.

our treatment thousands of patients, both in sanitarium and home practice, whose family physicians had declared that in order to save their lives they must submit to the knife without delay. With very few exceptions these people were cured by us without the use of a poisonous drug, an antiseptic or a knife. Several women who years ago were confronted with removal of the ovaries are today the happy mothers of healthy children. Many of our former patients who were treated by old school physicians for acute or chronic appendicitis and were strongly urged to have the offending organ removed, are today alive and well and still in possession of their vermiform appendices. During the last seventeen years I have treated hundreds of cases of appendicitis and so far we have not lost a case and not one has been operated upon. Other patients were threatened with operations for kidney, gall and bladder stones, fibroid and other tumours, floating kidneys, stomach troubles, intestinal and uterine disorders, not to mention the multitude of children whose tonsils and adenoids were to have been removed. All these one time "surgical" cases have escaped the knife and are doing very well indeed, with bodies intact and in possession of the full quota of organs given them by nature. Is it not better to cure a diseased organ than to remove it? On the other hand thousands of men and women operated upon for some local ailment which could have been cured easily by natural methods of treatment are condemned by inexcusable mutilation to life long suffering. Many, if not actually suffering pain, have been unnecessarily unsexed and in other ways incapacitated for the normal functions and natural enjoyments of life. When we learn that a major operation has been performed upon someone who consults us our barometer of hope drops considerably. We know from much experience that the mutilation of the human organism has a tendency to lessen the chances of recovery. Such patients are nearly always lacking in recuperative power. A body deprived of important parts or organs is forever unbalanced. It is like a watch with a spring or a wheel taken out. It may run, but never quite right; it is hypersensitive and easily thrown off balance by any adverse influence.

The Human Body a Unit

We are realising more and more that the human body is a homogeneous and harmonious whole, that we cannot injure one part of it without damaging other parts and often the entire organism. As previously stated, cutting in the vital organs means "cutting in the brain". It affects the functions of the nervous system most profoundly.

A physician in Vienna has written a very interesting book in which he shows that the inner membranes of the nose are in close relationship and sympathy with distant parts and organs of the body. He located in the nose one small area which corresponds to the lungs. By irritating this area with an electric needle he could provoke asthmatic attacks in patients subject to this disease. By anaesthetizing the same area he could stop immediately severe attacks of asthma and of coughing. Another area in the nasal cavity corresponds to the genital organs. The doctor proved that by electric irritation applied to this area abortions could be produced, and that by anaesthesia in the same area uterine haemorrhages could be stopped Another justification of my warnings against unnecessary surgical mutilations has come through the new system of zone therapy. This reveals in a startling manner the connection and interdependence on the nervous system in various parts. It shows that irritation and pains in distant parts of the body can be suspended or moderated by pressing certain spots on the fingers. These and many other facts of experience throw a wonderful light upon the unity of the human organism. You cannot injure one part of it without affecting in some degree its entire mechanism.

The evil after effects of surgical operations do not always manifest at once. On the contrary, the surgical treatment is frequently followed by a period of seeming improvement. The troublesome local symptoms have disappeared and after effects of the mutilations have not had time to assert themselves. But sooner or later the old symptoms return in aggravated form, or a new set of complications arises. The patient is made to believe that the first operation was a perfect success and that this later crop of difficulties has nothing to do with the former, but is something entirely new; or he is assured that the first operation did not go deep enough, that it failed to reach the seat of the trouble and must be done over again. And so the work of mutilation goes merrily on. The disease poisons in the body set up one centre of inflammation after another. These centres the surgeon promptly removes; but the real disease, the venereal, psoric or scrofulous taint, the uric or oxalic acid, the poisonous alkaloids and ptomaines affecting every cell and every drop of blood in the body — these elude the surgeon's knife and create new ulcers, abscesses, inflammation, stones, etc., as fast as the old ones are extirpated.

Those who have carefully studied the previous chapters will readily comprehend these facts. They will see that acute and sub-acute conditions represent nature's cleansing and healing efforts and that local suppression by knife or drug only serves to turn nature's corrective and purifying activities into chronic disease. I have uttered these warnings, especially against operations on the genital organs, ever since I started to lecture and write on this subject. Until a few years ago medical men would have condemned them along with other Nature Cure teachings as baseless, preposterous and malicious attacks upon a noble profession. But in the meantime surgical science has to some extent convicted itself of past malpractices. Surgeons now admit that cutting out the ovaries means "cutting in the brain", and that women robbed of these organs become the victims of nervous prostration and of insanity. Accidentally it was discovered that the terrible after effects on the nervous system, mind and emotional nature following the removal of the ovaries could be avoided if but a tiny part of the organs, not larger than a pea, were left. This reveals the immense importance of the secretions of the ovaries and of the other ductless glands in the economy of the body. If the secretions of a tiny part of these organs can exert such a powerful influence upon the human entity on all three planes of being, why not try to restore instead of destroying them? That this is easily possible we have proved in hundreds of such proposed surgical cases. The highest art of the true physician is to preserve and restore, not to mutilate or destroy. As bearing upon this discussion of surgical versus natural treatment, let us consider in detail the allopathic conception and handling of appendicitis, following this with the Nature Cure viewpoint and treatment.(1)

[1]
It would seem that the real sphere and function of surgery is in the repair of wounds and injuries and in the putting right as far as possible of congenital abnormalities and defects. Outside this it would seem to be wrong or at least a confession of failure or of ignorance; that is to say that we do not know how to cure or keep healthy a particular organ or part or that it has become so degenerated and diseased that to remove it is the lesser of two evils.

CHAPTER XIII

APPENDICITIS

Allopathic Description and Treatment

The disease is infective, the micro-organism usually at fault being the bacillus coli. In most cases the bacillus excites the disease only in presence of some injury to the mucous membrane of the appendix. Fæcal concretions or foreign bodies such as pins or grape seeds, may become the exciting causes of inflammation. Even without injury virulent bacilli may in some instances cause inflammation.

Symptoms. In an ordinary attack the initial symptoms are pain of sudden onset, at first over the whole abdomen but soon localized in the right iliac fossa; local tenderness greatest at McBurney's Point; elevation of temperature, furred tongue, constipation and vomiting. The muscles on the right side of the abdomen are rigid and frequently the right thigh is slightly drawn up. A definite swelling can usually be made out in the iliac fossa. When perforation into the peritoneum occurs, from ulcer or from gangrene, the symptoms are those of collapse, followed by those described under general peritonitis.

Treatment. (Allopathic): In all cases of appendicitis immediate operation is the best practice. Although complete recovery is the rule in ordinary cases without surgical interference, yet there is no foretelling that a perforation may not at any moment occur and cause a fatal peritonitis. Operation is of course necessary in the presence of abscess, and where there is generalized peritonitis it affords the only hope of recovery though the hope is but slender. Medical treatment finds a place only where opperation is refused or in anticipation of an operation. In such cases, hot fomentations, enemata to open the bowels, morphia for the relief of pain, fluid diet (chiefly milk), and absolute rest in bed, are the chief means of treatment.

From the Nature Cure Viewpoint

A propos of appendicitis and its prevalence the following story is told of Bill, the newsboy. He had been absent for some months from his favourite haunts and, on his return, was greeted by his mates with, "Hello Bill, we hear you had appendicitis". Bill replied, "Huh, appendicitis nothing — didn't have enough money for that — it was just stomach ache." Like many another joke this contains more truth than fiction. The time seems near when the vulgar throng will be spoken of not as the Great Unwashed but as the Great Unoperated. Already, at national conventions of physicians, at local gatherings, and in medical journals, the proposition has sometimes been made in all seriousness that appendectomy, together with the removal of tonsils, should be performed on all infants "in order to prevent affections of these organs later in life". Why not save our progeny all future trouble by scientifically and dextrously removing their heads?

The idea has prevailed among the laity that appendicitis is due in most cases to the lodgement of seeds and other foreign bodies in the appendix. This, however, is merely a plausible reply to importunate questioners. Actually seeds and other foreign bodies are found in less than one per cent of all cases operated upon for appendicitis. Dr. William Osler said: "Only two instances of foreign bodies in the appendix came under my observation in ten years' pathological work in Montreal; in one there were eight snipe shot and in another five apple pips." Moreover, according to the reports of prominent surgeons, not more than fifteen per cent of those operated upon for appendicitis really have this disease. The other eighty-five per cent are found to be suffering with inflammation in the caecum, ascending colon or small intestines. Sometimes the symptoms are caused by touches of peritonitis. The majority of such ailments are diagnosed and treated as appendicitis. This magic word has attained such hypnotic power over the public mind that it sends the patients, without question or remonstrance, straight to the operating table.

Surgeons say, "If it is appendicitis only an operation will save the patient's life". This we positively deny and have proved untrue in hundreds of cases. We have never had an operation for appendicitis performed on one of our patients and we have not lost a single case. Our own records and our reports to the Board of Health attest this fact. If our diagnosis be questioned, I answer that we have taken numerous cases which had already been treated for appendicitis by other physicians who claimed that operation was absolutely necessary. It may be argued: "Why make such a fuss over the useless vermiform appendix; it is but the remains of a part of the human anatomy which has become obsolete in the course of evolutionary developments". The truth is that in the meat eating mammalia the appendix is of a very small size or rudimentary. It is more fully developed in herbivorous animals, still more so in the fruit eating apes and most of all in man. This flatly contradicts the statement that the appendix is the remains of a defunct and degenerated organ. Instead of deteriorating, in the course of evolution, it has become more perfectly developed.

"What, then, are the uses of the appendix?" Dr. MacEwan, an English surgeon, who claimed to have performed more operations for appendicitis than any other surgeon in England, has entirely changed front on the question of operating and warned strongly against it. In an article on the subject he says:

"Observations of the interior of the caecum seen through defects in its walls showed that there were differences in the amount and fluidity of the secretion exuding from its mucous surface. When irritated mechanically the flow of exudate was greater and more fluid. At a variable interval after a meal — one or two hours — peristaltic effects in the colon ensued, resulting in the extrusion of its contents, and shortly after a clear thick fluid was poured from the secreting caecal surface, and in several instances was seen to exude in considerable quantity from the appendicular orifice. On one occasion quite a stream of fluid poured from the appendix just before the chyme began to pass through the ileo-caecal valve. When chyme passed through this valve it did so in small quantities at a time, and there were occasional pauses in which the ileo-caecal valve seemed to close — probably by reflex action. This fluid from the caecum and the appendix was invariably alkaline. Usually the flow from the ileo-caecal valve was slow, the material passing into the caecum in small quantities which slide over the orifice of the appendix and get smeared by the exudation from the general caecal cavity. It seems as though there were a control regulating the amount of material which passes from the small intestine into the caecum. If the valve by any means be rendered patent (open) the contents of the small intestine flow quickly into the caecum and a troublesome escape of semi-digested material ensues. When this agency is interfered with, caecal indigestion occurs, which generally ends in diarrhoea of partially digested matter but which occasionally leads to masses of matter gathering in the caecum and causing constipation, with subsequent fermentative action of a kind which is apt to result in irritation of the mucous membrane and appendix. The appendix is regarded as a mere diverticulum of the caecum and yet its vascular and nervous supply pertains more to that of the small intestine than that of the colon. When it is recollected that the circular muscles of the caecum are continuous with those of the appendix and that the longitudinal caecal bands themselves end on the appendix, it will be understood how easily the nervous apparatus of the appendix may initiate the larger movements of the caecum by first inducing movements in the appendix and how inhibition of these movements may cause caecal disturbance. The same agency, by control of the vascular supply, will regulate the exudation from the appendix, and that in accordance with the impulse received from the small intestine.

"Let us look now to the character and power of this exudation emanating from the appendix and cæcum. In the first part of the large intestine, and especially in the cæcum and appendix, the lymphatic follicles and the glands of Lieberkuhn are very numerous and well developed, the latter being larger, deeper and broader than the corresponding cells in the small intestine and the goblet cells which they contain are larger and more abundant. This all the histologists admit. So closely are those glands packed together in the cæcum that the united surface presented by them is immensely larger than the ridges between the glands, which is all that is left at this place for absorption. So that the histological structure would point to the cæcum and appendix being made for digestive purposes rather than absorption. The succus entericus which is exuded by these cells of Lieberkuhn is of great assistance in digestion. So powerful is it that while pancreatic juice alone took six hours to dissolve fibrin and had not even attacked the white of an egg in ten hours, the addition of succus entericus to the pancreatic juice dissolved fibrin in from three to ten minutes, and the coagulated white of egg in from three to six minutes. Taking the appendix apart, though there are individual differences, one sees in most appendices that the surface is covered with glands of Lieberkuhn in an active state of secretion during health. If one takes the appendix at an average of three and a half inches and lines that space with glands of Lieberkuhn encircling the interior it is seen that a considerable amount of succus entericus may be exuded from that surface alone, more especially as it is abundantly supplied with blood. Therefore the secretion of the appendix, viewed alone in this sense would be a valuable aid to digestion, and the excision of that organ, except in a hopelessly diseased condition, manifestly improper."

The Danger Spot in the Intestine

Why the cæcum is the danger spot in the intestinal tract can readily be understood. After food leaves the stomach it passes through the small intestine and enters the colon through the ileo-cæcal valve. The cæcum is a pouch formed by the lower end of the ascending colon, and lies below the level of the entrance of the small intestine into the colon or large intestine. From the cæcum the food residue passes upward through the ascending colon, laterally through the transverse colon, then downward and out through the descending colon, sigmoid flexure, rectum and anus. The reader will perceive that the ascending colon is the only part of the intestine in which the food residue has to move vertically upward. Therefore, by force of gravity or downward pressure, the fæces tend to accumulate in the cæcum and to distend it. Therefore it is the dangerous spot of the intestinal tract. If, in addition to this, there exists a tendency to sluggishness and constipation, the distension of the cæcum becomes very marked; food materials accumulate and give rise to fermentation and putrefaction. These morbid processes frequently result in inflammation of the walls of the cæcum, colon, adjacent small intestines and sometimes of the appendix. At other times the fœtid accumulations form encrustations. The secretions of the glandular structures in the appendix are then retained causing congestion, inflammation and abscesses with all the accompanying symptoms of fever, rapid pulse, sharp pains in McBurney's region, — in other words, the set of symptoms which are usually diagnosed as appendicitis.

From the foregoing it becomes apparent that the great majority of appendicitis cases are caused not by foreign bodies but by chronic sluggishness of the bowels. What does the surgeon do to cure this? Snipping off the appendix does not change the faulty habits and diseased conditions which produce the intestinal indigestion and constipation.

Several years ago a member of the French Academy of Science published statistics showing that appendicitis in different countries and in different classes of society increases in exact ratio with the consumption of meat. America leads the list in the prevalence of appendicitis and in the consumption of meat. Next in order come England, France and Germany. The disorder is much more prevalent among the well to do, meat eating classes of England, France and Germany than among the semi-vegetarian peasantry. The principal causes of constipation and therefore of appendicitis are meat, fish and fowl, eggs, coffee and white bread. Flesh foods taken in excess result in putrefaction. This favours the development of bacteria, inflammation and diarrhoea, which are followed gradually by atony and atrophy. We have learned in another volume of this series that an excess of nitrogenous and starchy foods, fats and sugars form disease producing substances in the human body. These pathogenic substances, together with zanthins of coffee and tea, first stimulate but later invariably benumb the organs of digestion. They not only make gall, kidney and bladder stones but also form encrustations in the bowels in the cæcum and appendix. These accumulations blockade the secretory glands and membranes, become a source of constant irritation and prevent the assimilation of food.

Why White Bread is Constipating

The germs of grains contain two powerful ferments called diastase and peptase. The diastase changes the starch of the grain into sugar. The peptase changes the gluten into proteose and peptones which serve as food for the growing sprout in similar manner as the yolk and white of egg serve as food for the chick. In whole grain flour these ferments are preserved. They take the place of yeast for the fermenting of the bread, turn the starch into dextrine and sugar and the gluten into proteose and peptones, thus predigesting the raw materials of the bread. They act on the flour in the same way as do the digestive ferments of the body. This is why whole grain meal "does not keep" and why it requires less yeast than does white flour for lightening. The latter in the milling process has been deprived of the germ which contains the diastase and peptase and has also been robbed of the hulls which contain the mineral salts and thus are the carriers of the vitamines. The small particles of hull in the whole grain meal serve as a natural stimulant to the peristalsis of the bowels. They loosen the starchy mass in the stomach and intestines and thus favour the penetration of the digestive juices.

White flour bread, pastry and other products deprived of the natural ferments and the hulls of the grain tend to form pasty, lumpy accumulations in the intestines. I have known horses to die from feeding on white bread. It formed solid lumps which caused intestinal obstruction and thus killed the animals. Is it any wonder human beings develop constipation and appendicitis when they try to digest foods which kill a horse? When the ordinary constipation producing meat—white bread—pastry—coffee diet begins to have the usual effects, drugs, laxatives and cathartics are taken to counteract the evil results. In accordance with the law of action and reaction these poisonous stimulants only hasten the chronic atrophy of the intestinal tract.

From the foregoing it becomes apparent that the best preventive of constipation and appendicitis is a well balanced vegetable diet containing liberal amounts of fruit and vegetables and whole grain cereal products. The seed bearing fruits, which have been accused of causing appendicitis, are in reality its best preventive. This is confirmed by practical experience. Constipation and appendicitis are practically unknown among those who live on a rational vegetarian diet, but the surgeon, well paid for snipping out the appendix, has no time to waste in preaching dietetics even if he knew how.[1]

Treatment of Acute Appendicitis

The treatment of acute appendicitis is the same as that of any other acute inflammatory feverish disease. The essentials are plenty of fresh air,

[1]
It should perhaps be noted that on one occasion appendicitis was contracted by a physician known to the editor who was a strict and life-long vegetarian. When, rightly or wrongly, an operation was performed it was found that a portion of denture which had broken off was lodged in the appendix.

absolute fasting, hydrotherapy and manipulative treatment. While fasting the patient may have as much water with dilute acid fruit juices of natural temperature as he desires. In every instance where I have been called to attend appendicitis patients who had been under treatment by physicians of other schools, I have had to remove either hot water compresses or ice bags. Both applications are positively harmful and destructive. Artificial heat may temporarily relieve congestion and pain, but at the same time it keeps up the heat in the affected parts. It does not do anything to promote heat radiation and thus favours abscess formation. The ice treatment chills and freezes the parts and thus checks and suppresses the inflammatory process, leaving the affected parts in a condition of destruction, or, in other words, of chronic disease. Rational treatment lies between the two extremes of heat and ice. It is strange that none of the other schools of healing have discovered this fact. The only natural and rational way is to use for the packs, compresses and ablutions, water of the ordinary temperature as it comes from the water supply. If the patient can endure it we apply the ordinary abdominal pack or trunk pack, with an additional wet compress over the seat of the inflammation. In serious cases throat packs and leg packs may be applied in addition to the trunk pack, in order to reduce high temperature and to divert the blood from the affected parts. If the patient is so sensitive that he cannot endure the application of packs or if the inflammation runs a mild course, compresses wrung out of water fresh from the hydrant may be spread over the abdomen. Of course the compresses must be renewed day and night whenever they become hot or dry. Neurotherapy, spinal inhibition, magnetic and mental treatment and the indicated homoeopathic remedies are valuable aids in the natural treatment. Absolutely essential, however, are complete rest, fasting, water with dilute fruit juices, and hydrotherapy. They will always be sufficient to produce a perfect cure, provided the natural remedies are applied from the start. No food of any kind should be taken not even milk or broth. Nature must be given a free hand. Any kind of food excites the peristalsis of the inflamed intestines, thereby preventing the healing processes. Food particles may become enclosed in the open sores and abscesses, thus causing delay, chronic irritation and "recurrent appendicitis". After all symptoms have subsided the fasting must be continued for several days, in many cases for a week or more, in order to prevent relapses and chronic after effects. By adhering to these simple rules we have cured every case which has come under our treatment. Fasting and cold water treatment keep the inflammatory processes below the danger point. They allow free heat radiation, prevent abscess formation and at the same time do not interfere with nature's purifying healing efforts.

91

What about Abscesses?

The question may be asked: "What would you do if an abscess has already formed?" Even then I would adhere to the same simple, natural treatment and trust to nature rather than to the surgeon's knife. That this is the best policy we have proved in a great many instances. Under the right treatment absorption of the abscess will take place or it will break in the direction of least resistance, usually into the cæcum, and discharge into the rectum or through an outlet in the abdominal walls. It is wonderful how nature in such cases, under proper treatment, seeks and finds the safest outlet. However, abscess formation, perforation, and peritonitis will not occur if the treatment is natural from the beginning. All these serious complications are the result of hot water treatment, ice packs, premature feeding or cathartics. Several cases have come under my treatment after abscess formation and perforation had taken place. The resulting peritonitis was easily controlled by the natural treatment. Most patients make good recoveries.

The Dangers of Surgical Treatment

In order to reach the seat of infection, abscess or perforation, the surgeon has to cut through many layers of tissues and then into the pus and germ-filled locality. Naturally the danger of infecting the peritoneal cavity is very great. Mother Nature herself ingeniously tries to minimize the danger of infection. I have several times heard surgeons remark upon the fact that abscesses are usually surrounded by strong fibrous walls in order to prevent rupture and to protect the organism from infection. This is an instance of nature's wonderful provision for the protection of health and life, for emergencies and for extraordinary demands upon the organism. Much as I admire Hahnemann, I cannot agree with him that "Nature is a poor healer". As a rule, the older, the more intelligent and experienced the physician or surgeon, the more he recognizes and trusts "vis medicatrix naturæ". The young man fresh from school enthusiastically cuts into everything that presents itself. His elders shake their heads and say, "Wait a while. See what nature will do."

In my experience one of the most remarkable cases of appendicitis, complicated with general peritonitis, was that of an elderly gentleman whom I shall call Mr. X. He had been suffering from diabetes for a long time. After seeking relief by medical treatment he was converted to Christian Science and for many years he and his family were staunch believers in Mrs. Eddy's teachings. The disease, however, gained on him steadily and in his last extremity he returned to allopathic treatment. When his physician candidly told him that there was no hope he came to us for examination and advice. The diagnosis from the iris revealed a large-itch spot in the pancreatic area. He remembered distinctly that in his youth he had suffered from a violent attack of "seven year itch" and that this had been suppressed with the usual sulphur-molasses and blue ointment treatment. Half a year of rational living and natural treatment put him in fine condition. Then, of course, "Science had done it" and he returned to "the flesh pots of Egypt". Later on Mr. X visited me occasionally and told me exultingly how Christian Science was making good in every way. "Oh doctor," he said, "if you only had Science with your Nature Cure, you would be alright. As long as I get my daily treatment from my "healer" I can enjoy my steaks and chops and hot cakes and coffee without the slightest inconvenience." Laughingly I answered: "Look out, Mr. X, you cannot cheat nature for ever. If you do not behave you will get your spanking in spite of 'Science'." So it proved. About six months later I received a message: "Come at once. Mr. X is dying." Attended by a nurse I hurried to his home and found him in a very precarious condition. The trouble had originated in a very serious attack of appendicitis. This had developed into abscess and general peritonitis. We at once applied cold packs and spinal inhibition, together with magnetic and mental treatment. Within half an hour we had the condition under control. The terrific pains had subsided and the patient was resting easily. He said, "Doctor for six days I have been in hell. I have suffered all sorts of pain in my life, but never anything like this. Through it all I had in attendance at one time or another six of the best Scientists in Chicago, but obtained no relief."

After the inflammation had somewhat subsided we tried to flush the bowels by enemas, but without result. We were forced to "trust to nature". On the twenty-eighth day they moved naturally and freely. From that time on, full recovery was only a matter of careful nursing. During the first few weeks his entire abdomen was covered with crusty looking eruptions, nature's cleansing efforts. There has been no return of the trouble. Mr. X is all right as long as he takes his "Science" with a liberal allowance of Nature Cure. He told me that after his recovery from diabetes and return to flesh diet, he suffered from constipation; that at times his bowels did not move for several days, often for a week at a time. When he mentioned this to his "healer" he was told, "Never mind, the Lord will take care of that". The Lord did take care of it until the filthy condition of the system brought about the attack of appendicitis. The healer who expected the Lord to make good for his own lack of common sense had been at one time a well known allopathic physician. Like many other people, not understanding the basic laws of health, disease and cure, he had swung from one extreme to another — from allopathic overdoing into Christian Science "nothing doing".

The Chronic After Effects of Appendicitis

It has been customary with surgeons to advise removal of the appendix even after the patient has recovered from an acute attack, in order to prevent recurrence. If appendicitis is cured in the natural way there will be no chronic after effects. Injudicious feeding, the use of drugs and surgical operations, however, may prevent perfect restoration of the affected parts and result in chronic appendicitis. I have already explained how food materials may invade wounds and abscesses and may become enclosed in them, causing permanent irritation. If the palm of the hand has a cut we do not continually close and open it; this would interfere with the healing process. The contact of food with the raw surfaces of the inflamed cæcum and appendix, in similar manner, interferes with healing. Surgical extirpation is by no means a guarantee for the non-recurrence of "appendicitis". I have observed in many cases that the worst attacks come after the removal of the organ. This was due to inflammation of neighbouring parts, weakened by the operation. We have learned that the appendix is a useful organ and that it performs important functions in the process of digestion. Its extirpation, therefore, involves a serious loss to the economy of the body. We find that people thus operated upon nearly always suffer more from digestive distrubances than they did before. There is more sluggishness, constipation and gas formation. The general tone of health is not as good as formerly and resistance is lowered. Major operations invariably mean a weakening of the tissues and saturation with poisonous antiseptics. The affected parts are, therefore, less resistant to deterioration and disease. That it is best to use Nature Cure first and not as a last resort is shown by the experiences of Mr. A, an Italian barber in my neighbourhood. His trouble started with chronic constipation and haemorrhoids. To correct the latter he was operated upon, but in consequence the rectum contracted to such an extent that another operation became necessary. Then the bowels did not move at all. One of the most prominent surgeons in this city performed another operation, removing the appendix. After that, enemas and the most powerful drugs had no effect upon the bowels. As a last resort, other experiments failing, the eminent surgeon made an opening through the abdominal wall into the ascending colon. Through this canal, by means of a silver funnel, warm water was poured into the intestines. This brought the desired result. When the man came to us for advice he had been pouring a pint or more of warm water into the intestine every day for two years. While this procedure moved the bowels, the wound was beginning to show signs of necrosis and he was told by physicians that there was grave danger of cancer. This finally brought him to Nature Cure. Under the natural regimen, within four weeks his bowels moved naturally and freely without irrigation from above. They have continued to do so ever since. At first he did not allow the wound to close, being afraid of a recurrence of his old troubles — constipation and intestinal obstruction. He kept the channel open artificially by daily inserting the funnel. When the bowels had acted normally for three months he allowed the wound to close. It healed perfectly and there has been no trouble since during a period of several years. I demonstrated this case before an assemblage of students and professors in a medical college. In the course of my remarks I said: "If it was possible to make the bowels move naturally and freely by four weeks of natural diet and treatment after three years of medical and surgical experimentation, how much easier it would have been in the beginning to accomplish the cure by natural methods. How much suffering, loss of time and money might have been avoided."

CHAPTER XIV

VACCINATION

The pernicious after effects of vaccination upon the system are similar to those of the various serum and antitoxin treatments. The discovery of vaccination is usually credited to the Englishman, Edward Jenner, about 1800. The doubtful honour, however, belongs in reality to an old Circassian woman who, according to the historian le Duc, in the year 1672 startled Constantinople with the announcement that the Virgin Mary had revealed to her an unfailing preventive against smallpox. Her specific was inoculation with the genuine smallpox virus. But even with her the idea was not an original one, because the principle of isopathy (curing a disease with its own disease products) was explicitly taught a hundred years before by Paracelsus, the great genius of the Renaissance of learning at the end of the Middle Ages. But even he was only voicing the secret teachings of ancient folklore, sympathy healing and magic dating back to the Druids and Seers of ancient Britain and Germany. The Circassian seeress cut a cross in the flesh of the applicant and inoculated the wound with smallpox virus. Together with this she prescribed prayer, abstinence from meat, and fasting for forty days. The fasting was undoubtedly the most efficient part of the treatment. Since at that time smallpox was a terrible and widespread scourge, the practice of inoculation was carried all over Europe.

Popular superstitions run a course very similar to that of epidemics. They have a period of inception, of virulence and of abatement, and they die as a natural result of their own falsities and exaggerations. It soon became evident that inoculation with the virus did not prevent smallpox, but on the contrary frequently caused it; and therefore the practice gradually fell into a state of innocuous desuetude, to be revived by Edward Jenner about one hundred years later in a modified form. He substituted cowpox virus for smallpox virus. Modern allopathy, in applying the isopathic principle, gives large and poisonous doses of virus, lymph, serums and antitoxins; while homoeopathy, as did ancient mysticism, applies the isopathic remedies in highly diluted and triturated doses only. From England vaccination gradually spread over the civilized world and during the nineteenth century the smallpox disease constantly diminished in virulence and frequency until today it has become comparatively rare. "Therefore vaccination has exterminated smallpox", say the disciples of Jenner.

Is that really so? Is vaccination actually a preventive of smallpox? This seems very doubtful, especially since the advocates of vaccination themselves do not believe it. If they truly did so why should they be afraid of "catching" it from those who are not vaccinated? If they are thoroughly protected, as they claim to be, how can they catch the disease from those who are not protected? In the years 1870-71 smallpox was rampant in Germany. Over 1,000,000 persons had the disease and 120,000 died. Ninety-six per cent of these had been vaccinated, and only four per cent had not been so "protected". Indeed most of the victims were vaccinated shortly before they took the disease. In 1888 Bismarck sent to the governments of all the German States an address in which it was admitted that numerous eczematous diseases, even those of an epidemic nature, were directly attributable to vaccination, and that the origin and cure of smallpox were still unsolved problems. In this message to the various legislatures the chancellor said: "The hopes placed in the efficacy of the cowpox virus as a preventive of smallpox have proved entirely deceptive." Realizing this to be a fact most of the German governments have modified or entirely rescinded their compulsory vaccination laws.

"But" our opponents insist, "you cannot deny that smallpox has greatly diminished since the almost universal adoption of vaccination." Certainly the disease has diminished. But the plague, the "Black Death", cholera, the bubonic plague, yellow fever and numerous other epidemic pests which until recently occasionally decimated entire nations have also diminished and, in fact, nearly disappeared. Not one of these epidemics was treated by vaccination. Why, then, did they abate and practically disappear? The answer is, because of the more general adoption of soap, bathtubs, all kinds of sanitary measures, such as plumbing, drainage and ventilation, and because of more hygienic modes of living. Many of us remember how yellow fever raged in Havana during the Spanish occupancy. Within a few months after the energetic Yankees took possession and gave the filthy city a good scouring, yellow fever had entirely disappeared — without any yellow fever vaccination.

The question is now in order, why of all the dreaded plagues of the past smallpox alone survives to this day? The answer is, because of vaccination. If scrofulous and syphilitic poisons were not artificially kept alive in the human body by vaccination, smallpox by this time would be as rare as cholera and yellow fever. In this connection it must be remembered that all vaccines, serums and antitoxins are alive with morbid (bacterial)

97

microzymes. Thanks to the oft-repeated compulsory vaccination of every citizen, young and old, we as a nation have become saturated with smallpox virus. Is it any wonder that occasionally this latent taint breaks out in acute epidemics? Undoubtedly the almost universal systematic contamination and degeneration of vital fluids and tissues, not alone with vaccine virus but also with many other serums, antitoxins and drug poisons, accounts in a large measure for the steady increase of tuberculosis, cancer, syphilis, infantile paralysis, insanity, and a multitude of other chronic destructive diseases unknown among primitive people that have not come in contact with the blessings of "Syphilization", mercurialization and vaccination. By weakening the system's reactionary powers against one disease, its reactionary powers against all diseases are weakened. In other words, creating in the body a form of chronic smallpox by means of vaccination favours the development of all kinds of chronic disease. If we quit sowing the seed we shall cease reaping the harvest. By the suppression of syphilis and by means of vaccination you are perpetuating smallpox.

It may be asked: "What has syphilis to do with smallpox?" They are in fact very closely related and are similar in appearance, symptomatology, and in their effects upon the organism, Dr. Cruwell, after having studied the subject thoroughly says: "Every vaccination with so-called cowpox virus means syphilitic infection. Cowpox is not a disease peculiar to cattle; it is always due to syphilitic or smallpox infection from the diseased hands of human beings. Cowpox pustules have been found only on the udders of milk cows which came in contact with human hands. Cattle roaming in pasture and prairie have never been affected by cowpox, nor have domesticated steers and oxen. If this disease were a disorder peculiar to cattle both sexes would be equally affected. Jenner's cowpox was caused by the diseased hands of the syphilitic milkmaid, Sarah Nehnes." Vaccination of healthy children and adults is often followed by a multitude of symptoms which cannot be distinguished from syphilis, viz: characteristic ulcers and eczematous eruptions, swellings of the lymphatic glands, atrophy of the mammary glands in women and in girls above the age of puberty, etc. This helps to explain the constantly growing demand for "bust foods" and "bust developers". A perfectly developed bust has become so rare that many hundreds of 'beauty doctors" and of business concerns that make a speciality of developing the flat-bosomed realize thousands of dollars annually. It is reasonable to assume that almost without exception the thousands of women who are thus treated have been vaccinated from one to three times before the age of puberty. When this is realized, and the fact that vaccination tends to dry up the mammary glands is taken into account, is it not time to pause and consider? Some years ago a disease similar to smallpox broke out among sheep in certain parts of Scotland. As a preventive the sheep were vaccinated. In the course of a few years it was noticed that a great many ewes were unable to nourish their lambs. With the discontinuance of vaccination this phenomenon ceased. Do not these facts help to explain why over fifty per cent of human mothers are now incapable of nursing their babies?

Looking Forward

At present the trend of allopathic medicine is undoubtedly toward the serum, antitoxin and vaccine treatment. Practically all medical research tends that way. Every now and then the medical journals and the daily papers announce new serums and antitoxins which are claimed to cure or create immunity to certain diseases. Suppose the research and practice of medicine are continued along these lines and are generally accepted; or as the medical associations would have it, are forced upon the public by law. What would be the result? Before a child reached the years of adolescence it would have had injected into its blood the vaccines, serums and antitoxins of smallpox, hydrophobia, tetanus, cerebro-spinal meningitis, typhoid fever, diphtheria, pneumonia, scarlet fever, etc. If allopathy were to have its way, the blood of the adult would be a mixture of dozens of bacterial extracts, disease taints and destructive drug poisons. The tonsils and adenoids, the appendix and probably a few other parts of the human anatomy would be extirpated in early youth under compulsion of the health departments.

Which is more rational and sensible: the endeavour to produce immunity to disease by making the body a swill pot for the collection of all sorts of disease taints and poisonous antiseptics and germicides, or to create natural immunity by building up the blood on a normal basis, purifying the body of morbid matter and poisons, correcting mechanical lesions and by cultivating the right mental attitude? Which one of these methods is more likely to be disease building — which health building? Just imagine what human blood will be like in coming generations if this artificial contamination with all sorts of disease taints and drug poisons is to be forced upon the people.

Why Vaccination Is Responsible for Many Acute and Chronic Diseases

We have learned that every inflammatory and feverish disease is a purifying and healing effort of nature. In accordance with this fundamental law of cure the organism tries to throw off through the sores and ulcers produced by vaccination not only the recently inoculated smallpox virus, but also other hereditary and acquired disease taints and systematic poisons. Allopathic physicians recognize this law and apply it in their practice. When they make use of "counter irritants" such as blisters, "Spanish Flies", belladonna plasters, leeches, cupping, etc., they endeavour to remove internal congestion and inflammation by creating artificial inflammation on the surface of the body. The Nature Cure physician accomplishes the same thing in a more natural way by wet packs and cold ablutions. The pus-like mass exuding from the smallpox, pustule or vaccination sore contains the virus not only of smallpox, but also of scrofula, psora, tuberculosis, syphilis, gonorrhoea, anthrax, lumpy jaw and whatever else there may be of hereditary and acquired disease taints and poisons in the system of the animal or human from which the virus is secured. Such filthy exudates are inoculated into the bodies of millions of innocent victims of a "scientific" superstition. When vaccination is followed by scrofulous or syphilitic eruptions, itchy eczemata, swellings of glandular structures, etc., in children or adults who before vaccination were free from these disorders, then people who ought to know better wonder where it all came from, "where the poor child caught it". Fathers and mothers have sometimes been accused by the family physician of transmitting syphilis to their offspring when, as a matter of fact, the foul vaccine poison which the doctor himself had inoculated into the child was the real cause of the suspicious sores and eruptions.

An Interesting News Item

The following item appeared in several Chicago dailies on May 17th, 1909, but was then promptly suppressed by those most deeply interested in upholding the practice of vaccination.

"The bureau of animal industry made public today a report which fastens the blame for the recent outbreak of hoof and mouth disease in Michigan, New York, Pennsylvania and Maryland on a contaminated strain of vaccine, which originally came from a foreign country. The disease was traced by inspectors of the bureau to calves that had been used for the production of virus. The report sets forth the belief that the epidemic, which cost the federal government $300,000 to suppress, was started by these calves at Detroit after they had been used for the production of vaccine. The vaccine with which they were inoculated was imported from Germany by Parke, Davis and Co., and contained an infection of hoof and mouth disease. These calves, after having been used in propagating vaccine, were sent to the Detroit stockyards to be disposed of in the market. Four days later three carloads of cattle from points in

Michigan reached the Detroit stockyards and some of them were put into pens that had been occupied by the vaccine calves. Some of these cattle were sold for slaughter at Detroit while the remainder were shipped to Buffalo and to other places where the disease was first observed some days later. It eventually spread to various places in Pennsylvania and New York and to one locality in Maryland.

Three separate series of experiments were made. Young cattle and sheep were inoculated with the vaccine virus obtained from the firms. The hoof and mouth disease was produced in these animals by the use of the vaccine of this particular strain, while other strains gave negative results. The disease was also transmitted from one animal to another through several series, in two instances being transmitted by natural modes of infection.

The investigation also indicated that the outbreaks of hoof and mouth disease in New England in 1902-3 were due to contaminated vaccine of Japanese origin.

Why are facts of such vital importance to the public and our farmers suppressed after the first publication in the daily press, and who is responsible for such suppression? To this day the public is left with the impression that the cause of these epidemics is unknown, The first point of significance in this report is that the companies concerned used a certain smallpox vaccine virus which was contaminated with hoof and mouth disease. In 1908 vaccine of this strain was used for the production of vaccine virus crops from calves. The procedure is as follows: The flanks of the animals are shaved, then long slits are made in the flesh. The seed vaccine is rubbed into these wounds. The poison thus inoculated spreads through the entire organism of the animal and thoroughly contaminates blood and tissues. Then nature endeavours to eliminate the morbid taints. The wounds in the sides of the animal become ulcerating sores. The revolting mass exuding therefrom is then prepared for the market and is used throughout the country for purposes of vaccination. The report further explains how it was positively proved that this particular vaccine virus was contaminated with the taints of hoof and mouth disease. In consequence of this, thousands of children in all parts of the country were infected through vaccination not only with vaccine virus but also with the cattle disease. While it is true that this virulent disease may not prove fatal to human beings, inoculation with the virus means certain contamination with another disease taint which in the human body may work insidious destruction in some other form, such as scrofula, tuberculosis, eczema, etc. Why should we take chances of contaminating the blood of the innocent with these and other vile poisons? It has been repeatedly claimed by different investigators that cowpox is not a disease peculiar to cattle, that oxen have never shown it; that it appears only on the udders of milch cows and originates there in syphilitic or other infection from the hands of milkers. This statement seems plausible; but whether it can be proved or not, the fact remains that cowpox as well as smallpox is a disease taint which should not be artificially propagated in the blood of human beings.

Never was humanity cursed by a blacker superstition than this, that disease can be cured and health maintained by the absorption of virulent poisons. Rational therapeutics will always eliminate morbid matter, not introduce it into the system. Without doubt, smallpox would be extinct in civilized communities as are the plague, cholera and yellow fever, if it were not kept alive and propagated by the morbid microzymes of vaccine virus. The trouble with these disease taints, as with the inorganic poisonous drugs, is that in most cases their work of destruction in the human organism is so slow and insidious that the after effects are not always traced to their true source. The anaemia, leukemia, scrofulosis, tuberculosis, eczematous eruption or ulceration of a syphilitic character are hardly ever traced by the usual methods of diagnosis to vaccination, antitoxin, serum or tuberculin treatment. Here also diagnosis from the iris of the eye is frequently of inestimable service in disclosing true cause and effect.

Another startling revelation is contained in the report of this incident. One would expect that the calves whose blood and tissues had been so thoroughly saturated with disease taints would be killed and their bodies consumed by quick lime. Instead, horrifying as it may be, they were sent back to the stock yards to be sold for meat in the market. It seems incredible that for a few dollars these wealthy and respected firms who pose as protectors and preservers of public health would foist these carcasses upon an unsuspecting public as foodstuff. Such commerce in vaccine veal undoubtedly has been going on for years and is probably flourishing still. While this epidemic of hoof and mouth disease was in progress I lectured on the subject before the "Open Forum" society. After I had finished my lecture a gentleman arose from the audience and asked permission to tell what he knew about the matter. His remarks were as follows: "I am one of the men sent here by the government in Washington to subdue the epidemic of hoof and mouth disease in the stockyards. I am aware that the facts concerning the causes of former epidemics, as related by Dr. Lindlahr, are well known to government officials, and there is strong evidence that the present outbreak (1914) originated in a similar way. It is also true that the facts are and were with-held from publication at the instigation of powerful influences who are interested in upholding vaccination. My present experience in the stockyards has also proved to me that Dr. Lindlahr is right when he says that every acute disease is a healing effort of nature and if treated right will make for cure. This is true even of hoof and mouth disease. As you probably know, several hundred very valuable high-bred animals on exhibition in this city became infected by the disease and were condemned to be killed. On account of their great value it was decided to make an effort to save them. Animals affected by this disease die from starvation, since the tongue becomes so inflamed and swollen that they cannot take food. We placed this bunch of cattle in a high, airy loft, kept them clean and fed them through rubber tubes stuck into their throats. After the inflammation in the mouth had run its course every one of them got well."

Is this not a remarkable confirmation of Nature Cure philosophy and practice? After this test had proved the easy curability of the disease, why were the farmers not informed of this wonderful discovery of a natural cure? Why was the ruthless and unnecessary destruction of thousands of valuable animals continued? The diseased animals would have done still better if instead of food nothing but water had been given. Undoubtedly, anthrax and other animal diseases could be cured in the same natural manner.

After Effects of Vaccination

A few years ago I happened to attend a public clinic in a Chicago medical college. One of the subjects was a strong, healthy looking girl about eighteen years of age. Although in general appearance she was the picture of health, her left hand was horribly affected. The thumb and parts of the inner surface of the hand were disfigured by destructive ulceration. These sores had begun to develop about six months previous to the clinical examination. The health record of the patient's family was excellent. For generations there had been no history of scrofulous or tuberculous disease on either side and the young woman herself had never in her life suffered from a serious ailment. All attempts of the assembled students and professors to find a cause for this condition of the patient's hand were futile. I approached the young woman and on looking into her clear blue eyes discovered that the region of the iris corresponding to the upper left arm disclosed a large dark spot inclosed by whitish lines — in iridiagnostic terms, a "closed lesion."

Closed lesions in the iris correspond to scar tissues in the body. As long as a wound, ulcer or catarrhal defect is open and active in the body it is represented in the iris by dark blackish shadings interwoven with white lines. When the lesion in the body is healed and closed this fact is recorded in the iris by the appearacne of a whitish frame around the dark shading. Thus a closed lesion in the iris stands for the formation of new tissues or "scar tissue" in the body. In the case of this young woman the region in the iris corresponding to the diseased hand exhibited the whitish clouds of acute inflammatory activity. The scar sign in the region of the upper arm and the peculiar ulceration of the hand suggested to me at once the idea of vaccination. Accordingly I asked her whether within the last year or two she had been vaccinated on the left arm and whether this had been followed by a large ulcerating sore which was "cured" by medicinal treatment. Somewhat surprised she confirmed every part of this diagnosis telling me that the year before, when returning from Europe on an ocean liner, she had been vaccinated, that a large sore had developed which was very slow to heal and was treated for some time with "salves from the drug store". Thereupon I gave it as my opinion to the clinic that vaccination and the suppression of the resulting ulceration were the direct cause of the tuberculous sore on the hand. My diagnosis created considerable hilarity among the allopathic students in attendance at the clinic. It seemed ridiculous to them that anything so thoroughly orthodox as vaccination could in any way be held responsible for such serious after effects, especially as the sores on the hand did not appear until six months after vaccination. Replying to this objection, I asked why luetic sores on the body and in the throat sometimes do not appear until six months or longer after the suppression of the original lesion on the genital organs has taken place, or why cancer does not develop in an organ affected by suppressed itch (as revealed in the iris of the eye) until many years after this suppression. To these questions orthodox medical science had, of course, no answer. The dean of the college, a liberal and discerning man, who was conducting this particular clinic, showed himself susceptible to an understanding of my point of view and said: "Dr. Lindlahr has given at least a very pertinent and plausible theory of this phenomenon, while you yourselves have given no explanation whatever. Therefore, gentlemen, please curb your hilarity and do some thinking."

Another interesting case illustrating the chronic after effects of vaccination is that of a Mr. B who came to us for consultation and treatment several years ago. For four years he had been suffering from a bad form of epilepsy. He had consulted with and been treated by the best physicians in Chicago, but without obtaining any relief. When I first examined his eyes I noticed in the region of the iris corresponding to the left arm a heavy, whitish streak which contained two black spots. This indicated an injury to the limb and a subacute condition. I asked the patient whether he had at any time sustained an injury to his left arm. This he denied, but after considerable questioning he said: "When the epileptic attacks come on I feel a pain in my left hand; this travels up the arm, and when it reaches the elbow I fall unconscious." Examining his iris again I asked whether the arm had been vaccinated. He replied that it had been about four years previously, that there had been very serious ulceration, that the arm had been greatly swollen and that he had been confined to bed for two weeks. He had never had epileptic fits before this and he began to have them shortly after.

Many people are suffering today from serious chronic affections of body and mind resulting from vaccination. These chronic after effects usually develop so slowly and insidiously that no one thinks of tracing them to their true cause. The diagnosis from the iris of the eye has exposed and explained many of these obscure cases. Allopathy, when asked about the causes of these and other serious chronic ailments, has but one answer, "Nobody knows"; and it assumes that nobody can know.

In this particular case we explain the sequence of events as follows: The vaccine injected into the arm caused blood poisoning of a kind. If the resulting ulceration had been allowed to discharge freely and fully, and if elimination had been encouraged by proper treatment instead of being hindered and suppressed by poisonous antiseptics, the blood would have purified itself and there would have been no chronic after effects. But the wounds were healed prematurely by the usual antiseptic treatment and the system was left in a poisoned condition. Diagnosis from the iris of the eye has revealed the fact that the epileptic centre is located in the cerebellum, just behind the left ear. In this connection it is significant that the vaccination was in the left arm. It was clear that the treatment to be applied had to be eliminative in character and this was what was done by the initiation of a course of natural treatment. During the sixth week, in accordance with the law of crises, a sore developed on the left arm in the same place where the ulceration had been four years earlier. The discharges from the arm acted as a fontanelle and safety valve through which nature eliminated the suppressed disease taint. After the sore had remained open for a few weeks it healed spontaneously. Since that time Mr. B has not had another epileptic attack. He has married and is now the happy father of several healthy children. According to medical science he was a "defective" who should have been sterilized for the protection of society.

In our Nature Cure practice we have met with many cases of tuberculosis, eczema, pernicious anemia, lockjaw, paralysis, etc., which were directly traceable to vaccination. Anti-vaccination societies also frequently report such cases. Last year (1908) in Chicago two deaths resulted from smallpox, but hundreds of serious diseases and fatalities were traceable to vaccination. In most cases, however, the detrimental after effects of vaccination are so insidious and obscure in their development that they are not easily traceable to their true cause — the smallpox or cowpox virus and its morbid microzymes. It remains for Iridology to bring proof positive of these hidden sequelae. Shortly after vaccination the colour of the iris

105

darkens, especially in the regions corresponding to the digestive and respiratory organs. This darkening of the colour is noticeable also in cases in which, according to common parlance, vaccination has "not taken". In fact, these persons often show in their eyes more serious defects than those in whom the regular sores developed. This means that, in accordance with the fundamental laws of cure, those who develop vaccination ulcers expel the poison through them, whereas children or adults who are already encumbered with scrofulous conditions and who are of weak vitality may have no purifying ulcerations because they are not able to develop them. Such people are retaining the poisonous infection, which results in greater deterioration of the organism in general and of the digestive and respiratory tracts in particular. The worst thing of all is that these "non takers" are frequently vaccinated again and again, although, to the great mystification of the medical fraternity, they continue not to "take". I have seen the report of a case in which a child was vaccinated ten times "without results", and then refused admission to the public schools because she was not properly vaccinated. Diagnosis from the eye would probably have revealed that the vaccination had in fact "taken" only too well, the child's body by that time being thoroughly saturated with the poison. The conclusion of the matter is that those with whom vaccination "takes" best generally retain the least of it, but those with whom it appears not to "take" may be the ones most seriously affected.

Diphtheria, as we know it, was first described by Bretonneau, a French physician, in 1820 some time after the general introduction of vaccination. Many conscientious and competent investigators claim that diphtheria in its present virulent form and frequency was not known before that time, and that diphtheria has faithfully followed vaccination from one country to another. Whether or not we can accept these radical charges in their entirety, this much is certain: diphtheria in its modern virulent form and frequency of occurrence seems to have been unknown in any country before the universal practice of vaccination. This can be explained by the fact that the vaccine virus, according to evidence furnished by diagnosis from the eye, locates and concentrates in the mucous membranes of the digestive tract and of the bronchi, throat and pharynx. It lowers the vitality of these parts and charges them with the poisons contained in the vaccine virus. At the first opportunity nature makes an heroic effort to throw off the scrofulous encumbrance. This opportunity may present itself when the next cold is "caught" — then the ordinary tonsilitis, pharyngitis or laryngitis may become a genuine diphtheria. We can readily conceive how the morbid soil created by the vaccine virus may produce microzymes which will develop into diphtheria germs. Sometimes we are told that this or that child had diphtheria, although it had never been vaccinated. To this we answer that many times the diagnosis of diphtheria is incorrect. It is always safer for the physician to diagnose the more serious disease, for if the patient recovers, the glory is so much greater. However, since the microzymes of diphtheria germs flourish in the bodies of vaccinated children and the air is polluted with them, why should not an unvaccinated child here and there succumb to the infection, especially when the blood of our children is hereditarily contaminated with the vaccine back to the third and fourth generation?

It is amusing to note the confusion of the public as well as of the scientific mind on the most simple questions of hygiene. The millionaire owner of a dozen palatial quick lunch rooms in Chicago is so deeply concerned about the health of his patrons that at stated intervals, under penalty of discharge, he compels every one of his employees to submit to vaccination; yet he sees no wrong in dealing out to his customers wholesale dyspepsia and nervousness in the form of cheap sausage, white bread, pie, tea and coffee. Where one person dies from smallpox, probably thousands die from the effects of the deadly quick lunch counter.

About two years ago I received the following letter from an address in Texas: "Dear Doctor: Allow me to submit to you the case of a young friend of mine. The patient is about twenty-one years of age. He was never sick in his life except with measles, and always enjoyed the best of health. A month ago on account of a supposed smallpox case in the neighbour-hood general vaccination was enforced. Mr. A, directly after vaccination, developed blood poisoning, and this resulted in cerebrospinal meningitis. This disease left him completely paralysed from the hips down. Water and fæces have to be removed artificially. Home doctors say that to move him would mean sure death. What do you think about the case, and would you advise us to bring him to you for treatment?"

To undertake the treatment of such a case seemed a risky thing, especially when the patient had to be transported over a thousand miles. The doctors at home had pronounced the case absolutely incurable and transportation out of the question. However, being entirely convinced of the efficiency of our simple, natural methods, I did not hesitate to assume the respons-ibility and wrote to the father to that effect. Within a week or two the patient came to our sanitarium. He was completely paralysed from the navel down. The urine had to be removed by the use of a catheter, and the bowels were emptied with great difficulty by enemas. Anterior poliomyelitis had undoubtedly been caused in this case by inflammation set up by vaccine virus, though the doctors at home tried to put the blame on a fall from a horse three months previously. Mr. A assured me positively that this fall had not injured him in any way. Having been a cowboy, he had had a great many falls more serious than this one. This case, being of recent origin, yielded with marvellous rapidity. Within two weeks after his arrival his bladder and bowels moved freely and he began to regain the use of his legs. After nine weeks he had regained full control over his lower limbs and began to talk of going home.

From the foregoing it will have become apparent that smallpox, like every other infectious disease, is a filth disease, that its microzymes grow in morbid soil only and that the smallpox eruptions are a sign of rapid elimination of hereditary and acquired disease taints. A good dose of smallpox may rid the system of more scrofulous, tuberculous and syphilitic poisons than could otherwise have been got rid of in a lifetime. Therefore smallpox is certainly to be preferred to vaccination. The one means the elimination of chronic disease, the other the making of it.

To many this may seem rash talk, but in this matter I can speak from practical experience. My eldest son was born at a time when both parents were heavily encumbered with hereditary and acquired disease conditions. At birth he weighed only two and a half pounds and his chance for life seemed very slight. The eyes were of a blackish blue, especially the outer portion of the iris, and this gradually condensed into a heavy scurf rim owing to the fact that nature's cleansing efforts in the form of skin eruptions were promptly suppressed with talcum powder and other home "remedies". For the first five or six years of his life he was a weak, sickly child, having one after another all of the common infantile ailments. However, we soon learned to treat these by natural methods and he was not vaccinated.

One day suspicious looking eruptions appeared, which soon spread all over the body. I called in two allopathic physicians to verify my diagnosis of smallpox, which they did unqualifiedly. We applied the natural treatment, which consisted of strict fasting, colon flushing and cold water applications. The child was kept day and night in wet packs — strips of linen wrung out of the water of natural temperature and covered with flannel bandages — which were changed whenever they became hot and dry. The face also was kept covered with cooling compresses. In addition to this I gave the indicated high potency homoeopathic remedies.

There was hardly a spot on the boy's body which was not covered with sores. However, constant renewal of the cold packs kept the temperature below the danger point and greatly alleviated the insufferable itching peculiar to the disease. My wife, her sister and myself by turns slept in the same room with the child without the least fear of infection, and although we had not been vaccinated since childhood we remained unaffected by the "contagious disease". The wet packs, of course, greatly furthered the processes of elimination and the disease practically ran its course in ten days. From that time on the sores healed rapidly and nothing remained to indicate the "ravages" of the disease but a telltale mark over the left eyebrow and a few similar scars on the boy's body. These also have now entirely disappeared. Under the natural treatment convalescence was rapid and complete, and soon after the eyes became much clearer and much lighter in colour. Since his recovery this boy has never had a sick day. He is now in his twenty-first year and well developed physically and mentally. As far as I could learn there was not another case of smallpox in Chicago and the vicinity at the time. If the infection theory be true, from whom did he "catch" the disease and why did not one of the many persons living in the same house become infected? My answer is: This acute eliminative process was nature's way of purifying the young body of inherited scrofulous and other disease taints.

With our younger boy we had a somewhat similar experience. When one year old he was taken with a severe attack of cerebrospinal meningitis. Every half hour or so his body was bent backward in the dreadful convulsions peculiar to this disease. Again I called in two allopathic physicians to confirm the diagnosis so that the facts might not be questioned in the future. In this case again nothing but natural treatment was used. For nine days it seemed a hopeless fight to everyone who had occasion to witness it. Then both eardrums "broke" and discharged pus and blood. From that time on all symptoms began to clear up rapidly, and on the eleventh day the child first took food. Previous to that he had not received so much as a drop of milk — nothing but cold water rendered slightly acid with fruit juices. For six weeks the discharge of pus and blood from the ears contined unhindered, but rather encouraged and promoted by natural methods of treatment and by the indicated homœopathic remedies. As in the case of the older boy, the physical and mental improvement and development following the disease were most gratifying. While before this eliminative crisis the child had seemed somewhat slow and dull, after the recovery he was much brighter and more active physically and mentally. Compare with this splendid recovery and subsequent improvement in general health the results which often follow the orthodox drug and serum treatment of spinal meningitis. According to statistics a high percentage of the patients die and the survivors are either paralysed or suffer some other form of chronic after effects. I claim that my two children eliminated in a few weeks more scrofulous and psoric taints and poisons from their systems through smallpox and meningitis than would have been possible otherwise in many years, or perhaps in a lifetime.[1] [2]

[1]
It is to be noted that hydrotherapy is the form of treatment above all others which is regarded by Dr. Lindlahr as the key to the successful and safe treatment of acute feverish diseases of all kinds. It is clear that he looks upon other forms of treatment

such as manual manipulation and homoeopathy as being supplementary to it, though often of great value and importance. If he is right the great fear which is engendered by epidemics of such things as smallpox especially in primitive countries is not well founded.

(2)

The picture presented by the theory and practice of vaccination and immunization has certainly changed somewhat since Dr. Lindlahr wrote. There are an enormous number of vaccines and serums used for the treatment and prevention of acute infectious diseases of all kinds. Some of these are conceived of as giving an active immunity by inducing a mild attack of the same or a similar disease and some as conferring a passive immunity by supplying the recipient with antibodies or antitoxins either to prevent the disease being contracted or by curing it when contracted. Moreover, the preparation of these substances has become highly complicated, technical and varied and the methods of administration too are varied, being sometimes by application to the skin, sometimes by injection and sometimes by mouth. The Nature Cure view has always been that such preparations are harmful, poisonous and suppressive even if they appear to be effective. The real point at issue is whether it is in fact possible and desirable by some means to create an immunity to specific diseases and, if so, how this should be done. The basic position of the Nature Cure school is that the really important thing is to create natural immunity to all diseases which is done by building up a positive condition of health and by paying due attention to hygiene. It has, however, been widely believed that it is or should be possible to confer a specific immunity to particular diseases. The homoeopaths have always used nosodes and other remedies in the treatment of infectious diseases and also for prophylaxis. The orthodox vaccine and serum treatments appear to constitute, as Dr. Lindlahr affirms, an aberration, distortion or misapplication of homoeopathic principles and methods. It is on genuine homoeopathic lines that we should seek to promote specific immunity when it is desirable to do so. These matters are further discussed in an appendix. (See Appendix II).

CHAPTER XV

THE DIPHTHERIA ANTITOXIN

In this country the antitoxin treatment for diphtheria is still in high favour, whereas in Germany where it originated many of the best medical authorities are abandoning its use on account of its doubtful curative results and the danger of certain after effects. According to the advocates of the treatment the antitoxin is a "certain" cure for diphtheria, but it is doubtful whether this claim is borne out by the actual facts. The Health Bulletins sent regularly to every physician in the City of Chicago by the Health Department show a considerable number of deaths from cases treated with antitoxin. Considering the great uncertainty of medical statistics, I am not prepared to affirm whether or not the antitoxin treatment actually has reduced the mortality percentage, but we of the Nature Cure School claim and can prove that the hydropathic treatment of diphtheria insures a much lower percentage of mortality than does any other treatment.

The crucial point to be considered is the after effects of the different methods of treatment, and I make the following claims:

(1) That the antitoxin, being itself a powerful poison, may be and often is the direct cause of paralysis, or of death due to heart failure.

(2) That diphtheria treated with antitoxin may be and often is followed by paralysis, heart failure or lifelong invalidism of some kind after the patient has recovered from the diphtheria itself.

(3) That these undesirable after effects of diphtheria do not occur when the disease is treated by natural methods, but that they are the result of the antitoxin treatment and its suppressive effect upon the disease.

To prove these claims I submit the following facts: I have in my possession clippings from newspapers from various parts of the country stating that death has followed the administration of the diphtheria antitoxin for prevention or "immunization" in persons not actually suffering from the disease.

Several of these cases created quite a sensation in Germany about twenty years ago. Dr. Robert Langerhans, the superintendent of a Berlin hospital, was a strong advocate of the antitoxin treatment and was responsible for its being officially recommended for free distribution in the city of Berlin. Shortly after this his cook was taken off to hospital with suspected diphtheria, and he administered antitoxin to his son, a child of eighteen months, as a protective precaution. The child shortly afterwards developed symptoms of blood-poisoning and died of heart-failure within twenty-four hours. About the same time another Berlin doctor's child with a slight sore throat was given a prophylactic injection which was followed by a severe and protracted illness.

In this connection, remarks made by Dr. William Osler in his "Practice of Medicine" are of interest. "Of the sequelae of diphtheria, paralysis is by far the most important. This can be experimentally produced in animals by inoculation of toxic material produced by the bacilli. The paralysis occurs in a variable proportion of all the cases, ranging from 10 to 15 and even to 20 per cent. It is strictly a sequel of the disease, coming on usually in the second or third week of convalescence . . . It may follow very mild cases; indeed the local lesion may be so trifling that the onset of the paralysis alone calls attention to the true nature of the disease . . . The disease is a toxic neuritis, due to the absorption of the poison. Of the local paralyses the most common is that which affects the palate . . . Of other local forms perhaps the most common are paralyses of the eye muscles . . . Heart symptoms are not uncommon . . . Heart failure and fatal syncope may occur at the height of the disease or during convalescence, even as late as the sixth or seventh week after apparent recovery."

It appears to me that the mystery of these sequelae can easily be explained. It is certain that a mere sore throat, not serious enough to be diagnosed as diphtheria, cannot produce paralysis or heart-failure; but we know positively that the antitoxin can do it and does it. The cases to which Dr. Osler refers may safely be assumed to have received the antitoxin treatment, because it is administered on the slightest suspicion of diphtheria, and indeed even to perfectly healthy persons "for purposes of immunization."

In my own practice, I am frequently consulted by chronic patients whose troubles date back to diphtheria "cured" by antitoxin. Among these I have met with several cases of idiocy and insanity, with many cases of partial paralysis, infantile paralysis and nervous disorders of the most serious nature, also with other forms of chronic destructive disease. In the iris of the eye the effect of the antitoxin on the system shows a darkening of the colour. In many instances, the formerly blue or light-brown iris assumes an ash-grey or brownish-grey hue. One of my secretaries had clear blue eyes up to her tenth year. About that time she had several attacks of diphtheria and a severe "second" attack of scarlet fever which were treated and "cured" under the care of an allopathic physician. She does not remember whether she was given antitoxin, but recalls that her throat was painted and her body rubbed with oil and that she had to take a great deal of medicine. Since that time her eyes have turned brown. They show plainly the reddish-brown spots of iodine in the areas of the brain, the throat, and other parts of the body. The effect upon the iris of the eye would be very much the same whether the attack of diphtheria had been suppressed by antitoxin or by the old-time drug treatment. A significant fact in this connection is that, while Mrs. C was with us, following natural methods of living and under the effects of the treatments which she took regularly for several months, her eyes became much lighter and in places the original blue became visible under the brown. The nerve rings in the region of the brain, which were very marked when she first came to us, became less defined. Corresponding improvement took place in her general health and especially in the condition of her nerves.

In regard to my claim that undesirable after effects do not occur under treatment by natural methods, I wish again to call attention to the fact that for fifty years the Nature Cure physicians in Germany have proved that their treatment of diphtheria is not followed by paralysis, heart failure or the different forms of chronic, destructive diseases. This has been confirmed by my own experience.

At this point I must diverge for a moment to show that I am not alone in being strongly opposed to vaccination and in being convinced that there is a connection between vaccination and diphtheria. An eminent Californian physician of the orthodox school, Dr. Tenison Deane, the holder of many public, hospital and academic appointments, became convinced that vaccination was "the greatest mistake ever made, the enormity of which can never be equalled nor half appreciated" and eventually wrote a book entitled "The Crime of Vaccination". In this book he gives a case history which led him to start the investigations and study which led him to his conclusions. The history is as follows: "In June 1889 the author was spending his vacation on the ranch of a wealthy farmer. It was a large farm, fifteen miles from the nearest town and with no immediate neighbours. The farmer had a wife and seven children. The foreman, a negro, had a wife and five children. None of them had ever been vaccinated. Six of them were selected and vaccinated by the author: The farmer's wife, age 43 years, the farmer's daughter age 6, the farmer's sons ages 8 and 25, the negro foreman age 46, his son age 12. All the rest were left out and were not afterwards vaccinated. On August 1, 1890, the farmer, his wife and five children went to the mountain ranch forty miles away, taking with them the foreman, his wife and five children. There had been no diphtheria in the town nor any in their neighbourhood. The mountain ranch was an uninhabited virgin pine forest district with pure water where they took up their camp.

"Three weeks later an epidemic of sore throat and canker sores developed among the children. Farmer's daughter, seven years old, son nine years old, and the foreman's son thirteen years old developed very serious throat and constitutional symptoms and were taken to the home ranch, where a doctor was sent for. Diphtheria was the diagnosis. The farmer's wife also developed diphtheria. All the rest who had not been vaccinated cured rapidly of their sore throats. The farmer's daughter, seven years old died. The farmer's son nine year's old did not recuperate for one year. The farmer's wife, 44 years old, had paralysis and sequelae, which lasted over one year. The foreman's son, thirteen years old, became very weak and did not return to normal health.

"In 1893, the farmer's son, 29 years old died in Los Angeles from tubercular intestinal trouble; in 1900, the foreman, at 57 years of age died of tubercle or cancer of the larynx; in 1902, the foreman's son, 25 years old, died of tuberculosis; in 1909 the farmer's wife, 63 years old, died of cancer; in 1911, the farmer's son, 30 years old died of tubercular meningitis. The farmer died of old age. All the rest are living and in perfect health, nor have they ever been vaccinated. No tuberculosis has shown in any of those living, nor is there any family history of tuberculosis. All who were vaccinated in 1889 are now dead.

"In view of the foregoing, what unutterable silliness the present anti-tuberculosis crusade and the elaborate 'cancer research.' On these, millions are spent yearly, countless dumb brutes are tortured, and human beings are experimented on with every nostrum conceivable to modern medicine! And all the while the state manufacture of cancer and consumption (as well as other diseases) goes briskly forward. It is a tragedy, repeating itself year after year, as people are forced to be vaccinated on various pretexts. School attendance, the chance to earn your bread, to go about your business — these are made dependent on getting vaccinated whenever health boards see fit to order."

This book of Dr. Tenison Deane's is of great interest and significance both because it is a confirmation of Nature Cure philosophy from an orthodox source and because the writer clearly sees that it is the long term effects of vaccination which are so serious rather than any immediate reactions.

Nature Cure in Germany and America

That it is possible to cure all kinds of serious acute disease by drugless methods of healing, has been proved by Nature Cure practitioners in Germany, nearly all of whom were men who had never attended medical school. For over half a century many thousands of them have been practicing the art of healing, in all parts of Germany. With hydrotherapy and other natural methods they have treated successfully typhoid fever, diphtheria, smallpox, appendicitis, cerebrospinal meningitis and all other acute diseases. It is a significant fact that, in spite of the most strenuous opposition and appeals to the lawmaking powers on the part of the regular school of medicine, the lay practitioners could not be prevented from practising the natural methods of treatment in law and police ridden Germany. Moreover, the number of Nature Cure practitioners, most of them laymen, has tended to increase and is undoubtedly due to the success of the methods they employ. This success has been demonstrated in spite of all kinds of opposition and attempted restriction, for while the Nature Cure practitioner is generally permitted to treat those who come to him for relief, he does not have the right, as does the allopath, to cover his mistakes with six feet of earth. If one of his patients dies, a doctor has to be called in to testify to the fact and issue a death certificate. Though lay practitioners of natural methods have sometimes been brought before the courts both in Germany and elsewhere, the evidence in their favour and the harmlessness of their methods have made it virtually impossible for convictions to be obtained against them.

In America, though medical critics have questioned the efficacy of our methods, I have, during the last seventeen years, treated and cured all kinds of serious acute disease without resorting to allopathic drugs and in no instance was surgery needed. In a very extensive practice I have not in all these years, lost a single case of appendicitis, typhoid fever, smallpox, scarlet fever, etc., and only one case each of cerebrospinal meningitis, lobar pneumonia and diphtheria. These are the facts which may be verified through the records of the Health Department of the City of Chicago. I leave it to my readers to judge whether Nature Cure philosophy is inspired by blind fanaticism and based on ignorance and inexperience, or whether it is justified in the light of scientific facts and demonstrated by experience.

I here give the main part of the contents of a letter which I received: "Dear Dr. Lindlahr. On the 11th of November last, our boy, aged thirteen years, was taken ill with diphtheria . . . I called at your office and asked your advice. You replied 'wet packs, no food except fruit juices, colon flushing, spinal treatment and — no antitoxin.'

"We called an osteopathic physician, who at once sent a specimen from the boy's throat to the city laboratory, where it was pronounced diphtheria. A physician from the Board of Health came and quarantined us and inquired if we had used the antitoxin treatment. When my wife replied 'No', he said 'I suppose you know that the percentage of deaths of those who do not have it is very high.' She said 'Yes, I know, but we do not intend to use it.'

"The boy had all the acute symptoms, was drowsy, with headache, and on the second day his temperature went to 105 degrees. We applied the wet body pack and by night had reduced his temperature to 100 degrees. With the aid of the osteopathic treatment, which he had each night, the boy slept well all through the illness. On the fifth day, the membrane spread from his throat to his nose, and his temperature rose again; but the wet body packs again reduced it so that it was never again over 100 degrees. The boy was bright, his mind was clear, he was able to read, and after the first week was able to play chess. The only unfavourable symptom he had at all was an irregular pulse. He took no medicine and no food except fruit juices. We used occasionally the tepid water enema. On the tenth day he took a little lamb broth, but refused it the next day, and again asked for fruit juices. It was not until two weeks had passed that his appetite returned and he began to eat. He lost flesh, but he did not lose strength in the same degree — he was able to go to the bathroom each day unaided.

During all this time his only attendant was his mother and the osteopathic physician who came daily. The boy has fully recovered and has suffered no bad results that often follow such diseases . . . In contrast I would like to cite the case of a neighbour of ours whose little girl died of the disease under the antitoxin treatment. She recovered from the diphtheria, but her heart failed and she died suddenly. They had a regular M.D. and a trained nurse. Her mother took ill, but recovered. The father told me that their drug bill amounted to 75 dollars . . . Sincerely yours, Hinton White."

This letter and numerous similar evidences go to prove the curability of diphtheria by natural methods. In this case, as in many others, I gave directions for treatment verbally and over the telephone without having seen the patient personally. Once more I must repeat that hydropathic treatment will give good results in all forms of acute disease.

CHAPTER XVI

SUPPRESSIVE SURGICAL TREATMENT OF TONSILITIS AND ENLARGED ADENOIDS

In many larger cities, physicians and nurses, by order of state boards of health, are regularly visiting the public schools. They examine the children, gather statistics and give hygienic and medical advice to teachers and parents. The idea is a good one and will be productive of much benefit, provided that the advisers themselves are rightly informed. Unfortunately this is not always the case.

A large proportion of school children are nowadays afflicted with chronic tonsilitis and with inflammation or hypertrophy of the adenoid tissues, which are located in the nasal pharynx. When these abnormal conditions are discovered, the parents are at once advised to have the offending tonsils and adenoids removed. Frequently we are consulted by parents about the advisability of having these operations performed. The explanation which I give to these enquiries is as follows. The tonsils are excretory glands which nature has created for the elimination of impurities from the body. Acute, sub-acute and chronic tonsilitis accompanied by enlargement and cheesy decay of the tonsils means that these glands have been habitually congested with pathogenic matter, that they have had more work to do than they could properly attend to. These structures constitute however, a valuable part of the drainage system of the organism. If the blood is poisoned through overeating and faulty food combinations, or with scrofulous, venereal or psoric taints, the tonsils are called upon with other organs to eliminate these morbid taints. Is it any wonder that frequently they become inflamed and subject to decay? What, however, is to be gained by destroying them with iodine or extirpating them with the surgeon's wire snare? Were the drains in your house too small to carry off the waste, would you seal or remove them? This, however, is what is actually being done. The surgeon says: "The swollen tonsils and adenoids are closing up the nasal breathing passages; especially at night the child breathes through the mouth. This may cause all kinds of chronic ailments, deformations of the chest, changes in the facial expression, sometimes marked alteration in the mental condition and in certain cases stunting of physical and mental development. The removal of the tonsils will bring back quick relief from all these troubles; why then delay the simple operation"?

It is true that "drying up" or extirpating the tonsils will give instant local relief. The voice and the breathing will become unobstructed; the Eustachian tube, which forms an air passage from the mouth and ears, will open and the parents and the family physician will rejoice over the splendid results of the "trivial" operation. But, as usual, they take into consideration the first effects only; the secondary and lasting ones are regarded and treated as new diseases. In case of any morbid discharge from the body, whether through haemorrhoids, open sores, ulcers or through tonsils, scrofulous glands, etc., a fontenalle has been established to which and through which systemic poisons make their exit. If such an outlet be blocked by medical or surgical treatment, the morbid matter is forced to seek another escape or else accumulate somewhere in the system. Fortunate is the patient when such an escape can be established, because in whatever part of the system morbid excretions, suppressed by medical treatment, concentrate, there will be found the seat of chronic disease. After the tonsils have been extirpated, the morbid matter which they would have eliminated usually finds the nearest and easiest outlet through the adenoid tissues and nasal membranes. These now take up the work of vicarious elimination and in their turn become hyperactive and inflamed. Sometimes it happens that the adenoid tissues become affected before the tonsils. In that case, also, relief is sought through surgical treatment, and then the process is reversed; after the adenoids have been removed, the tonsils become inflamed. When both tonsils and adenoids have been extirpated, the nasal membranes in turn become congested and swollen. Often the mucoid elimination increases to an alarming degree and frequently polypi and other growths appear; or the turbinated bones soften, swell and obstruct the nasal passages. Thus again the patient becomes a "mouth breather". But in vain does nature protest against local symptomatic treatment. When the nasal organs take up the work of vicarious elimination, the same mode of treatment is resorted to. The mucous membranes of the nose are now swabbed and sprayed with antiseptics and astringents or "burned" by cauterizers, electricity, etc. The polypi are cut out, and frequently parts of the turbinated bones as well, in order to open up their air passages. Now surely, it is felt, the patient must be cured. But, strange to say, new and more serious troubles are apt to arise. The posterior nasal passages and the throat now become affected by chronic catarrhal conditions and there is much annoyance from phlegm and mucous discharges dropping into the throat. These catarrhal conditions frequently extend to the mucous membranes of the stomach and intestines.

When the drainage system of the nose and the naso-pharyngeal cavities has been seriously impaired, the impurities must either travel upward into the brain or downward into the glandular structures of the neck and thence into the bronchi and the tissues of the lungs. If the trend be upwards to the brain, the patient grows nervous and irritable or becomes dull and apathetic. Frequently a child is reprimanded, even punished for laziness and inattention when it is not responsible. In many instances the morbid matter affects certain centres in the brain and causes nervous conditions, hysteria, St. Vitus' dance, epilepsy, etc. In children the impurities frequently find an outlet through the ear drums in the form of pus discharges. This frequently averts inflammation of the brain, meningitis, imbecility, insanity, or infantile paralysis. I have frequently traced serious attacks of mastoiditis directly to the extirpation of the tonsils and adenoids. In such cases the surgeon trephines the skull and treats the mastoid cells with antiseptics, thereby suppressing the inflammation. I have never applied such destructive treatment and have never lost a case.

If, on the other hand, the trend of the suppressed impurities and poisons be downward, it often results in hypertrophy and degeneration of the lymph glands of the neck. In such cases the suppressive treatment, by drugs or knife, is again resorted to. The scrofulous poisons, suppressed and driven from the diseased glands in the neck, now find lodgement in the bronchi and lungs where they accumulate and form a luxuriant soil for the propogation of the bacilli of pneumonia and tuberculosis. In other cases the vocal organs become seriously affected by chronic catarrhal conditions, abnormal growths and, in later stages, by tuberculosis. Many a fine voice has been ruined in this way.

Prevention and cure of all these ailments lie not in local symptomatic treatment and suppression by drugs or knife, but in the rational and natural treatment of the body as a whole. First of all, antitoxins, vaccines and serums must be avoided because the morbid microzymes of these preparations breed scrofulous conditions and all sorts of chronic diseases. Then the diet must be regulated in accordance with the principles of natural dietetics. The young bodies must be toned up, and elimination through the skin must be stimulated by air and sun baths and cold water treatment. Massage and neurotherapy must correct the spinal lesions, remove the pressure from nerves and blood vessels and increase the activity of the internal organs of elimination and assimilation. Under such general constitutional treatment, elimination will be distributed evenly, the membranes and the glandular structures of nose and mouth will be relieved and will resume their normal structure and function. Herein lies the natural, rational cure for tonsilitis, adenoid vegetations, mouth breathing and kindred diseases. That this is not mere vagary is proved by the fact that in hundreds of cases of tonsilitis and kindred ailments treated during the last seventeen years, we have not in a single instance resorted to surgical treatment. As the regeneration of the system through natural living and treatment proceeded, the affected organs became normal.

CHAPTER XVII

PART I. WOMAN'S SUFFERING

"Woman's physical suffering" is so universal among civilized races that the very phrase has become proverbial. That woman should suffer severe pain, especially during the menstrual period, at the climacteric and in childbirth, is looked upon as unavoidable and as a matter of course. The fact that the women of primitive races in Africa, in South America, and in the Arctic circle and on our western plains are practically exempt from these chronic ailments indicates that the cause must lie in artificial habits of living and in the unnatural treatment of disease common among civilized races. Many are beginning to recognize these truths.

The various forms of female troubles usually begin to manifest at the age of puberty when normal menstruation should commence. In many instances this flowering of the sex life is abnormal from the beginning. Frequently it is irregular, very painful, too profuse, too scanty or entirely absent. These conditions in themselves do not constitute disease but are the effects of abnormal conditions in the system, caused by abnormal prenatal influences, by wrong management of the infant, unnatural habits of living later in life, and by the suppressive treatment of acute and subacute diseases. Violations of nature's laws, which constitute the primary cause of disease, have been described in other parts of this volume. Prominent among them are wrong food combinations over rich in negative disease producing substances which clog the system with pathogenic materials. This leads to defective elimination through skin, intestines and kidneys. The impurities then seek an outlet through catarrhal conditions of the tonsils, adenoids and nasal passages. These eliminative efforts of nature are promptly suppressed by the extirpation of tonsils and adenoids and by the destruction of the nasal membranes by means of poisonous antiseptic sprays and cauterizers. When the impurities congest the lymphatic glands in the neck these are frequently extirpated by the surgeon's knife; when, as described in Chapter XI, elimination is attempted through the membranous linings of the bronchi and digestive tract in the form of colds, catarrhs, purgings, etc., the work of suppression is persistently continued until the organism in self-defence starts trying to eliminate these systemic poisons through the membranous linings of the genital organs by means of the menstrual discharge and through leucorrhea.

The menstrual function has been established by nature to bring about conditions suitable for the fructifying and implantation of the ovum, but she uses it also for the purification of the organism from pathogenic matter. If these impurities happen to be of an irritating, poisonous nature they may cause inflammatory and painful conditions of the genital organs. Leucorrhea, like all other catarrhal conditions, is a form of elimination and at the back of it is systemic poisoning. The system is overloaded with pathogenic matter and the organs of elimination through overwork and continued irritation have become so clogged and inactive that they cannot keep a clean house. Then one of two things will happen. Either nature must find an outlet for the morbid encumbrances through the membranous linings of the internal tracts, or life will become impaired or extinct through the accumulations of impurities in the body.

What is the orthodox treatment of leucorrhea? It is generally antiseptic and astringent douches and curetment. These methods not only suppress nature's purifying efforts, but are in themselves positively destructive. The poisonous antiseptics and astringents saturate not only the tissues of the womb but also of the neighbouring organs, benumb and paralyze natural function and disorganize normal structure. In other words they embalm the tissues and in time destroy the sex function.

This is a matter to be considered in connection with the growing practice of birth control which often consists in douching with poisonous germ killers and astringents. Such unnatural practices will result in time in permanent sterility, degeneration of tissues and tumour formation. The retention of the impurities which nature is trying to get rid of through menstrual and leucorrheal discharges results in acute and chronic inflammation of the uterus, Fallopian tubes and ovaries. These symptoms are in turn suppressed, if possible, by the same form of local treatment.

Curetment in itself is a barbarous mutilation of the cradle of life. The surgeon dilates the neck of the womb, inserts sharp hooks in its interior and drags the womb to the mouth of the vagina. He then scrapes the internal walls of the organ with a spoonlike instrument, tearing off the tender membranes in order to force nature to build new ones. He does not stop to consider whether, under the diseased condition of the system, they will be any better than the old ones. The entire procedure is unnatural and barbarous. The pulling of the womb to the entrance of the vagina may result in permanent weakening and stretching of the ligaments and muscles supporting it. Frequently it causes the rupturing of adherent tissues and internal haemorrhages. The cureting itself often results in serious injury to the membranes of the uterus. It happens not infrequently that the spoon of the curet penetrates the walls of the uterus or badly lacerates the openings of the Fallopian tubes. The retention of the impurities caused by cureting may set up serious subacute or chronic inflammation, ulceration and hardening of the internal tissues of the womb, and chronic metritis, only too often resulting in the formation of polypi, benign or malignant tumours. Obstruction of the Fallopian tubes frequently follows, and this interferes with the discharge of the ova from the ovaries into the uterus. Many women tell me that they were curetted in order to facilitate conception. What an absurdity! In menstruation and in childbirth nature opens the blood vessels of the womb from within out, through a natural process. The dilatation of the neck of the womb and the scraping away of internal membranes is done forcibly in violation of nature's ways. Women have come to us in the most wretched condition of health, ruined physically, mentally and spiritually through a dozen or more curetments. One sufferer had been curetted twenty-one times, hoping every time that "this would be the last one" and "bring about good health". How would this be possible, considering the normal structure and natural functions of the generative organs?

When acute and chronic inflammation, ulcers, abscesses, endurations, adhesions and tumours develop as the result of long continued suppressive treatment, what then? Surgical extirpation of the affected parts and organs is held to be the only remedy. Far from being a cure this makes a cure forever impossible and can only be justified on the ground that organs have become useless and might just as well be removed. However, Nature Cure physicians are proving in everyday practice that acute and chronic inflammation can be cured, that adhesions can be dissolved and tumours absorbed, providing they be not too large, by natural methods of living and treatment.

Shortly after I began to practice, there was brought to me for examination a woman whose ovaries were in a condition of acute inflammation owing to gonorrheal infection from her husband. He believed that he had been cured of the infectious disease by allopathic suppression. In fact, he had been assured by the physician who treated him that it was perfectly safe for him to marry. Soon after marriage, however, his wife developed acute inflammation of the vagina and this extended to the ovaries. Before she came to me, arrangements had been perfected for the surgical removal of the ovaries. The operation was to take place on the following day. They had been assured that this was absolutely necessary in order to save the woman's life. After consultation with me she was placed under our care and treatment. At the end of the fifth month the woman was discharged as cured. Since that time she has had three children. They were brought up in harmony with the teachings of Nature Cure and are in perfect health and splendidly developed physically and mentally. The mother wrote to me a few years ago, "I am the happiest woman in the world. I cannot express to you sufficiently my gratitude for saving me from the dreadful fate of an unsexed woman." This is only one case of hundreds which we have treated and cured during the last eighteen years and in no single case were the affected organs extirpated. Extirpation cuts at the very foundation of life; not only does it deprive a woman of the joys of motherhood, but it leads to physical, mental, and emotional defectiveness and abnormality and often to life-long suffering and doctoring, to premature death or, possibly, insanity.

The orthodox treatment for these abnormal conditions also consists of surgical operations, shortening of the round ligaments of the womb, cutting adhesions which hold the womb in an abnormal position, stitching of the womb to the frontal walls of the abdomen, etc. This sort of treatment is purely local, symptomatic and suppressive — not in any way curative. The sagging of the womb and other genital organs, sometimes resulting in protusion of the neck of the womb from the mouth of the vagina, is caused by general weakness of the system, particularly by a weakened, relaxed and prolapsed condition of the stomach and intestines. It is the sagging down of the stomach and intestines, usually loaded with old accumulations of fæcal matter, which pushes down the genital organs into the bottom of the pelvis. This interferes with the free movement of the womb and crowds it into abnormal position resulting in the bending or kinking of the organ upon itself forward or backward and in abnormal pressure upon the bladder or the rectum. These adhesions and flexions of the womb may interfere with menstrual or leucorrheal discharges or with the entrance of the procreative germ. Such abnormal pressure on the genital organs may also result in irritation, inflammation and the formation of adhesions and tumours. These conditions may be aggravated by subluxations, curvatures or ankyloses of the spinal vertebrae which produce pressure or irritation of nerves passing out between the vertebræ, irritation and inflammation of the digestive and pelvic organs, resulting in weakness and atrophy and in a flabby relaxed condition of the digestive and genital organs. It is a fact known to every observing physician that over fifty per cent of all civilized women have some kind of misplacement of the genital organs and that only a comparatively small number of these cases result in local disturbances, indicating that misplacement alone does not always create serious trouble. It is ridiculous to assume that the small, flabby uterus of an anaemic woman can obstruct the rectum and cause serious disease; but the idea that it can has been used as a talking point to bring people to the operating table.

Another cause contributing to woman's suffering is unsuitable clothing, though this is less so than it once was. The main evil effects are the result of tight clothing and high heeled shoes. The old fashioned very tight corset has been abandoned but the use of constricting bands and belts is often sufficient to cause unnatural compression of and pressure on the many organs lying within the circumference of the waist line. Such constriction always interferes more or less with the circulation of the blood, lymph and nerve currents between the upper and the lower parts of the body, thereby causing congestion in the organs of the abdominal and pelvic cavities; and congestion when not properly treated is, as we have learned, the first step toward inflammation and its manifold destructive consequences. As far as possible clothing should be suspended from the shoulders. A normally developed body, not weakened by the corset or waist band habit, does not require support. All artificial bracing and supporting of the body is weakening rather than strengthening.

Cuplike or ring shaped pessaries have been designed to support and to press upwards the prolapsed womb, but these contrivances eventually serve to aggravate and to increase the weakness of the organs. Through abnormal pressure and irritation they can cause acute and chronic inflammations, lasting malformations, or benign and malignant tumours. This is so obvious that it seems incredible that men who pride themselves on their scientific knowledge should advocate their use. Likewise, it stands to reason that shortening of the ligaments and fastening of the womb to the abdominal wall will not overcome the causes of these abnormal conditions. They will not invigorate and strengthen the weakened abdominal organs and raise them to their normal positions, removing the abdominal pressure on the genital organs. The only way this can be done is by building up the system generally by removing the three primary manifestations of disease, and especially by invigorating the abdominal organs through curative exercises and manipulative treatment.

While studying Nature Cure in Europe I took special courses in Thure-Brandt massage. By means of this internal manipulative treatment, adhesions, displacements, weakness of ligaments and muscles can be corrected without knife or drugs. During my first years in practice I frequently resorted to internal manipulative treatment with good results, but I found that this was not always necessary. I learned that correction of spinal and pelvic lesions and consequent removal of pressure and irritation on the nerves, the cure of chronic constipation and malnutrition by pure food diet and hydrotherapy, the strengthening of the pelvic nerves and muscles by active and passive movements and exercises were fully sufficient to correct the local symptoms in a natural manner.[1]

When surgical procedures are used rather than natural treatments the end results for the patient are apt to be very unhappy. When the misplaced womb is torn loose by the knife, in order to be kept in the new position it must be stitched to the frontal abdominal wall. This stretches the organ and prevents its natural movements, resulting frequently in serious nerve strain and irritation. Often the womb will not stay fixed; it breaks loose and relapses into the same abnormal position. Granted that it remains fixed, woe to the woman if she becomes pregnant. The womb cannot assume the constantly changing positions of pregnancy, and either abortion or malformation of the foetus, together with great suffering, can be the result. The operation has done nothing to correct unnatural habits of living or to purify the system of its scrofulous, venereal and psoric taints, or of drug and food poisons. These gather in the parts weakened and irritated by the surgeon's knife, where they set up new inflammations, ulcerations and, only too often, malignant tumours. As a result one operation follows another. We cannot cut in the genital organs without "cutting in the brain". The nervous system is a unit and, next to the brain, the genital organs represent the most complex and sensitive nerve centres. The two are intimately connected. Mutilations in the genital nerve centres almost invariably mean affections of the brain and of the nervous system in general. It is almost axiomatic that a woman whose uterus or ovaries have been operated on is afterwards mentally abnormal. Nervousness, irritability, and only too often nervous prostration and insanity are the sequelae of operative treatment. There are some signs that this is now beginning to be realized in medical circles which is leading to somewhat less surgery and to a more conservative type of it.

The Climacteric or Change of Life

Under our artificial methods of living, the climacteric, or change of life, has become the bugbear of womanhood. It seems to be universally assumed that this period in a woman's life must be fraught with manifold sufferings and dangers. It is taken as a matter of course that during these changes in her organism a woman is assailed by serious physical, mental and psychic ailments which may endanger her sanity and often her life. Like rheumatism, neurasthenia, neuralgia, and hundreds of other medical terms, "change of life" is a convenient phrase to cover the doctor's ignorance. No matter what ailments befall a woman during the years from forty to fifty, be the causes ever so obscure, the diagnosis is easy. "You

[1]
There is undoubtedly a place in natural therapeutics for the use of internal as well as external manual procedures. There have been and still may be some osteopaths and others who have specialized in this kind of work, but there may well be a danger of the expertise being forgotten.

are in the climacteric, you are suffering from the change of life", says the doctor, and the patient, satisfied, resigns herself to the inevitable.

Frequently, women come to us for consultation, and after reciting a long series of troubles conclude with the remark: "Of course, doctor, I'm in the change, and I know that lots of these things are natural at my time of life." However, among primitive races suffering incident to the change of life is practically unknown. The same is true in a lesser degree of the peasant population of Europe. The causes of it must, therefore, be sought in the artificial modes of living peculiar to our hyper-civilization and in the unnatural suppressive methods of treating disease. Let us examine the specific causes of the climacteric. Aside from their other physiological functions, the menses are for women a monthly cleansing crisis through which nature eliminates from the system considerable amounts of waste and morbid matter which under a natural regimen of life would be discharged by means of the organs of depuration, viz., the lungs, skin, kidneys and bowels. The more natural the life, and the more normal the woman's physical condition, the shorter and less annoying and painful will be the menstrual periods. Through unnatural habits of eating, drinking dressing, breathing, and through equally unnatural methods of medical treatment, the kidneys, skin and bowels have become inactive and be-numbed. As long as vicarious monthly purification by means of the menses continues, the evil results of the torpid condition of the regular organs of depuration do not become so apparent. The organism has learned to adapt itself to this mode of elimination. But when, on account of the organic changes of the climacteric, menstruation ceases, then the systemic poisons (pathogen) which formerly were eliminated by this monthly purification, accumulate in the system and become the source of all manner of trouble. All tendencies to physical, mental or psychic disease are greatly intensified. The poisonous taints circulating in the blood over-stimulate or else depress the brain and the nervous system. As a conse-quence, mental and psychic disorders are of common occurrence; the more so because the waning of the sex functions is accompanied by a tendency to negativity and hypersensitiveness.

The obvious way to avoid or cure the ailments of the climacteric and to re-establish the equilibrium of the organism, lies in restoring the natural activity of the organs of elimination. This is what Nature Cure accompli-shes easily and successfully with its natural methods of treatment. Air and sun baths, water treatments and massage bring new life and activity to the enervated skin. Pure food diet, neurotherapy, curative gymnastics, homoeopathic or herb remedies restore the natural tonicity and functioning of the stomach, liver, kidneys, and intestines. Psycho-therapy systematic-ally practised may also have a part to play. When the natural equilibrium of the organism is thus restored there is absolutely no occasion for the troubles of the climacteric. We have proved this in hundreds of cases. As kidneys, skin, and bowels begin to function normally and freely, physical and mental conditions commence to improve until, one after another, the symptoms disappear.

In contrast to this common-sense kind of treatment, the orthodox medical treatment is almost entirely symptomatic. The sluggish organs of elimination are prodded by poisonous cathartics, laxatives, diaphoretics, cholagogues and tonics, all of which, after temporary stimulation, leave the organs in a more weakened, and the system in a more poisoned, condition. If brain and nerves are irritated and aching, sedatives and hypnotics are given to stupefy them into insensibility. If the heart action is weak and irregular, it is whipped up by poisonous stimulants; if too fast it is benumbed by sedatives and depressants. Thus, instead of removing the underlying causes, every symptom is promptly suppressed. Drug poisons are added to the waste and morbid matter which are already clogging the channels of life. Under such unnatural treatment, in many instances the victims go from bad to worse. Flushes, headaches, rheumatic and neuralgic pains, melancholia, irritability, mental aberration, partial paralysis and a multitude of other symptoms appear and gradually increase in severity. When the family physician has arrived at the end of his wits, the surgeon has his innings. He, in turn, leaves the patient in a still worse condition of chronic suffering. These experiences are so common that the manifold troubles of the climacteric are regarded as unavoidable and as a matter of course. Here, as in countless other instances, it is the treatment which prevents the cure. If the efficiency of common-sense natural treatment were more widely known, how much unnecessary suffering could be avoided. The rational treatment of the various ailments of the female organs will be described.

PART II. THE EFFECTS OF SUPPRESSION OF VENEREAL DISEASES

Another good illustration of suppression may be found in the allopathic treatment of venereal diseases. Almost invariably the drug treatment suppresses these diseases in the stages of incubation and aggravation, thus locking them up in the system. The venereal taints and germs, however, are living things which grow and multiply until the body has been completely permeated by them. Then they must find an outlet somehow and somewhere, and consequently they break out in the manifold so-called "secondary" and "tertiary" symptoms. The drug poisons which are used to "cure" (suppress) these symptoms, greatly aggravate the disease. They create conditions in the system infinitely worse than the venereal diseases themselves. Thus the acute, easily curable stages of these ailments are changed into the dreadful and obstinate chronic conditions. It is in this way that venereal diseases are made hereditary and transmitted to future generations.

In the light of my own experience in the treatment of these conditions, I make the following claims:-

(1) Venereal diseases are not necessarily chronic in their progressive development.

(2) They are essentially acute and self-limited, but may become chronic through neglect or through suppressive drug treatment.

(3) The chronic, so-called secondary and tertiary manifestations of venereal diseases, such as ulceration of bones and fleshy tissues, gummata of the brain, sclerosis of the spinal cord, arthritic rheumatism, degeneration and destruction of other parts and organs of the body, are not so much the result of the original gonorrheal or syphilitic infection, as of the destructive drug poisons which have been taken to cure or rather to suppress the primary lesions and acute inflammatory symptoms.

(4) Venereal diseases in the acute inflammatory stages are easily and completely curable by natural methods of living and treatment.

(5) Venereal diseases treated and cured by natural methods during the acute inflammatory stages are never followed by any chronic after-effects or secondary or tertiary manifestations whatsoever.

(6) When venereal diseases have reached the secondary and tertiary stages, they are still curable by natural methods of living and of treatment, providing there is left sufficient vitality to respond to treatment and providing the destruction of vital parts and organs has not advanced too far. Hundreds of cases of well-developed locomotor ataxy, paresis, and other so-called secondary and tertiary diseases of the brain and nervous system, of bony and fleshy tissues, and of vital organs have been cured by our natural methods of treatment. It is self-evident, however, that the treatment and cure of the chronic conditions require more patience and perseverence than the cure of acute conditions not tampered with and suppressed by drugs.

(7) Venereal diseases treated and cured by natural methods are never followed by chronic after-effects. On the other hand, mercury, iodine, quinine, and coal-tar poisons produce all the so-called secondary and tertiary symptoms of syphilis in people who never in their lives were afflicted with venereal disease, but who have taken or absorbed these drug poisons in other ways . . . These facts are proven beyond doubt by diagnosis from the eye. All destructive poisons taken in sufficient quan-

tities will in time reveal their presence and exact location in the body through certain well-defined signs or discolourations in the iris. These poisons undermine the structures of the body and deteriorate vital parts and organs so slowly and insidiously that the superficial observer does not trace and connect cause and effect.

Medical men may say to all this that the Wasserman and Noguchi tests furnish positive proofs of syphilis in the system. These chemical tests are supposed to reveal with certainty the presence of venereal taints in the body, — at least the public is left under this impression. I am convinced, however, that in many instances the "positive" Wasserman or Noguchi tests are the result of mercurial poison instead of syphilitic infection. In a number of cases where these tests proved "positive", that is, where, according to the theory of allopathic medical science, they indicated a luetic condition of the system, the subjects had never in their lives shown any symptoms of syphilis, nor, as far as they knew, had they ever been exposed to infection, but every one of them showed plainly the sign of mercurial poisoning in the iris of the eye. The history in these cases indicated that the subjects had taken a considerable amount of mercury in the form of calomel or of other medicinal preparations for diseases not of a leutic nature, or had been "salivated" by coming in contact with the mercurial poison in mines, smelters, mirror factories or workshops of other kinds. This leads me to believe that, sooner or later, medical science will have to admit that the Wasserman and Noguchi tests reveal, in many instances at least, the effects of mercurial poisoning instead of that of syphilis. And this would not be surprising since it is well known that mercury has very similar effects upon the system as does syphilis.

It takes the mercurial poison from five to ten and even fifteen years before it works itself into the brain and spinal cord, and there causes its characteristic destruction of brain and nerve tissues which manifest outwardly as locomotor ataxy, paralysis agitans, paresis, apoplexy, hemiplegia, epilepsy, St. Vitus dance, and different forms of idiocy and insanity. Mercurial poisoning is also in many instances the cause of deafness and blindness. When the symptoms of mercurial destruction begin to show, then they, in turn are suppressed by preparations of iodine, the "606", or other "alteratives", and so the merry war goes on: poison against poison, Beelzebub against the Devil, and the poor suffering body has to stand it all. In this way the system is periodocally saturated with the most virulent poisons on earth, until the undertaker finishes the job. And this is miscalled "scientific treatment". There never was invented by cruel Indian or fanatical inquisitor worse torture than this. They mercifully finished the sufferings of their victims within a few hours or, at worst, days; but this torture inflicted on human beings in the name of medical science continues for a lifetime. It means dying by inches under the most horrible conditions for ten, twenty, thirty years or longer.

In this connection it may be well to quote the testimony of Professor Farrington, one of the most celebrated homoeopathic physicians of the nineteenth century. He says, in his "Clinical Materia Medica":- "The various constitutions of dyscrasia underlying chronic and acute infections are, indeed, very numerous. As yet, we do not know them all. We do know that one of them comes in gonorrhea, a disease which is frightfully common, so that the constitution arising from this disease is now rapidly on the increase ... This is because allopathic physicians, and many homoeopaths as well, do not properly cure it. I do not believe gonorrhea to be a local disease. If it is not properly cured, a constitutional poison which may be transmitted to the children is developed. I know, from years of experience and observation, that gonorrhea is a serious difficulty, and one, too, that complicates many cases that we have to treat. The same is true of syphilis in a modified degree. Gonorrhea seems to attack the nobler tissues, the lungs, the heart, and the nervous system, all of which are reached by syphilis only after a lapse of years."

Concerning the destructive after-effects of mercury, Professor Farrington has this to say:- "The more remote symptoms of mercurial poisoning are these. You will find that the blood becomes impoverished. The albumin and fibrin of that fluid are affected. They are diminished, and you find in their place a certain fatty substance, the composition of which I do not exactly know. Consequently, as a prominent symptom, the body wastes and emaciates. The patient suffers from fever which is rather hectic in its character. The periosteum becomes affected, and you then have a characteristic group of mercurial pains, bone pains worse in changes of the weather, worse in the warmth of the bed, and chilliness with or after stool. The skin becomes of a rather brownish hue; ulcers form, particularly on the legs; they are stubborn and will not heal. The patient is troubled with sleeplessness and ebullitions of blood at night; he is hot and cannot sleep; he is thrown quickly into a perspiration, which perspiration gives him no relief. The entire system suffers also, and you have here two series of symptoms. At first the patient becomes anxious and restless and cannot remain quiet; he changes his position; he moves about from place to place; he seems to have a great deal of anxiety about the heart, praecordial anguish, as it is termed, particularly at night. Then, in another series of symptoms, there are jerkings of the limbs, making the patient appear as though he were attacked by St. Vitus' dance. Or, you may notice what is more common yet, trembling of the hands, this tremor being altogether beyond the control of the patient and gradually spreading over the entire body, giving you a resemblance to paralysis agitans or shaking palsy. Finally, the patient becomes paralyzed, cannot move his limbs, and he presents a perfect picture of imbecility. He does all sorts of queer things. He sits in the corner with an idiotic smile on his face, playing with straws; he is forgetful, he cannot remember even the most ordinary events. He becomes disgustingly filthy and eats his own excrement. In fact, he is a perfect idiot.

"Be careful how you give mercury; it is a treacherous medicine. It seems often indicated. You give it and relieve; but your patient is worse again in a few weeks and then you give it again with relief. By and by, it fails you. Now, if I want to make a permanent cure, for instance, in a scrofulous child, I will very seldom give him mercury; should I do so, it will at least only be as an intercurrent remedy".([1])

[1]
The second part of this chapter is to some extent out of date in that the use of mercury in medication has now practically ceased. It would appear that there is now a general realization of its harmfulness. Poisonings from heavy metals such as mercury and lead do occur but they are generally due to industrial processes or to accidents or pollutions of one kind or another. However, Lindlahr is undoubtedly right in laying emphasis on the particular dangers of metals when taken into the body and retained there. Some metals such as zinc, silver and gold are still extensively used in medicaments and trouble can be produced by such things as aluminium cooking vessels and amalgam in dentistry. The study of provings in a good homoeopathic materia medica would appear to indicate that many substances are capable of producing long term effects on the body very similar to those of mercury. On the other hand it may well be that the substitution of antibiotics for mercurial and other powerful drugs in the treatment of venereal and other diseases may be leading to a decline in some of the worst chronic diseases particularly of the central nervous system (e.g. Locomotor ataxia).

CHAPTER XVIII

CANCER

For many years it has been admitted that the regular orthodox treatment of cancer by means of drugs, surgical operations, X-Rays, radium, etc., is, to say the least, highly unsatisfactory. Indeed it has been established that, in many cases, if not in all, such treatments and extirpations increase the malignancy and size of recurrent or secondary growths. The truth of the matter is that cancer is not a local ailment but a manifestation of constitutional disease. It must also be realized that the more skilled the allopathic school becomes in the suppression and in the prevention of acute diseases by drugs, knife, X-Rays, serums and vaccination virus, the greater will be the increase in dyspepsia, nervous prostration, insanity, locomotor ataxia, paresis, cancer, secondary and tertiary syphilis, tuberculosis and many other so-called incurable diseases. These scourges are most prevalent in countries which are looked upon as advanced, prosperous and enlightened and in which there are plenty of drug stores. In such countries the doctor is called for every passing ailment. Colds, catarrhs, diarrhoeas, skin eruptions and every other form of acute elimination must be treated promptly and thoroughly with antiseptics, antipyretics, antitoxins, and all sorts of other "antis". Antiseptic lotions, soaps, tooth-powders, etc. are constantly applied to kill germs and to prevent infection. On the other hand, wrong living habits, food poisoning, alcohol, nicotine, vaccine and antitoxins systematically poison the human organism, and when nature endeavours, by means of acute reactions, to free the system of morbid accumulations, she is thwarted by suppressive treatment. These practices repeated from generation to generation must lead finally to deterioraton of blood and tissues and to the development of hereditary taints. That is why "cancer loves a shining mark".

It is generally acknowledged that cancer is not contagious; that it can be transmitted only by means of transplantation of the cancer cells themselves into the flesh of healthy individuals and that even then it "takes" only in a small percentage of cases. These observations, based on experiments carried out mainly on rats and mice, confirm my claim that in order to develop cancer or any other chronic destructive disease a certain diathesis or diseased condition of the body is needed. In order to develop tuberculosis or cancer something more is necessary than the tubercle bacillus or the cancer cell; there must be that in the system on which these "parasites" (or rather their microzymes) live and thrive. If the cancer cell of its own accord could create cancer every animal inoculated with it would develop the fatal disease. The cancerous growth in itself is only a symptom of the disease; the real disease is the constitutional taint (the morbid matter which develops normal microzymes into cancer cells) which stimulates and feeds the malignant growth; therefore a real cure can consist only in eliminating from the system the poisons which irritate the cells and stimulate them into unlimited multiplication.

Extirpation by drugs, knife or freezing only removes the local manifestations of a constitutional taint or miasm. Malignant tumours grow only in "bad blood"; their favourite breeding places are to be found in scrofulous and psoric constitutions, especially where hereditary conditions are aggravated by food and drug poisoning or where spinal lesions irritate the nerves and the tissues which these nerves supply. What, then, can be gained permanently by destroying the local growth, when the disease soil from which it springs, or the spinal irritation, still remains? Our claim that cancer is a constitutional disease is further confirmed by the admission that cancer, or the tendency to it, is hereditary, as has been shown by experiments on mice.

In this last connection it is interesting to note that Hahnemann, the father of homoeopathy, recognized the hereditary transmission of disease taints and proclaimed it in his theory of psora. He taught that the ordinary itch eruptions (scabies) are accompanied by the elimination of internal scrofulous taints, which, in turn, are a survival of the ancient leprosy. He asserted that systematic suppression of the external lepra continued throughout the ages, gradually transformed this external skin disease into the internal psora, which manifests occasionally on the surface in the acute forms of itch, lice, crab-lice, hives, itchy eczemata, etc., and internally as tuberculosis, cancer, sarcoma, asthma and other chronic destructive diseases. For a hundred years, Hahnemann's theory of psora has been scouted and ridiculed by the allopathic schools, and even among homoeopaths but few have accepted his theory. Now we are confronted by the remarkable fact that, at this late date, the diagnosis from the eye confirms the observations and speculations of the great genius of homoeopathy. After the suppression of itch eruptions, lice, or crab-lice, there appear, in certain parts of the iris, spots ranging in colour from light browns to dark red. These "itch spots" indicate the localities in the body in which the suppressed disease taints have concentrated. These suppressions represent not only the psoric taints which nature was trying to eliminate through the eruptions and parasites, but also the poisons contained in the bodies of the parasites and the drug poisons which were used to kill them. It has been proved that the bodies of the parasites contain a poisonous taint called by homoeopaths, psorinum. When the minute animals burrowing in and under the skin are killed by drug treatment, the morbid taints in their bodies are absorbed by the human organism and added to the psoric taints which nature was trying to eliminate. Thus, after suppression, the organism is cumbered with three poisons instead of one; first the hereditary and acquired scrofulous and psoric taints which the tissues were throwing off into the blood stream and which the blood stream was feeding to the parasites on the surface; second, the morbid taints contained in the bodies of the parasites and, third, the drug poisons used as suppressants.

These facts explain why the itch spots in the eye frequently indicate serious chronic, destructive diseases in the corresponding parts of the body; why in asthma and tuberculosis we often find itch spots in the lungs; why cancer of the liver is indicated by itch spots in the liver area, etc. That itch or psora is actually at the bottom of the cancerous diathesis is attested by the fact that all cancer patients whom we have treated and cured have, with two exceptions, broken out with itchy, burning eruptions at one time or another during the natural treatment. The bodies of most of these patients were inflamed with fiery eruptions from head to foot for days and often weeks. We allow these healing crises to run their course unhindered and unchecked; we rather encourage them by air and sun baths, cold water treatment and homoeopathic remedies. When the parasites have consumed the poisonous taints on which they feed, they depart as they came, no one knows whence or whither. For the removal of lice we prescribe only water and comb; even antiseptic soaps must be avoided lest they kill the parasites burrowing in the skin and flesh.

When during the last few years, I asserted that we could cure cancer by natural methods of treatment, my claims were scouted and ridiculed. Many a poor sufferer has missed his chance of recovery because he believed that his only possible chance lay in a surgical operation. Now comes considerable evidence from orthodox medical sources and laboratories that cancer is curable in principle, that it sometimes cures itself spontaneously and that in certain animals it can be cured with reasonable certainty. A number of dogs who had contracted cancer or who had been rendered cancerous by inoculation were cured by having most of the blood in their bodies drained off and having transfused in its place blood from animals which had proved resistant to inoculation. This confirms our assertion that cancer is not a local ailment but a constitutional disease. However, we of the Nature Cure school say that it is not necessary to pump the diseased blood out of the organism. In natural methods of living and treatment we possess the means of purifying and regenerating the blood while it is in the body, and we have proved this in a number of cases. It is obvious, however, that the earlier the disease is treated by natural methods, that is, before the breaking down process is far advanced, the easier and quicker will be the cure. I maintain that external cancers in the first stages of development, that is, before they have grown to large proportions, belong to the easily curable forms of disease. Cures become more difficult when the tumours affect internal vital parts and organs, but even then we have been successful in many cases.

I cannot refrain from illustrating my deductions by telling of one typical case taken from our clinical records. About six years ago there came to us a Polish woman whose head, on the right side, was covered by an enormous cancerous growth. She gave us the following history of her case: At first she had a large wen on the right side of her head. This was removed by a beauty doctor. The wound healed, but soon after opened and formed an ugly sore. This was treated surgically in hospital. After a while the wound opened again and became more virulent than before. Skin grafting was now resorted to in order to cover the large exposure of raw flesh, yet the wound refused to stay cured, and two more operations were performed in the same hospital. Powerful antiseptics were used to cauterize the sores and they were burned with hot irons. This was done so thoroughly that a piece of bone became charred and worked out during our course of treatment; it resembled a piece of charcoal. After the fourth operation, when the entire side of the head was covered by a cancerous mass, she was dismissed as incurable. She then came under our treatment and after five months the sores had entirely disappeared and the wounds, including the hole in the skull, were covered with new sound skin. During the treatment, the patient passed through the usual crises in the forms of catarrhs, coughs, diarrhoeas, itchy skin eruptions, etc. After the wounds on the head had healed perfectly, she began to use meat and coffee. Within a few weeks the scars reopened and began to bleed. She then confessed that she transgressed our rules. After returning to the natural regimen and treatment, the wounds closed again. Later on she repeated the same experiment with the same results. Since then there has never been a recurrence of her trouble and today she is in perfect health. She has never had occasion to employ doctors since she was with us. In the meantime she has married, and now has three healthy children.

More recently certain discoveries by Dr. H. C. Ross of London England, have confirmed again my claims that cancer is not at all of local and accidental origin, but that it is constitutional, and that it may be caused by the gradual accumulation in the system of certain toxins which develop in decaying animal matter. One day, while experimenting in his laboratory, Dr. Ross brought living cells into contact with a certain aniline dye on the slide of a microscope, and noticed that they began at once to multiply by cell division (proliferation). He realized that he had made an important discovery and continued his experiments under the microscope in order to find out what other substances would cause cell proliferation. He found that certain xanthines and albuminoids derived from decaying animal matter were the most effective for this purpose and induced more rapid cell proliferation than any other substances he was able to procure. He obtained these "alkaloids of putrefaction" as he called them, from blood which had been allowed to putrefy in a warm place. He found that albuminoids derived from decaying vegetable substances did not have the same effect. His discoveries led him to believe that the "alkaloids of putrefaction" produced in a cut or wound by the decay of dead blood and tissue cells are the cause of the rapid multiplication of the neighbouring live cells, which gradually fills the wound with new tissues. If this is so it would seem to provide a rational explanation of the method by which the natural repair of injured tissues takes place. However, Dr. Ross applied his theory further to the causation of benign and malignant growths, reasoning that the "alkaloids of putrefaction" produced in or attracted to a certain part of the body by some local irritation are the cause of the rapid, abnormal multiplication of cells in tumour formations. In benign tumours the abnormal proliferation takes place slowly, and they do not tend to immediate or rapid decay and deterioration. In malignant tumours the "wild" cells, created in immense numbers (from microzymes feeding on psoric taints and systemic poisons), decay almost as rapidly as they are produced because the abnormal growths are devoid of normal organization. They have no established, regular blood and nerve supply, nor are they provided with adequate venous and lymphatic drainage. They are, therefore, cut off from the orderly life of the organism and doomed to rapid deterioration. The processes of decay of these tumour materials liberate large quantities of "alkaloids of putrefaction", and these in turn stimulate the normal healthy cells with which they come in contact to rapid, abnormal multiplication. The malignant growth, therefore, feeds on its own products of decay, in addition to the systemic poisons and morbid materials already contained in the blood and tissues of the body. These morbid products permeate the entire system. They are carried by the circulation of the blood into all parts of the body. This explains why cancer is a constitutional disease, why it is, as I stated it, "rooted in every drop of blood". It also explains why cancer, or rather the disposition to its development (diathesis), is hereditary.

If the original cancerous growth is removed by surgical intervention, X-rays, the electric needle, cauterization, or any other form of local treatment, the poisonous materials (alkaloids of putrefaction) in the blood will set up other foci of abnormal, "wild" proliferation. Medical science has applied the term "metastasis" to such spreading and reappearing of malignant tumours after extirpation.

The findings of Dr. Ross also throw an interesting light on the relationship between cancer and meat eating. Is it not understandable that in a digestive tract filled most of the time with large masses of partially digested and decaying animal food enormous quantities of "alkaloids of putrefaction" are created? These are absorbed into the circulation, attracted to every point where exists some form of local irritation, and then stimulate the cells in that locality to abnormal proliferation. It is true that vegetarians are to a small extent afflcted with cancer; but it must be remembered that vegetarians may be affected hereditarily with psoric and scrofulous taints, that a high protein vegetarian diet may be disease producing as well as a meat diet, and that a natural diet without treatment may not be sufficient to eliminate the cancer soil. Alkaloids of putrefaction are constantly produced in every animal and human body. They form in the excretions of living cells and in the decaying protoplasm of dead cells, and if the organs of elimination do not function properly, these morbid materials will accumulate in the system and produce morbid microzymes.(1)

[1]
The contention in this chapter that cancer should be regarded as a constitutional and not a local disease and that it should be treated by general measures involving a vigorous application of all natural methods of treatment in combination, is undoubtedly sound. Most of modern cancer research because it does not recognize that cancer is a manifestation of biochemical and cytological breakdown in the system as a whole would appear to be condemned to futility. However it does seem that there are certain special methods and lines of approach which are of value in the study and treatment of cancer. It appears that malignancy is linked to a disturbance in the functioning and balance of the endocrine system and that the system of endocrinotherapy based on the ideas of Dr. Jules Samuels has been successfully used in cancer treatment. Another method which appears to have been used with great success is the Grape Cure as set forth by Johanna Brandt and Basil Shackleton. Little is now heard of the work of the American William Koch but he does appear, by a profound study of biochemistry, to have elaborated a preparation by which cancer could be successfully treated. The basis of this treatment, as I understand it, is that in malignancy there is a breakdown of the oxidation processes in the body and that a very subtle and attenuated preparation can be injected into the bloodstream which acts as a catalyst and which activates and restores the oxidation mechanism. It also seems to be established that malignancy is associated with too much sodium and too little potassium in the body and that when this balance is upset it should be corrected by a drastic reduction of the salt intake and the use of foods rich in potassium.

CHAPTER XIX

THE TREATMENT OF THE "CHRONIC"

Nature Cure is constantly criticized and avoided because it is believed to take so long. It is, in fact, the swiftest cure in existence. One reason why this false idea has grown up is that it is usual that we are asked to deal with advanced cases of so-called incurable diseases. As long as there remains a particle of faith in the medicine bottle, the knife or the metaphysical formula of the mind-healer, people prefer these "easy" methods which require no effort on their part, rather than the Nature Cure treatment which necessitates personal exertion, self-control, the changing or giving up of cherished habits. This is what most of us evade as long as we can.

The fear of cold water seems to be particularly prevalent and undoubtedly it has kept thousands from Nature Cure and thereby from the only possible cure for their chronic ailments. Actually, this foolish fear is entirely groundless. It is one of our fundamental principles of treatment never to do anything that is painful to the patient. We always regulate the coldness of water and the force of manipulations to the sensitiveness and endurance of the subject. Beginning with mild, alternately warm and cool sprays, which are pleasant and agreeable to everyone, we gradually increase the force and lower the temperature until the patient is so inured to cold water that the "blitz guss" becomes a delightful and pleasurable sensation. There is certainly no finer tonic than cold water, no more exhilarating sensation than that produced by the skillful application of alternating douches and the "blitz".

The spirit of Father Kneipp, the pioneer of hydrotherapy and champion of the cold water treatment, has descended upon his followers in the Nature Cure movement and they realize the importance of hydrotherapy if real and lasting cures are to be effected. Some of our friends, notably among the osteopaths, chiropractors and naprapaths, have only a pitying smile for our arduous labours in this field. They ask, "why fool with cold water and drive patients away, when pleasant manipulations bring the business and get the results?" In a number of cases a longer or shorter course of manipulative treatment may be sufficient to produce marked primary improvement, but it is not usually enough to launch the chronic

139

patient into a healing crisis because it does not remove the underlying causes of the disease. Furthermore, if a healing crisis be produced under manipulative treatment the physician, if he does not understand the law of crisis, may suppress the healing crisis. If after a while the latent chronic condition again manifests in external symptoms, the patient returns for another course of treatment which is not likely to produce any more permanent cure. There are, it is true, some chronic diseases or conditions which are directly caused by lesions of the spine or other bony structures or by defects in bodily structure, posture or mechanics. In such cases correction by manipulative treatment may produce a cure within a few weeks. But notwithstanding the views very generally expressed in osteopathic and chiropractic teachings and texts, the majority of chronic ailments have their origin in other causes. In most such cases the existing spinal lesions are themselves the result of other primary disease conditions which must be overcome before the spinal lesions will remain corrected. The mode of treatment depends upon the object that is to be accomplished. If it is to make the patient "feel better" with the least possible expenditure of time, money, personal effort and self control on his part and the least amount of exertion on the part of the physician or "healer", then manipulations or metaphysical formulas may be in order. But if the object is to cure actually and permanently a deep seated chronic disease, all methods of natural treatment, intelligently combined and adapted to the individual case, are required in order to accomplish satisfactory results.

In the treatment of chronic disease it must be remembered that the first sign of improvement does not mean a cure. Diagnosis from the iris of the eye, borne out by every day practical experience, discloses the fact that symptomatic manifestations of disease are due to underlying constitutional causes; that the chronic symptoms are nature's feeble and ineffectual efforts to eliminate from the system scrofulous, psoric or syphilitic taints and the disease products resulting from food and drug poisoning, or to overcome the destructive effects of surgical mutilations. An abatement of symptoms is, therefore, not always a sign of real or permanent cure. The latter depends on the elimination of the hereditary and acquired constitutional taints and poisons. When, under the influence of natural living and treatment, the body of the chronic becomes sufficiently purified and strengthened, a period of marked improvement may set in. All disease symptoms gradually abate, the patient gains strength both physically and mentally and feels as though there were nothing the matter with him any more. But the eyes tell a different story. They show that the underlying constitutional taints have not been fully eliminated — the weeds have not been pulled up by the roots. This can normally be accomplished only by healing crises, by nature's cleansing and healing activities in the form of inflammatory and feverish processes. Anything short of this must be regarded as preliminary improvement or "training for the fight", but not a cure. Treatment should be continued until hidden constitutional taints and drug poisons are thoroughly eliminated from the system.

Frequently we have been severely criticized for accepting for treatment seemingly hopeless chronic cases, but if we should dismiss those of our patients who, from the orthodox and popular point of view, are considered incurable, there would not remain ten out of a hundred. Yet our total failures are few and far between. Many such seemingly hopeless cases have come for treatment month after month, in several instances for a year or more, apparently without any marked advance; yet today they are in the best of health. The word "chronic" in the vocabulary of the old school of medicine is synonymous with "incurable". This is not strange, for since the medical and surgical symptomatic treatment of acute diseases creates the chronic conditions, it certainly cannot be expected to cure them. Nature Cure achieves results in the treatment of chronic diseases because its theories and practices are entirely opposite to those just described.

Since, then, Nature Cure offers to the so-called incurable the only hope and the only possible means of regaining health, why not give him a chance? Many times apparently hopeless cases have responded most readily to our treatment, while more promising ones offered the most stubborn resistance. Even with the best possible methods of diagnosis it is hard to determine just how far the destruction of vital organs has progressed or how deeply they have been impregnated with drug poisons. Therefore it is often an impossibility to predict with certainty just what the outcome will be. This can be determined only by a fair trial. In many cases the patients become discouraged and ask: "Why do others recover so quickly when I show such slow improvement? This cure seems all right for some diseases but evidently it does not fit my case." This is defective reasoning. True Nature Cure fits every case because it includes everything good in natural healing methods. In stubborn cases Nature Cure is not to blame for the slow and unsatisfactory results; the difficulty lies in the character and advanced stage of the disease — in failure to turn to natural methods soon enough. In the following chapters I shall briefly outline the natural method of diagnosis, prognosis and treatment of chronic diseases.

CHAPTER XX

DIAGNOSIS AND PROGNOSIS

The allopathic school of medicine lays more stress upon correct diagnosis than upon treatment. This is the natural result of looking upon all chronic disease as incurable. Many times have I seen the presiding professor in a clinic spend an hour or more analysing minutely the anatomical, physiological and psychological aspects of a case. To my question . . . "What is the cause of the trouble?" he would answer "Nobody knows". "What can we do for him?" "Nothing". "The case is incurable. Give him a Placebo".

Our professor on Diseases of the Eye, Ear and Nose was doing postgraduate work in Vienna. In one of his letters he wrote as follows: "This is certainly the greatest place in the world for doctors, but I doubt whether it is for patients. All that the doctors seem interested in is to see their diagnosis verified on the postmortem table. Treatment is of secondary importance." This attitude may be contrasted with that which we of the Nature Cure School seek to take towards diagnosis and treatment of chronic diseases. We claim that we make more thorough examinations and give more minutely accurate diagnoses and prognoses of disease in all its forms than does any other school of medical science, but from our point of view diagnosis is of relatively small importance in the treatment and cure of any particular disease. To us, curing is far more vital than diagnosing. Naturally, we are often asked the question: "How can you cure if you do not first determine what is the disease?" To this we answer: "The unity of disease is a fact in Nature. All disorders can be traced back to three primary manifestations, namely: (1) Lowered vitality; (2) Abnormal composition of blood and lymph; (3) Accumulation of waste materials, morbid matter and poisons." It then follows that, whoever succeeds in correcting these three underlying causes, thereby removes whatever disease originates from them.

To illustrate: Suppose a stranger should come to me and say: "Doctor, I am suffering from some serious chronic disease. Can you cure me without the customary examination?" I should reply: "If that is your wish I shall gladly treat you. And furthermore, I am confident of excellent results, if in the nature of the case improvement be possible." In accordance with

142

the primary law of disease, I would first instruct the patient how to avoid all loss of vitality in his habits of thinking, feeling, eating, drinking, bathing, breathing, working, resting, and in his sex life. I should then instruct him how to regulate his meals and combine his foods in such a way as to take in the minimum of disease producing and a maximum of blood building and purifying food elements. By blood building and purifying food elements I refer to the juicy fruits and fresh, leafy vegetables. I would apply all methods of natural treatment which tend to make the skin, bowels and kidneys more active and alive. I would use good, old fashioned massage to "squeeze" the morbid matter out of the tissues into the venous and lymphatic circulation and to stimulate the inflow of red arterial blood with its freight of oxygen and other elements of nutrition. Next in order would be Swedish movements and the best suited manipulative treatment based on our principles of neurotherapy tending to correct spinal and other mechanical lesions in bony structures, muscles, ligaments and connective tissues. I would teach him how to distinguish discordant and destructive from harmonious and constructive thinking and feeling, and how to help himself by positive, optimistic affirmations and suggestions.

In response to these teachings and treatments the patient's condition would gradually improve and he would steadily advance toward the enjoyment of perfect health. The only conditions which might prevent this happy consummation would be (1) vitality so lowered as to make response to treatment an impossibility; (2) destruction of vital organs beyond the possibility of repair; or (3) mechancial obstructions such as congenital malformation, large tumours, stones, etc., which might have to be removed by surgical operation.

These statements are not made to discourage thorough examination, diagnosis and prognosis, but to show the wonderful possibilities and the simplicity of the Nature Cure philosophy and practice. It is quite true that thorough examination gives the physician a much better understanding of abnormal conditions with which he must contend, and thereby greatly facilitates efficient treatment. Moreover, the patient is entitled to a correct diagnosis and to a rational and reliable prognosis. Such explanation, in conformity with the findings in the case, confirms his faith in the physician and secures his hearty co-operation.

Nature Cure Diagnosis

In our methods of examination and treatment we combine all that has proved true and efficient in all systems, from the oldest to the most advanced, whether "orthodox" or "irregular", provided it conforms to the fundamental laws of cure. This is what makes Nature Cure philosophy and practice the only true eclectic system of treating human ailments.

While our physical and laboratory examinations are made in accordance with the most advanced methods of the regular school of medicine, our interpretation is often at wide variance with the established theories of the old school.

The diagnosis from the iris of the eye is of great interest and importance to us, not only because it gives accurate information about causes of disease which cannot be diagnosed in any other way, but also because these wonderful records confirm the fundamental principles of Nature Cure philosophy and practice. This fact must be strongly impressed upon the mind of the reader so that it may not be lost sight of in studying the interesting revelations of the signs in the iris. However, we do not claim to be able to read in the iris all the details of disease and of specific pathological conditions. Yet I do claim emphatically that this science contains so much of paramount importance in the diagnosis and treatment of disease that the conscientious physician and even the intelligent layman cannot afford to ignore or discredit it. Thus while we do not depend on this method of diagnosis alone, by combining it with all other approved methods of examination we find that one elucidates and confirms the others. Thus, we find that we very rarely fail in giving a reliable diagnosis and prognosis of a case which has undergone systemic examination by our combined methods, iridiagnosis, spinal examination, medical examination and laboratory tests.([1])

([1])
It may be noted that since Dr. Lindlahr's time considerable advances have been made in various forms of electronic and radionic diagnostic techniques. These can be very valuable in addition to and perhaps, in some cases, as a substitute for iridiagnosis.

It should be noted that the acceptance of the Nature Cure viewpoint that Disease does not come as the result of bad luck or chance but because of the violation of the laws of Health, does not rule out the undoubted fact that accidents can be and are a very frequent cause of diseases of many kinds in a more or less direct way. Any practitioner who has acquired the skills necessary to examine the body framework from the postural and mechanical point of view and to investigate the past history of the cases which come to him will become aware of how often the ill health of a patient can be traced back to some accident or injury which so upset the mechanical functioning of his body framework and so interfered with the blood and nerve supply to various parts and organs that a general lowering of vitality has taken place and particular organs and parts have ceased to function properly and have begun to deteriorate. The success of good manipulative therapists of various schools has been based on their ability to correct these postural and mechanical defects and so bring about improvement and cure.

"For the explanatory chart of Iridiagnosis see frontispiece"

CHAPTER XXI

THE TREATMENT OF CHRONIC DISEASE

The old school of medical science defines acute diseases as those which run a brief and more or less violent course, and chronic diseases as those which run a protracted course and have a tendency to recur. Nature Cure attaches a broader and more significant meaning to these terms. This has become apparent from my discussion of the causes, the progressive development and the purpose of acute diseases in the preceding pages. From the Nature Cure viewpoint, the chronic condition is the latent, constitutional disease encumbrance, whereas acute disease represents nature's efforts to rectify abnormal conditions, to overcome and eliminate hereditary or acquired morbid taints and systemic poisons and to re-establish normal structure and functions.

To use an illustration: In a case of permanent or recurrent itchy psoriasis, the old school physician would look upon the itchy skin eruption as the "chronic disease", while we see in the external eczema an attempt of the healing forces of nature to remove from the system the inner, latent hereditary or acquired psora, which constitutes the real chronic disease. It stands to reason that the exterior eruptions should not be suppressed by any means whatever, but that the only true and really effective method of treatment consists in eliminating from the organism the inner, latent psoric taint. After this is accomplished the external 'skin disease' will disappear of its own accord. As another illustration of the radical difference in our respective points of view, let us take haemorrhoids (piles). The allopathic doctor considers the local haemorrhoidal enlargement in itself the chronic disease, while the Nature Cure physician looks upon haemorrhoids as one of nature's efforts to rid the system of certain morbid encumbrances and poisons which have accumulated as the result of sluggish circulation, chronic constipation, defective elimination through kidneys, and from any other causes. These constitutional abnormalities, which are the real chronic disease, have got be treated and corrected, and when this has been done, the haemorrhoidal enlargements and discharges will take care of themselves. It is, therefore, absolutely irrational, and frequently followed by the most serious consequences, to extirpate the piles or suppress the haemorrhoidal discharges, and thereby to drive these concentrated poison extracts back into the system. In a number of cases we have traced paralysis, insanity, tuberculosis, cancer and other forms of chronic destructive disease to the forcible suppression of haemorrhoids.(1)

Chronic disease, from the viewpoint of Nature Cure philosophy, means that the organism has become permeated with morbid matter and poisons to such an extent that it is no longer able to throw off these encumbrances by vigorous, "acute" eliminative effort. The chronic condition, therefore, represents the slow, cold type of disease, characterized by feeble, ineffectual efforts to eliminate the latent morbid taints and impediments from the system. These efforts may take the form of open sores, skin eruptions, catarrhal discharges, chronic diarrhoea, etc., etc. If acute diseases are treated in harmony with nature's laws, they will leave the body in a purer, healthier condition. But, if the treatment is wrong, if under the old school methods fever and inflammation (nature's methods of elimination) are checked and suppressed with poisonous drugs, serums and antitoxins, or if, instead of purifying and invigorating cells and tissues, the affected parts are extirpated with the surgeon's knife, nature is not allowed to get rid of the disease matter and poisonous taints and morbid encumbrances remain in the organism. In this way originate the worst forms of chronic disease which now afflict civilized races. The truth of this assertion is proved by the fact that the most destructive chronic diseases are not found among any of the primitive peoples of the earth, as the negroes in Africa and Australia and the Esquimaux of the arctic regions. They are not found among people who do not use drugs. The different forms of venereal disease, cancer, tuberculosis, many forms of paralysis and paresis, etc., are unknown in those countries whose inhabitants live in harmony with nature. The reason is that these people have not learned to suppress nature's acute purifying and healing efforts by poisonous drugs and surgical operations.

Let us now study the actual conditions of the cells, tissues and organs of the body in chronic disease. We know that the human body is made up of millions of minute cells of living protoplasm, and that the life of the protoplasm and especially of the germ plasm is inherent in the microzymes. Though these cells are so small that they have to be magnified under the microscope several hundred times before we can see them, they are individual living beings which grow, eat, drink and throw off waste matter, just like the larger conglomerate cell which we call "man". Each one

(1)
It should be noted that haemorrhoids can be caused wholly or mainly by sacro-iliac subluxations and other pelvic and low back lesions which produce a disturbance of the circulation and a congestion in the veins.

of these little cells has its own business to attend to, whether it be digestion, assimilation, elimination or the performance of any of the thousand and one functions and activities which make up the metabolism of the human organism. If these little beings are well individually, the man is well. If they are starved or ailing, the entire man is similarly affected. We know now that the health of the cell depends upon the well being of its micro-zymes. The whole depends upon the parts. It is our duty to provide the most favourable conditions of living for the cells which make up the individual human organism. If we do that there will be no occasion for disease. "Natural immunity" will be the result.

Herein lies the vital difference between the attitude of Nature Cure and that of the allopathic school towards disease. The latter spends all its efforts in fighting the disease symptoms, while the former confines itself to creating healthy conditions in the habits and surroundings of the patient in the belief that the disease symptoms will then take care of them-selves and will disappear because of non-support. It is the practical application of the injunction "Resist not evil but overcome evil with good".

Under the influence of wrong habits of living and the suppressive treatment of diseases, all forms of waste and morbid matter (the faeces of the cells), together with food, drink and drug poisons, accumulate in the system, injure the cells and obstruct the minute spaces between them. These morbid encumbrances impinge upon and clog the blood vessels, the nerve channels and the other tissues of the body. This is bound to interfere with the normal functions of the organism and in time leads to deterior-ation and organic destruction.

In this connection we wish to call attention to a difference in viewpoint which there seems to be between Osteopaths and Chiropractors and followers of the Nature Cure school. The former tend to attribute disease very much to "impingement" or abnormal pressure upon nerves and blood vessels resulting from dislocations and subluxations of the vertebrae and of other bony structures. They do not usually take into consideration the impingement upon and obstruction of nerve channels and blood vessels all through the system caused by local or general encumbrances of the organism with waste matter, morbid products and poisons that have accumulated in cells and tissues.

Every individual cell must be supplied with food and with oxygen. These it receives from the red arterial blood. The cells must also be provided with an outlet for their waste products. This is furnished by the lymphatic and venous circulations which constitute the drainage system of the body. If drainage is defective, the effect upon the organism is similar to the effect produced when drains are obstructed and sewage is forced back into the

147

building. Furthermore, every cell must be in unobstructed communication with the nerve currents of the body. Most important of all it must be in touch with the sympathetic nervous system through which it receives the life force which vivifies and controls all involuntary functions of the cells and organs. Each individual cell must be supplied with two sets of nerve connections, one to convey its sensations and needs to "headquarters", the nerve centres in brain and spinal cord; the other to carry impulses from the cranial, spinal and sympathetic centres to the cell, governing and directing its activities. For instance, if the cell be hungry, thirsty, cold or in pain, it telegraphs these sensations to headquarters in the brain or spinal cord, and from there directions necessary to comply with the needs of the cell are sent forth in the form of nerve impulses to the centres controlling the circulation, the food and heat supply, the means of protection etc. This circuit of communication from the cell over the afferent nerves to the nerve centres in the brain or spinal cord, and from these centres over the efferent nerves back to the cell or other cells is called "the reflex arc".

Let us use an illustration: Suppose the fingers come in contact with a hot iron. The cells in the finger tips experience the sensation of burning pain. At once this sensation is telegraphed over the afferent nerves to the nerve centres in the brain and spinal cord. In response to this call of distress the command comes back over the efferent nerve filaments: "Withdraw the fingers". At the same time the impulse to withdraw the fingers is sent over the motor nerves to the muscles which control the movements of the hand. If the means of communication between the different parts of the organism are obstructed or cut off entirely, the individual cell is bound to deteriorate and to die, just as a person lost in a barren wilderness and cut off from his fellow men must perish. In warfare it is well known that if one of the contending armies succeeds in cutting off the food supply or the telegraphic communication of the other army with its headquarters, the activities of the enemy are seriously handicapped. So the waste materials in the system, the disease taints, narcotic and alcoholic poisons, etc., obstruct the nerve passages and thus interfere with the functioning of the cell by cutting off its means of communication.

What has been said will serve to elucidate and emphasize the necessity of perfect cleanliness, inside as well as outside the body. It justifies the dictum of Kuhne, one of the pioneers of Nature Cure, "Health is cleanliness." Anything that in any way interferes with or obstructs the circulation of vital fluids and nerve currents in the system is bound to create abnormal conditions and functioning which constitute disease. When the morbid encumbrances and obstructions in the organism have reached the point where they seriously interfere with the nourishment, drainage and nerve supply of the cells, the latter cannot perform their activities properly, nor can they rid themselves of the impediment. They may be compared to individuals who are forced to live in unwholesome surroundings and who cannot do their best work under these unfavourable conditions. In this way originates chronic disease, which means that cells have become incapable of arousing themselves to acute eliminative effort in the form of inflammatory febrile reactions. In my lectures I sometimes liken the cell thus encumbered with morbid matter and poisons to a man buried in a mine under the debris of a "cave in" in such a manner that it is impossible for him to free himself of the earth and timbers which are pulling him down In such a predicament the man is unable to help himself. His fellow workers or his friends must come to his aid and remove the obstructing masses so that he may be able to free himself. This is a good illustration of the condition of the cells of the body in chronic disease. They also have become unable to help themselves and need assistance until they can once more arouse themselves to self-help by means of acute eliminative effort.

What can we do to help them? We must endeavour, in the first place, to furnish the cells with the right nourishment. We must abstain from everything that may be injurious to the body in food and drink so as to relieve the cells of all unnecessary work. Whatever one may think of vegetarianism as a continuous mode of living, a little consideration will make it plain that a rational vegetarian diet is the "sine qua non" in the cure of chronic diseases. It builds up the blood on a normal basis, excludes all food and drink poisons and thereby gives the organism an opportunity to throw off the old accumulations of waste and morbid materials. In chronic disease, every drop of blood and every cell of the organism is affected. In order to produce a cure, the old tissues must be broken down and removed and new tissues built up. The more thorough the change in diet, the greater and more rapid will be the changes for the better in cells and tissues. especially if only pure and eliminating foods are used. For these reasons it is advisable to omit meat from the dietary. All animal flesh contains the morbid excretions and other waste products of the animal organism, and this means additional work for the cells already overburdened with systemic poisons.

Secondly we must work for elimination. Cold water applied to the surface of the body is the most powerful stimulant to the circulation. It pulls and pushes the blood through the system. One actually feels the blood rushing through the arteries and veins with greater force. The cold water treatment makes the skin more alive and active, stirs up and accelerates the circulation throughout the system and thus promotes the elimination of systemic poisons through the skin. This stimulating effect of cold water has been proved by counting the number of red blood corpuscles in a drop of blood before and after the application of the cold "blitz guss". In some instances they were found to have doubled in number. This does not mean that in an instant twice as many red blood corpuscles had come into existence; but it does mean that before the cold "guss" one half of them were dozing lazily in corners. The cold water stirred them up, forced them into circulation, made them travel and attend to business.

Thirdly, it must be remembered that another powerful means of promoting elimination is thorough, systematic massage. The deep kneading, twisting, rolling and stroking actually squeezes the stagnant morbid matter and the waste products out of the tissues into the circulation, to be carried off through the venous drainage. This allows the red blood with its nourishment and fresh supply of oxygen to flood the cells and organs. Massage, too, is very effective as a means of regulating the blood supply in the system. In every chronic disease there is obstruction or congestion in some part of the organism, causing high blood pressure in the interior of the body and insufficient blood supply to surface and extremities. Massage distributes the blood quickly and evenly. In most cases if not in all neurotherapy is of great importance. Hardly a person can be found today whose spine and body framework is not abnormal in one way or another, just as there is not a perfectly normal human iris. Impingement on nerves and blood vessels should be corrected by expert manipulation. Neurotherapy removes abnormal pressure upon nerves and blood vessels, reduces tension and steps up energy, establishing a free and abundant flow of nerve and blood currents. Air and light baths, by stimulating the skin in a natural manner to increased activity, also to the attainment of the various good results just described.

Physical exercise comes next in importance. Corrective and curative movements and gymnastics combined with deep breathing promote the combustion (oxidation) of morbid materials and in this way facilitate their elimination from the system. Life itself is dependent upon breathing. The Life Force enters the body with every breath we draw. Show me a man with well, full breathing lungs and I will show you a man with good vitality.

Last but not least among the natural methods of treating the cell in chronic disease we must mention the right mental and emotional attitude. Fear and anxiety and all kindred emotions as it were congeal the nerve matter and so shut off the supply of nerve force. The cells actually starve and freeze. On the other hand, the emotions of hope, confidence, and cheerfulness relax and open blood vessels and nerve channels and allow the free and unobstructed inflow and circulation of fluids and of vital energy.

When, through natural methods of living and treatment, the morbid encumbrances have been removed sufficiently to provide and maintain normal blood supply, better venous and lymphatic drainage and the unobstructed flow of nerve currents, when lesions of the body structure have been corrected by skilful adjustment and when, through the right mental attitude, a free and abundant inflow of Life Force has been established, then the cells and tissues of the body become once again able to arouse themselves to an acute eliminative effort and the organism is ready for a healing crisis.

To recapitulate:- the objects to be obtained in the treatment of chronic disease are: (1) to economize vitality; (2) to promote assimilation; (3) to promote the elimination of waste and morbid matter; (4) to correct mechanical lesions; (5) to adjust and harmonize mental and emotional conditions. In the following chapters the laws and principles underlying healing crises and their periodicity will be fully described and also the practical application of the different methods of natural treatment.

CHAPTER XXII

CRISES

Crisis in the ordinary sense of the word means change, either for better or for worse. In medical parlance the term "crisis" has been defined as "a decisive change in the disease, resulting either in recovery or in death". We of the Nature Cure School distinguish between "healing crises" and "disease crises", according to the character and tendency of the acute reaction. If an acute disease is brought about through the accumulation of morbid matter to such an extent that the health or the life of the organism is endangered, in other words, if the disease conditions are forcing the crisis, we speak of disease crisis. But if acute reactions take place in the system because conditions have become more normal, because the healing forces have gained the ascendancy and forced the acute inflammatory processes, we refer to them as healing crises.

Healing crises are simply different forms of elimination by means of which nature endeavours to remove the latent chronic disease encumbrance from the system. The most common forms of these acute purifications are acute catarrhal colds and hemorrhoidal discharges, boils, ulcers, abscesses, open sores, skin eruptions, diarrhoeas, haemorrhages, abnormal perspirattion and all sorts of inflammatory processes. Healing crises and disease crises may seem very much alike. Patients often tell me: "I have had this before. I call it an ordinary cold (or boil or fever)." This may be true. The former disease crisis and the present healing crisis may be similar in their outward manifestations; but they are taking place under entirely different conditions.

When the organism is loaded to the danger point with morbid matter it may arouse itself in self-defence to an acute eliminative effort in the shape of cold, catarrh, fever, inflammation, skin eruption, etc. In these instances, the disease conditions bring about the crisis and the organism is on the defensive. These are disease crises. Such unequal struggles between the healing forces and pathogenic conditions sometimes end favourably and sometimes fatally. On the other hand, healing crises develop because the healing forces are in the ascendancy and take the offensive. They are brought about through natural methods of living and treatment, and always result in improved conditions.

152

A simple allegory may assist in making clear the difference between a healing crisis and a disease crisis. For years a prize fighter holds the championship because he keeps himself in perfect physical condition and before every contest spends many weeks in careful training. When he faces his opponent in the ring, he has eliminated from his organism as much waste matter and superfluous flesh and fat as possible by strictly regulated diet and a great deal of vigorous exercise. As a consequence, he comes off victorious in every contest and easily maintains his superiority. These victories in his career, like healing crises in the organism, are the result of training and preparation. The prize fighter in the one case and Vital Force in the other are on the offensive from the beginning of the struggles and have the advantage from start to finish. Rendered over confident by long continued success, our champion gradually permits himself to drift into a weakened physical condition. He omits his regular training and indulges in all kinds of dissipation. One day, full of self conceit and underestimating the strength of his challenger, he enters the ring without adequate preparation and is ingloriously defeated by a man who, under different circumstances, would not be a match for him. So, in the case of a patient in a disease crisis, fatal termination may be due to excessive accumulation of waste and morbid matter in the system, to lowered vitality and to lack of preparation. Victory or defeat in acute reactions, as well as in the "ring", depends upon right living and preparatory training. In the healing crisis, vitality is the stronger and gains victory in the struggle; in the disease crisis disease conditions have gained the ascendancy and bring about the defeat of the healing forces.

Under conditions favourable to human life, a body endowed with healthy blood and tissues and good vitality cannot be affected by acute disease. Such an organism is practically immune to all forms of inflammatory febrile reactions. They always indicate that there is something in the system which nature is trying to correct or to get rid of, namely, pathogenic matter.[1]

In the catechism of Nature Cure I have defined healing crises as follows:

[1]
There is undoubtedly a distinction between healing and disease crises and in old and chronically ill people an acute crisis is often the prelude to the end of life. However, in the ordinary clinical situations which arise, it would often seem difficult to say whether a crisis is a disease crisis or a healing crisis and it would appear that one may easily be turned into the other by the way in which it is dealt with — that is to say it may either be something which leads to betterment or to deterioration according to the treatment given. Moreover a certain complication arises from the fact that certain acute diseases are communicable and tend to occur in epidemics. Lindlahr is no doubt right that an acute reaction is a manifestation of energy and that it is normally not undertaken by the body unless it can be carried through to a successful conclusion. This is particularly so when the crisis is a stage in a process of cure or betterment induced by initiation of

A healing crisis is an acute reaction resulting from the ascendancy of nature's healing forces over disease conditions. Its tendency is towards recovery, and it is, therefore, in conformity with nature's constructive principle. The possibility of producing healing crises and thereby curing chronic ailments depends upon the following conditions:- (1) The patient must have sufficient vital energy and power of reaction to respond to the natural treatment and to a change of habits. (2) The destruction and disorganization of vital fluids and organs must not have advanced too far. Some patients become frightened at the idea of crises. They exclaim: "I came here to get well, not to grow worse". However there is no occasion for alarm. Healing crises occur in mild form only because under the influence of natural living and treatment, nature has the advantage in the fight. The healing forces of the organism have gained the ascendancy over the disease conditions. Nature, in fact, never undertakes a healing crisis until the system has been prepared for it, until the organism is sufficiently purified and strengthened to conduct the reaction to a favourable termination. Furthermore, it is well to remember that crises cannot be avoided, because it is through fevers and inflammatory processes that nature effects the cure, — that she decomposes pathogen into simpler compounds suitable for elimination.

On the other hand, if a patient is possessed of good vitality, is not too heavily encumbered with pathogenic materials, and if the organs of elimination are in good working order, the purification and adjustment of the organism may proceed gradually without the occurrence of marked reactions or crises. When the morbid encumbrances consist largely of highly complex ptomaines, leukomains and alkaloids which resist neutralization by alkaline mineral elements, then nature has to resort to bacterial activity and inflammatory processes in order to reduce these pathogenic materials to simpler compounds suitable for elimination through the natural channels.(1)

Healing crises, when properly conducted, are never fatal to life. The

natural treatment and habits of living. It does seem, however, that in some cases, as the result of infection in an epidemic or otherwise an acute crisis may be induced at a time and in circumstances which take the body at a disadvantage. In such a case danger may be greater and treatment require to be more skilful and rigorous.

(1)
Later in Chapter XXIX Dr. Lindlahr discusses the chemical composition of the different forms of waste with which the body has to cope. He argues here that when these morbid encumbrances are of a complex kind fever and bacterial action may be the only way in which they can be eliminated. On the other hand it seems that the wise physician can to a great extent bring about improvement and health in chronic conditions by a process of lysis rather than crisis. There is evidence that good homeopathic physicians do in fact do this.

only danger lies in suppressing these acute reactions by drugs, knife or other means. If acute reactions are suppressed, the constructive healing crisis may be changed into a destructive disease crisis. Therefore we earnestly warn our patients never to interfere in any way with a healing crisis lest the chronic condition become worse than before. When nature, with all the force inherent in the human organism, has finally worked up to the point of a healing crisis, another defeat by a new suppression may beyond her powers of endurance and recuperation. Fatal collapse may then be the result.

Our explanations of the natural laws of cure and of natural therapeutics are often greeted by old school physicians and students with remarks like the following: "You speak as if you had the monopoly of eliminative treatment and of the production of crises. With our laxatives, cathartics, diuretics, diaphoretics and tonics, we are accomplishing the same thing. What is more effectual for stimulating a sluggish liver and cleansing the intestinal tract than calomel followed by a dose of salts? What will produce more profuse perspiration than pilocarpin; or what is a better stimulus to the kidney than squills or buchu? Can we not by stimulants and depressants regulate heart action to a nicety? We accomplish all this in a clean, scientific manner, without resorting to unpleasant dieting and to the applications of douches, packs, and manual treatments. Isn't it more dignified and professional to write a Latin prescription? How much better the impression on the laity than soaking and rubbing?"

Let us see if these statements be true, whether laxation, urination or perspiration produced by poisonous drugs is identical in character and in effect with the elimination produced by healing crises brought on through natural living and natural methods of treatment. Mercury, in the form of calomel, is one of the best known cholagogues. It is a favourite laxative and cathartic of allopathy. The prevailing idea is that calomel acts on the liver and intestines; but in reality these organs act on the drug. All laxatives and cathartics are poisons; if it were not so, they would not produce their peculiar, drastic effects. Because they are poisons, nature tries to eliminate them from the system as quickly and thoroughly as possible. In order to do this, the excretory glands and membranes of the liver and the digestive tract greatly increase the amount of their secretions and thereby produce a forced evacuation of the intestinal canal. Thus the system, in the effort to eliminate the mercurial poison, expels also the other contents of the intestines. This may effect a temporary cleansing of the intestinal tract, but it does not and cannot cleanse the individual cells throughout the body of their impurities. Besides, "action and reaction are equal and opposite". In accordance with the law of action and reaction, the temporary irritation and over-stimulation of the sensitive membranes of the digestive organs are followed by corresponding weakness and exhaustion, and if this procedure be repeated it becomes habitual. As atrophy progresses the dose of the purgative must be increased in order to accomplish the desired result and this, in turn, hastens the degenerative changes in the system. Such enforced artificial purging may flush the drains and sewers but does not cleanse the inner chambers of the house. The cells in the interior remain encumbered with morbid matter. A genuine and truly effective house-cleaning must start in the cells and must be brought about through the initiative of the vital energies in the organism, through healing crises and not through stimulation by means of poisonous irritants.

When, under a natural regimen of living and of treatment, the system has been sufficiently purified, adjusted and vivified the cells themselves begin the work of elimination. This is what takes place: the morbid matter and poisons thrown off by the cells and tissues are carried by means of the venous circulation to the organs of elimination, the bowels, kidneys, lungs and skin, and to the mucous membranes lining the interior tracts, such as the nasal passages, the throat and bronchi, the digestive and genito-urinary organs, etc. These organs of elimination become overcrowded with the rush of morbid matter and the accompanying congestion and irritation cause the acute inflammatory processes and feverish symptoms characterizing the various forms of colds, catarrhs, skin eruptions, diarrhoeas, boils and other acute forms of elimination which we call healing crises. In other words, what the old school of medicine calls the disease, we look upon as the cure. Acute elimination brought about in this manner is, as previously explained, nature's method of housecleaning. It is a true healing crisis, the result of purification and increased activity from within the cell, produced by natural means.

At this point the old school physician may continue the argument somewhat as follows: "You claim that you bring about your acute reactions by natural means only, and that these are never injurious to the organism. What difference does it make if the circulation is stimulated and elimination increased by a cold water spray or by digitalis? The cold water stimulation produces a reaction ju‹t as digitalis does and the one must therefore be as injurious as the other." The answer to this is that the stimulating effect produced by digitalis is the first action of a highly poisonous drug; the second, lasting, effect is weakening and depressing. On the other hand, the first action of a cold water spray is depressive; it sends the blood into the interior of the body and leaves the surface bloodless. The sensory nerves at once report this sensation of cold to headquarters in the brain, and immediately the command is telegraphed to the vasomotor centres which control the circulation: "Send blood to the surface". As a result, the blood is carried to the surface and the skin becomes warm and rosy. In this case the stimulation is the second and lasting effect of the water treatment, from which there is no further reaction unless the patient be in a very weakened condition. Then the treatment must be modified accordingly. Similarly, the stimulation produced by exercise, massage, neurotherapy, or the exposure of the nude body to light and air, is natural stimulation produced by harmless natural means. It is entirely due to the fact that conditions in the system have been made more normal.

Drugs, stimulants and tonics, when they do produce an artificial, temporary stimulation, do not change the underlying abnormal condition in the organism. Likewise, the flushing of the colon with water, the use of laxative herb teas and decoctions, or forced sweating by means of Turkish or Russian bath , though not as dangerous as inorganic minerals and poisonous drugs, cannot be classed among the natural means of cure. These agents, which by many persons are looked upon as natural treatment, irritate the organs of elimination to forced abnormal activity without at the same time arousing the cells in the interior of the body to natural elimination. Dr. H. Lahmann, one of the foremost scientists of the Nature Cure movement, made a series of interesting experiments. From certain patients he gathered the natural perspiration produced by ordinary exercise in the sunshine. These excretions of the skin were evaporated and analyzed and were found to contain powerful toxins. When, however, profuse sweating was produced in the same patients by high temperature of the hot air box or the electric light cabinet, their perspiration, when evaporated and analyzed, was found to contain only small amounts of toxins. Thus Dr. Lahmann proved that sweating and the elimination of disease matter are two somewhat different processes, that artificially induced sweating does not eliminate disease matter to any great extent and that the organism cannot be forced by irritants and stimulants and artificial means, but eliminates morbid matter only in its own natural manner and when it is in proper condition to do so. In a lesser degree this applies also to fasting. Under certain conditions it becomes a necessity but it may easily be abused and overdone as will be discussed in a later chapter. That the medical profession does not understand the principle of natural elimination is proved by the fact that in cases where the system works up to some form of natural elimination in the way of purging, catarrhal discharges, skin eruptions, etc., they forthwith suppress these purifying processes by poisonous drugs and other agents.(1)

[1]
In spite of what is said here it can be contended that there is a place in natural therapeutics for the limited and intelligent use both of sweating and of colonic lavage. For

To the question: "Do we never fail?", the answer is that we certainly do, but we believe that our failures are usually due to the fact that the sick, as a rule, do not consider Nature Cure except as a last resort. The methods and requirements of Nature Cure appear at first so unusual and exacting that most people seek to evade them as long as they have the least faith in the miracle working power of the poison bottle, a metaphysical healer or the surgeon's knife. When health, wealth and hope are entirely exhausted, then the chronic sufferer grasps at Nature Cure as a drowning man clutches at a straw. But even though ninety per cent of the cases which come to us are of the apparently incurable type, our total failures are few and far between. If there is sufficient vitality in the body to react to natural treatment and if the destruction of vital parts and organs has not advanced too far, a cure is possible. Often the seemingly hopeless cases yield the most readily. Our success is due to the fact that we do not rely on any one method of treatment, but combine in our work everything that is practical and beneficial in all different systems of natural healing.

Everywhere in nature and in the world of man we find the Law of Crises in evidence. This proves it to be a universal law, ruling all cosmic relations and activities. Wars and revolutions can be regarded as the healing crises in the life of nations — of social and political life. Heresies and reformations are the crises of religion. In strikes, riots and panics we can recognize the crises of commercial life. The earth itself has in the distant past repeatedly changed the configuration of her continents and oceans by great cataclysms and geological crises. When the sultry summer air has become pregnant with poisonous vapours and miasms, atmospheric crises, such as rainstorms and electric storms, cool and purify the air and charge it anew with life giving ozone. In like maner will healing crises purify the disease laden bodies of man.

Emanuel Swedenborg gives us a wonderful description of the law of crises in its relationship to the regeneration of the soul. I quote from the chapter in which he describes the working of this law, entitled: "Regeneration is Effected by Combats in Temptation". "They who have not been instructed concerning the regeneration of man think that man can be regenerated without temptation. But it is to be known that no one is regenerated without temptation; and that many temptations succeed, one after another. The reason is that regeneration is effected for an end, in order that the life of the old may die, and the new life which is heavenly be insinuated. It is evident, therefore, that there must be a conflict"

instance, pyretic baths can be used not only to produce perspiration but also to restore the tone and functioning of the skin and superficial tissues. Similarly, colonic irrigation can be done in a way which will not only clean out the bowel but will also help to restore its muscular tone and peristaltic functioning.

(healing crisis); "for the life of the old man resists and determines not to be extinguished; and the life of the new man can only enter where the life of the old is extinct. Whoever thinks from an enlightened rationale, may see and perceive from this that a man cannot be regenerated without combat, that is, without spiritual temptation; and further, that he is not regenerated by one temptation, but by many. For there are many kinds ot evil which formed the delight of his former life, that is, of the old life. These evils cannot all be subdued at once and together; for they cleave tenaciously, since they have been inrooted in the parents for many ages back" (the scrofula of the soul) "and they are therefore innate in man, and are confirmed by actual evils from himself from infancy. All these evils are diametrically opposite to the celestial good" (perfect health) "that is to be insinuated and which is to constitute the New Life."

Thus Swedenborg, the inspired philosopher of the North, draws a vivid picture of what we call healing crises in their relation to moral regeneration. We cannot help recognizing the close agreement of physical and spiritual crises. This appears to demonstrate the continuity and correspondence of Natural Law on the different planes of being. We of the Nature Cure school know that this great Law of Crises dominates the cure of chronic disease. The cure invariably proceeds through the darkness and chaos of healing crises to the ultimate goal of perfect health, periods of marked improvement alternating with acute eliminative activity until perfect regeneration has taken place.

CHAPTER XXIII

PERIODICITY

In many forms of acute disease, crises develop with marked regularity and well defined periodicity. This phenomenon has been observed and described by many physicians. It is not so well known, however, that under the treatment of chronic diseases by natural methods crises develop in accordance with certain laws of periodicity. This periodicity is governed by the septimal law, or the law of sevens, which seems to be the basic law governing the vibratory activities of this planet. The law of sevens dominates the life of individuals and of nations and of everything that lives and has periods of birth, growth, fruitage and decline. The law of sevens governs the days of the week, the phases of the moon, the menstrual periods of the woman. Every observing physician is aware of its influence on feverish, nervous and psychic diseases.

Over two thousand years ago Pythagoras and Hippocrates distinctly recognized and proclaimed the laws and crises of periodicity in their bearing on the cure of chronic diseases. They taught that alternating, well defined periods of improvement and of crises were determined and governed by the law of periodicity or the law of numbers. The following quotations are taken from the Encyclopedia Britannica:

"But this artistic completeness was closely connected with 'the third cardinal virtue' of Hippocratic medicine — the clear recognition of disease as being equally with life a process governed by what we should now call natural laws, which could be known by observation and which indicated the spontaneousness and normal direction of recovery, by following which alone could the physician succeed."

"Another Hippocratic doctrine, the influence of which is not even yet exhausted, is that of the healing power of nature. Not that Hippocrates taught, as he was afterwards reproached with teaching, that nature is sufficient for the cure of diseases; for he held strongly the efficacy of art. But he recognized, at least in acute diseases, a natural process which the humours went through . . . being first of all crude, then passing through coction or digestion, and finally being expelled by resolution or crisis through one of the natural channels of the body. The duty of the physician was to foresee these changes, 'to assist and not to hinder them' so that 'the sick man might conquer the disease with the help of the physician'. The times at which crises were to be expected were naturally looked for with anxiety; and it was a cardinal point in the Hippocratic system to foretell them with precision. Hippocrates, influenced as is thought by the Pythagorean doctrine of numbers, taught that they were to be expected on days fixed by certain numerical rules, in some cases on odd, in others on even numbers . . . the celebrated doctrine of 'critical days'. It follows from what has been said that prognosis, or the art of foretelling the course and event of the disease, was a strong point with the Hippocratic physicians. In this perhaps they have never been excelled. Diagnosis or recognition of the disease, must have been necessarily imperfect, when no scientific nosology, or system of disease, existed, and the knowledge of anatomy was quite inadequate to allow of a precise determination of the seat of the disease; but symptoms were no doubt observed and interpreted skilfully. The pulse is not spoken of in any of the works now attributed to Hippocrates himself, though it is mentioned in other works of the collection."

"In the treatment of disease, the Hippocratic school attached great importance to diet, the variations necessary in different diseases being minutely defined . . . In chronic cases diet, exercises and natural methods were chiefly relied upon."

The author of this article in the Britannica does not see that it is the modern orthodox "scientific nosology or system of disease" which is largely responsible for obscuring the simplicity and precision of the Hippocratic philosophy of disease and cure. These truths, with other wisdom of the ancients, were lost in the darkness of latei times and modern medicine tends to look upon the claims and teachings of the Hippocratic school as "superstition, without foundation in fact". However, the great sages of antiquity, drawing upon a source of ancient wisdom, proclaimed many truths. Every case of chronic disease treated by natural methods proves the reality and stability of the law of crises. It is strange to anyone who knows, that this all important and self-evident law is practically unknown to the disciples of the regular schools.

In accordance with the law of periodicity, the sixth period in any seven periods is marked by reactions, changes, revolutions or crises. It is, therefore, looked upon by popular superstition as an unlucky period. Friday, the sixth day of the week, is regarded as an unlucky day — Friday "hangman's day"; according to tradition the Master, Jesus, was crucified on Friday. Counting from the first sixth or Friday period in any given number of hours, days, weeks, months, years or groups of years, as the case may be, every succeeding seventh period is characterised by crises. This explains why thirteen is considered an unlucky number. It represents the second critical or Friday period. However, there is really no cause for this superstitious fear of Friday and the number thirteen. It is due to a lack of understanding of nature's laws. By intelligent cooperation with these laws we may turn the critical periods in our lives into "healing crises" and beneficial changes. We should not fear the crisis periods of the larger life and the changes in our outward circumstances which they may bring any more than we should fear crises in the physical body. A thorough understanding of the nature and purpose of healing crises in acute and chronic diseases has taught me the nature and purpose of evil in general. It has made me understand more clearly the meaning of "Resist not Evil" and of the saying: "We are punished by our sins and not for our sins." It has shown me that evil is not a punishment or a curse, but a necessary complement of good; that it is corrective and educational in its purposes; that it remains with us only so long as we need its salutary lessons.

The evil of physical disease is not due to accident or to the arbitrary rulings of a capricious Providence, nor is it always "error of mortal mind". From the Nature Cure philosophy and its practical application we have learned that, barring accidents and conditions or surroundings unfavourable to human life, it is caused in every instance by violation of the physical laws of our being. So long as transgressions of the physical laws of our being result in hereditary and acquired disease encumbrances, we must expect reactions which may either become disease crises or healing crises. Therefore we should not be afraid of changes and crisis periods but cooperate with them. Then they will result in improvement and further growth. Many of our patients formerly looked upon their diseased conditions as great misfortune and undeserved punishment; but since it brought them in contact with Nature Cure philosophy and showed them the necessity of complying with the laws of their being, they now look upon the former "evil" as the greatest blessing in their lives, because it taught them how to become the masters of fate instead of remaining the playthings of nature's destructive forces.

We find that our primary division of time into weeks consisting of seven days is in accord with the septenary law. But it is interesting to note that the years in a life time also appear to arrange themselves in groups of seven and in cycles of seven times seven. The first, or Sunday period, includes the first seven years of life. This is the birthday period characterized by the weakness and helplessness of the newborn and its entire dependence upon parents or guardians. The second, or Monday period, includes the years from eight to fourteen. This is the age of childhood still

162

characterized by weakness and dependence but reason, willpower and self-control should now have developed to a sufficient degree to impose on the individual the obligation of personal responsibility. In other words, with the completion of the seventh year the child becomes to a certain extent morally responsible. This age is also best adapted for the acquisition of the simpler forms of useful knowledge. The third, or Tuesday period, reaches from the fifteenth year until the twenty first. This is the period of youth, or adolescence, and should also be spent under the guidance and protection of parents or guardians. It is still a period of immaturity and should be utilized for the further acquisition of knowledge and for active preparation for the business of life. Nearly all civilized countries take cognizance of the completion of the third period by fixing the legal age at twenty one at which time the person is regarded as qualified to take care of himself.

The fourth (Wednesday) period from the twenty second to the twenty eighth year, is characterized by the beginning of the independent struggle for existence. During this time the normal person seeks to establish himself firmly in some line of work, business or profession. During the fifth (Thursday) period from the twenty ninth to the thirty fifth year, a person should succeed in establishing himself firmly enough to be able to found and support a family and thus to fulfill one of the primary purposes of existence, the reproduction of the species.

Nature, however, does not intend us to continue indefinitely in the security of a well established routine of life and therefore during the sixth or Friday period from the thirty sixth to the forty second year there tends to be a time of reactions, changes or "crises". With the achievement of primary objectives comes unrest and the striving for the satisfaction of new ambitions, and for the attainment of higher ideals. Success in a financial way on a small scale tends to lead to larger undertakings and more risky speculations. The attainment of financial independence gives rise to political ambitions, to the desire for distinction in other fields of endeavour or to the awakening of altruistic and philanthropic impulses. This sixth period is, therefore, often characterized by sudden upheavals and changes in business affairs and home surroundings and the taking up of new lines of endeavour. Frequently also this is a time of changes in physical conditions, brought about by the development of disease crisis resulting from wrong living and wrong treatment of minor ailments in the past. All these changes and reactions in the affairs of life naturally involve unrest, uncertainty, losses, deprivations and the necessity for fresh starts, reconstruction on a new basis and all the anxiety and concentrated effort which this requires. The sixth period is therefore often considered unlucky, but if we understand its true significance we should not so regard it. The experiences which we may consider "unlucky", unfortunate or destructive may well be necessary for the further development of our latent faculties, capacities and powers and for the strengthening of our physical, intellectual and moral fibre. I am convinced that an optimistic conception of the nature and purpose of seeming misfortunes, trials and tribulations is the right one and I have seen this verified in many thousands of cases.

During the seventh period the effects of the sixth or crisis period continue and adjust themselves. It is a period of reconstruction, of recuperation and rest and thus the best preparation for a new cycle of sevens which begins with the fiftieth year. In this connection it is interesting to note that the Mosaic Law recognized the law of periodicity and fixed upon Sunday as the first day of the week and upon Saturday (the Sabbath) as the last or "rest" day in which to prepare for another period of seven days. It is now very generally thought that the normal span of human life should be as much as one hundred and fifty years. This would constitute three cycles of forty nine years each, the first corresponding to youth, the second to maturity and the third to fruition.

The Law of Sevens in Febrile Diseases

If we apply the law of periodicity to the course of acute febrile or inflammatory diseases we find that the sixth day from the beginning of the first well defined symptoms marks the first "Friday" period or the first crisis of the disease, and that every seventh day thereafter is also distinguished by aggravations and changes either for better or for worse.(1)

The Law of Sevens in Chronic Diseases

Applied to the cure of chronic diseases under the influence of natural methods of living and of treatment, the law of crisis and periodicity

(1)
This discussion of periodicity in connection with acute disease has been amplified by Mackinnon as follows:- With regard to the treatment of acute diseases, barring pleurisy and typhoid fever, a time period of two weeks is involved. In cases of pleurisy and typhoid the time period is seven weeks. Just as soon as a temperature appears, the first thing to do is to apply a body pack, from the armpits to the lower level of the abdomen. This pack should be changed every three hours during the day-time. The body should be sponged from head to foot with cold water immediately the pack is removed. Follow this with the fresh pack. Dilute fruit juices such as orange, grape-fruit and prune should be the only nourishment. Water or fruit juice should be taken about every hour during waking time. This keeps water moving towards the kidneys which is important. When a temperature shows up, as a general average, it follows this pattern: First three days the temperature stays up; second period of two days in tends to drop down, perhaps to normal; sixth day it tends to rise again and this is a dangerous day especially if natural methods have been ignored; on the evening of the seventh day the temperature tends to fall below normal. The second week is the recuperative period. In pleurisy and typhoid days are replaced by weeks. In other cases it is imperative that the patient stays in bed for a period of seven days, otherwise there is apt to be a relapse. If there is an indication of a diphtheritic condition it would be well to begin with the use of a whole sheet pack. The time for this should be from two to three hours. Then follow with the body pack.

manifests as follows: When a chronic patient, whose chances of cure are good, is placed under proper (natural) conditions of living and treatment he will, as a rule, experience five weeks of marked improvement. The sixth week, if conditions are favourable, usually marks the beginning of acute reactions or healing crises. This means that the healing forces of the organism have grown strong enough to begin the work of acute elimination. By all sorts of acute reactions, such as skin eruptions, diarrhoeas, feverish, inflammatory and catarrhal conditions, boils, abscesses, muco-purulent discharges etc., nature now endeavours to remove the latent, chronic disease taints from the system.

The allopathic school of medicine looks upon these acute reactions as the disease; we of the Nature Cure School recognize them as milestones on the road to cure. The entire structure of allopathy is built upon a misconception of the true nature of disease. At this fundamental point the ways of the old school and the Nature Cure school part, never to meet again.

Many allopathic physicians who read the foregoing statements will indignantly deny their truthfulness. They will claim that the old school of medicine also regards acute reactions as manifestations of nature's eliminative activity and that it endeavours to promote the same by all possible means. We are aware that in many instances the teachings of the allopathic school acknowledge, theoretically at least, the eliminative character of acute diseases. But how does practice agree with theory? Skin eruptions and boils are "cured" with metallic and other ointments; coughs, mucous discharges and diarrhoeas are arrested by opiates and astringents; fevers and inflammations are subdued by quinine, coal tar products or the ice bag; headaches and pains of all kinds are stopped by morphine, cocaine, phenacetin, salicylates etc.; excited nerves and restless brain are paralyzed and stupefied with bromide and chloral; syphilitic ulcers and gonorrheal discharges are checked by cauterization, drying powders or strong antiseptic injections; scrofulous glands and goitres are "absorbed" by iodine; diseased tonsils or inflamed appendix are extirpated with the surgeon's knife; — and so on, ad infinitum. Are such suppressive tactics calculated to induce and promote elimination?

The character of healing crises and the time of their occurrence in any given case can often be accurately predicted by means of the diagnosis from the iris of the eye, — from nature's records in the iris. But the best of all methods of diagnosis is the cure itself, because weak spots and morbid taints in the organism are revealed through the healing crisis. Frequently we hear from a patient in the throes of crises: "These are the same old aches and pains that I had before. This is not a crisis." He has lost sight of the fact that healing crises are nothing more nor less than a coming-up-again of old disease conditions, an acute manifestation of ailments which had become chronic through neglect or suppression. Of course, therefore, they are "the same old aches and pains" but the difference now is that they are now running their course under different conditions because the patient is now living in harmony with nature's laws. Nature is, in fact, "tearing down the old and building up the new." The old schools of healing often proclaim Mother Nature a "poor healer", but we of the Nature Cure school believe that the power which created this complex mechanism knows also how to preserve and repair it. Every healing crisis passed under natural conditions assisted by natural methods of treatment leaves the body purified and strengthened and nearer to perfect health.

Another question we frequently hear is: "Do healing crises develop in every chronic disease under natural treatment?" Our answer is: "If the condition of the patient is not favourable to a cure, that is, if the vitality be too low and the destruction of vital parts too far advanced, the healing crises may be proportionately delayed or may not occur at all. In such cases the disease symptoms will increase in severity and complexity and become more destructive instead of more constructive until the final crisis. The end may come quickly or the patient may decline gradually toward the final termination.

Again, patients ask us: "Through how many crises shall I have to pass?" We tell them — just as many as you need; no more, no less. So long as there is anything wrong in the system, crises will come and go; but each crisis, if successfully passed, is another milestone on the road to perfect health. It is intensely interesting to observe in how orderly and intelligent a manner nature proceeds in her work of healing and repair. One problem after another is taken up and adjusted. First of all the digestive organs are put into better condition because further progress depends upon proper assimilation and elimination. The bowels must act freely and naturally before any permanent improvement can take place. A treatment which fails to accomplish this first preliminary improvement will surely fail to produce more important results. In this connection it is significant that nearly all our patients, when they come under our care, are suffering from stubborn constipation in spite of (or on account of) lifelong drugging.

The greatest difficulty in our work lies in conducting our pateints safely through the crisis periods. The first, preliminary improvement is often so marked that the patient believes himself already cured. This feeling of mental elation and physical well being is usually the sign that the first general improvement has progressed far enough to prepare the system for a healing crisis. Therefore, I emphasise that the first improvement is not the cure and that it is only the preparation for the real fight which is soon to begin. In fact, within a few days the same patient is often down in the slough of despond. His digestive organs may be in a wretched condition, he may be nauseated, his tongue coated, and he may be suffering from headache or one of a multitude of other symptoms, according to his individual condition. Many of the old aches and pains may come again with renewed force. Moreover, healing crises, representing radical changes in the system, are always accompanied by physical and mental weakness and often by great mental depression and a feeling of strong revulsion from the natural regimen and everything connected with it. The patient may think that, after all, Nature Cure is not for him, that he is growing worse instead of better. In these critical times it requires all our powers of persuasion to keep the depressed and discouraged one from giving up the fight and "taking something" to relieve his distress. He insists that "something" must be done for him and cannot understand how he will ever get out of his "awful condition" without some good strong medicine. If our patients were not continually and thoroughly instructed regarding the laws of crisis and of periodicity and if we did not encourage them to persevere many would not hold out during these critical periods. This explains why so many people fail to be cured and it also explains why natural living and self-treatment often do not meet with the desired results if carried on without the instruction and guidance of a competent, experienced Nature Cure physician. However, every crisis which is conducted to a successful conclusion in accordance with nature's laws, with or without help, becomes an inspiration to the sufferer who follows her guidance and assists her with intelligent effort.

CHAPTER XXIV

THE TRUE SCOPE OF MEDICINE

One able to read the signs of the times cannot help observing the powerful influence which Nature Cure philosophy is already exerting upon the trend of modern medical science. In Germany the younger generation of physicians has been forced by public demand to adopt the natural methods of treatment, and the German government has introduced them into the medical departments of the army and navy. In English speaking countries the foremost members of the medical profession are beginning to talk straight Nature Cure doctrine, to condemn the use of drugs and to endorse unqualifiedly the Nature Cure method of treatment. As an illustration I quote from an article on "Medicine" by Sir William Osler in the Encyclopedia Americana. (Vol. X.)

"The new school does not feel itself under obligation to give any medicines whatever, while a generation ago not only could few physicians have held their practice unless they did, but few would have thought it safe or scientific. Of course, there are still many cases where the patient or the patient's friends must be humoured by administering medicine where it is not really needed, and indeed often where the bouyancy of mind which is the real curative agent, can only be created by making him wait hopefully for the expected action of medicine; and some physicians still cannot unlearn the old training. But the change is great. The modern treatment of disease relies very greatly on the old so called "natural" methods, diet and exercise, bathing and massage, — in other words, giving the natural forces the fullest scope by easy and thorough nutrition, increased flow of blood, and the removal of obstructions to the excretory systems or the circulation in the tissues. One notable example is typhoid fever. At the outset of the nineteenth century it was treated with "remedies" of the extremest violence, — bleeding, blistering, vomiting, purging, and the administration of antimony and mercury. and plenty of other heroic remedies. Now the patient is bathed and nursed and carefully tended, but rarely given medicine. This is the result partly of the remarkable experiments of the Paris and Vienna schools in the action of drugs, which have shaken the stoutest faiths; and partly on the constant and reproachful object lessons of homoeopathy. No regular physician would ever admit that the homoeopathic preparations, "infinitesimals", could do any good as curative agents; and yet it was perfectly certain that homoeopaths lost no more of their patients than others. There was but one conclusion to draw, — that most drugs had no effect whatever on the diseases for which they were administered."

Sir William Osler is one of the greatest medical authorites on drugs now living. He was formerly professor of materia medica at the Johns Hopkins University of Baltimore, and now is Regius Professor of Medicine at Oxford. His books on medical practice are in use in universities and medical schools throughout the English speaking world. His views on drugs and their real value as expressed in this article should be an eye opener to those good people who believe that we of the Nature Cure school are altogether too radical, extreme, and somewhat "cranky". However, what Sir William says regarding the "New School" is true only of a few advanced members of the medical profession. On the rank and file the idea of drugless healing has about the same effect as a red rag to a bull. There are few physicians in general practice who would not lose their bread and butter if they attempted to practice drugless healing on their patients. Both the profession and the public need a good deal more education along Nature Cure lines before rational methods can become general.

It is interesting to note that in his article Sir William admits the efficacy of mental therapeutics and therapeutic faith as curative agents and ascribes the helpful effects of medicine to their stimulating influence upon the mind rather than to any beneficial action of the drugs themselves. With regard to the origin of the modern treatment of typhoid fever, however, he is certainly wrong. The credit for the introduction of hydropathic treatment of this disease does not truly belong to the "remarkable experiments of the Paris and Vienna schools". In fact, these schools and the whole medical profession fought this treatment for many years. For thirty years Priessnitz, Bilz, Kuhne, Father Kneipp and many other pioneers of Nature Cure were persecuted and prosecuted, they were dragged into the courts and tried on charges of malpractice and manslaughter for using their sane and natural methods. Not until Dr. Brandt of Berlin wrote an essay on the good results obtained by the hydropathic treatment of typhoid fever and it had in that way received orthodox baptism and sanction, was it adopted by advanced physicians all over the world. Through this the mortality of the disease has been reduced from over 50 per cent under the old drug treatment to less than 5 per cent.

Unfortunately the average medical practitioner has not yet learned that the same simple fasting and cold water treatment used so effectively in the cure of typhoid fever, is just as effective in the treatment of every other

169

form of acute disease as, for instance, scarlet fever, diphtheria, smallpox, cerebro-spinal meningitis, appendicitis etc. Therefore, we hold that there is no necessity for the employment of poisonous drugs, serums and antitoxins for these purposes.

I would also take Sir William to task on what he says about the effects of homoeopathic and other medicines. The effect of homoeopathic medicine is not, as he implies, altogether negative and homoeopaths lose fewer patients than allopaths on account of the effectiveness of their remedies. Moreover, when he says that most drugs have no effect whatsoever, he makes a serious misstatement. While they may not contribute to the cure of the disease for which they are given, they are often very harmful in themselves. Almost every virulent poison known to man is found in allopathic prescriptions. It is now definitely established by diagnosis from the iris of the eye that these poisons have a tendency to accumulate in the system, to concentrate in certain parts and organs for which they have a special affinity and there to cause irritation and actual destruction of tissues. The greater part of all chronic diseases is created or complicated by the suppression of acute diseases by means of drug poisons and through the destructive effects of drugs themselves. This is coming to be realized by advanced physicians in Europe and America. However, it also seems to me that Osler "pours out the baby with the bath" in that his opinion regarding the ineffectiveness of drugs is entirely too radical. There is a legitimate scope for medicinal remedies in so far as they build up the blood on a natural basis and serve as tissue foods. Many people who have lost their faith in old school methods of treatment have swung to the other extreme. In fact, Osler himself has been and can be accused of being a "medical nihilist". We of the Nature Cure school do not absolutely condemn the use of all medicines. We do condemn the use of drugs in so far as they suppress acute diseases or healing crises, which are nature's cleansing and healing efforts; but, on the other hand, we realize that there is a wide field for the helpful application of medicinal remedies in so far as they act as foods to the tissues of the body and as neutralizers and eliminators of waste and morbid materials.(1)

(1)
This quotation from the writings of Sir William Osler and Lindlahr's discussion of it are of very great interest in the light of developments since that time. Sir William was a person of imposing stature as a man, as a scholar and teacher and as a physician, and he exercised a great influence on the development of medical practice and teaching in his time. This influence was on the whole a very good one, but there is a certain justice in the contention that he ended up by being something of a nihilist. He "debunked" and swept away much that was bad and in particular had little use for the crude and powerful drug medication which was common in his early days or for vaccination. He did not, however, have much to put in the place of what he criticized or destroyed except that he was a firm believer in good hygiene, good nursing and a human and common sense approach to patients. He was not tempted, as might have been, to take steps either

In every form of chronic disease there exists in the system an excess of certain morbid materials and a deficiency of certain mineral constituents, "organic" salts, which are essential to the normal functions of the body. Thus in anaemic diseases the blood is lacking in iron which picks up the oxygen in the air cells of the lungs and carries it to the tissues, and in sodium, which combines with the carbon dioxide that is constantly being liberated in the system and conveys it to the organs of depuration, especially the lungs and the skin. (In point of fact, oxygen starvation is sometimes due as much to the deficiency of sodium and the consequent accumulation of carbon dioxide in the system as to the lack of iron in the blood, as assumed by the old school of medicine). Foods or medicinal remedies which supply this deficiency of iron and sodium in the organism tend to overcome the anaemic conditions.

The great range of uric acid diseases, such as rheumatism, calculi, arterio-sclerosis, certain forms of diabetes and albuminuria, are due on the one hand to the excessive consumption of acid producing foods, and on the other to a deficiency in the blood of certain alkaline mineral elements, especially sodium, magnesium, lithium and potassium whose office is to neutralize the acids which are created and liberated in the processes of starch and protein digestion. In another chapter I have explained the origin and progressive development of uric acid diseases and in our volume on "Natural Dietetics" there is additional proof that practically all diseases are caused by or are complicated with acid conditions in the system. Any foods or medicines which provide the system with sufficient quantities of the acid binding, alkaline mineral salts prove good medicine for all forms of acid diseases. Lime, potassium, phosphorus and silicon are needed to impart textile strength and stamina to the bony and fleshy tissues of the body. The mineral constituents necessary to the vital economy of the organism should, however, be supplied in the live, organized form, as will be explained more fully later.

From what I have said it becomes apparent that it is impossible to draw a sharp line of distinction between foods and medicines. All foods which

---

towards homoeopathy or towards the vigorous application of Nature Cure methods. Had he been so the history of medicine since his time might have been very different. As it was the rooms which he left swept and garnished have been filled with much that is new and strange. The picture in connection with drugs has greatly changed since the time of Osler and Lindlahr who were roughly contemporaries. The chemotherapy of today is infinitely more varied and more subtle than the old and there has been added to it the discovery and elaboration of anti-biotics. It would perhaps be hard to say whether this is a change for the better or for the worse. The amount of anti-biotics and inorganic drugs now being used is truly staggering, but it is possible that some preparations can sometimes be used temporarily in emergencies in ways which are justifiable and helpful and which may even save life. Iridiagnosis is perhaps the best way of revealing what substances are harmful to the body and what are not.

serve the above named purposes are "good medicines", and all non-poisonous herb extracts and homoeopathic remedies that have the same effect upon the system are, for the same reason, good "foods". The medicinal treatment prescribed by the Nature Cure school consists largely in the proper selection and combination of food materials. This must be so. It stands to reason that nature has provided within the ranges of natural foods all the elements which man needs in the way of food and medicine. But it is quite possible that, through continued abuse, the digestive apparatus has become so weak and abnormal that it cannot function properly, that it cannot absorb and assimilate from natural foods a sufficient quantity of the elements which the organism needs. In such cases it may be very helpful and, indeed imperative to prescribe the organic mineral salts in the forms of fruit, herb and vegetable juices, extracts and decoctions. Among the best food remedies are extracts of leafy vegetables such as lettuce, spinach, Scotch kale, cabbage, Swiss chard, etc. These vegetables are richer than any other foods in the salts of positive mineral elements. The extract may be prepared from one or more of these vegetables according to the supply on hand or the tolerance of the digestive organs and the taste and preference of the patient. They should be ground to a pulp in a vegetable grinder, then pressed out in a small fruit press. One or two teacups per day will be sufficient to supply the needs of the system for mineral salts. This extract should be prepared fresh every day.

The "Tissue Remedies" first prepared by Schuessler, one of the pioneers in the Nature Cure movement, are refined triturations of the positive mineral elements needed by the human organism. However, they remain in the inorganic mineral state and therefore cannot supplant the organic mineral salt combinations prepared in the best possible form in nature's own laboratory in the fruits, vegetables, cereals and dairy products.

The Difference between Organic and Live Organized Matter

Professor Béchamp, the discoverer of microzymes, has pointed out distinctly the difference between organic and live, organized substances. He taught that what chemists call "organic" matter consists of various combinations of carbon with other elements of matter, while "live organized" substances are those which contain live microzymes. He says in his book on "The Blood": "The distinguishing of organic matter reduced to the condition of definite proximate principles (that is to say, of the organic matter of the chemists, which is not living) from natural organic matters, such as they exist in animals and plants; that is to say, of the organic matter of physiologists and of anatomists, which is reputed living or as having lived, lies in this. The proximate principles are naturally unalterable, do not ferment even when they are left in contact with a limited quantity of ordinary air, in water at a physiological temperature; on the other hand, natural organic matters, under the like conditions or absolutely protected from atmospheric germs, invariably alter and ferment."

This distinction made by the great scientist between the "organic" and "live organized" substances to me is as interesting and important as the discovery of the microzymes. It confirms what I have frequently claimed, that nature's live foods and medicines in vegetable and animal matter cannot be imitated and substituted by the chemist in the laboratory. The organic matter of the chemist is not alive with microzymes whose ferments produce all the great changes in the normal metabolic processes of the living body. In order to produce live, organized foods and medicines the chemist should have the power to produce microzymes. While I admit that the so-called organic compounds are less destructive than inorganic minerals like mercury, arsenic etc. in the crude, earthy form, it is also true that the carbohydrate and protein compounds produced by the chemist in the laboratory cannot take the place of nature's living foods and medicines in vegetable, animal and human protoplasm. It is for this reason that the Schuessler "Tissue Foods" never take the place of the products of nature's own laboratory, because they are not even organic substances. The claims of Professor Béchamp are proved by the fact that organic or proximate food substances (both are identical in nature) cannot sustain life. It has been proved by scientists of the Nature Cure school, long ago, that animals fed on chemically pure starch, white sugar or other organic or proximate food elements die sooner than animals who receive nothing but water. The obvious explanation now is that organic compounds do not contain the microzymes whose ferments are necessary to "digest" the food materials.

This brings us to another point in connection with the chemistry and physiology of digestion. Formerly it was assumed that all the ferments which digest the foods are produced by the body. Now it might appear that to a large extent the ferments which digest the foods are produced by the microzymes in foods themselves, provided, of course, that the foods are of the live, organized kind.[1]

[1]
There are various forms and degrees of cooking, processing and refining to which food can be subjected and these vary considerably in their effects. The idea here put forwards that microzymes in the food eaten or ferments derived from them play an important part in the processes of digestion adds very much to the argument in favour of consumption of much food in the raw state. However, much of the harm which is done

Thus our attitude towards the use of medicinal remedies is that we do not hesitate to prescribe homoeopathic medicaments (which as we shall further explain in another chapter, produce their results because they work in harmony with the laws of nature), herb juices and extracts, which assist in the elimination of morbid matter and in building up blood and lymph on a normal basis. Such remedies supply the organism with the mineral elements in which it is deficient, in the live, organized, easily assimilable form and they increase its fighting power against disease without in any way inflicting injury upon it. Here lies the legitimate scope of medicine. On the other hand we reject all drugs or medicines which tend to hinder, check or suppress nature's cleansing and regenerating processes. We never prescribe anything in the least degree poisonous. We avoid all anodynes, hypnotics, sedatives, antipyretics, laxatives, cathartics, and like harmful agents. Judicious fasting, cold water applications, manipulative treatment, and, if necessary, warm water injections in case of constipation, will do everything that is claimed for poisonous drugs.

Physicians of various schools, diet experts and food chemists have for many years been divided on the question as to whether mineral substances which in the live form enter into the composition of the human body may safely be used in foods and medicine in the inorganic form. The medical profession is almost unanimous in holding that it is permissible and "good practice" to do so, and nearly every allopathic medical prescription contains some such inorganic substance or, worse, one or more virulent mineral poisons, such as mercury, arsenic, phosphorus, etc. So far the discussion about the usefulness or otherwise of inorganic minerals as foods and medicines has been largely theoretical. Neither party has had positive proofs for its contentions. Now, however, nature's records in the iris of the eye appear to settle the question once and for all. One of the fundamental principles of the science of iridiagnosis is that nothing shows in the iris by abnormal signs or discolourations except that which is abnormal in the body or injurious to it. When substances which are uncongenial or poisonous to the system accumulate in any part or organ of the body in

---

to food comes not so much from conservative cooking as from refining and processing which removes from it most or all of the alkaline minerals and vitamins, leaving only acid forming substances and throwing the body chemistry out of balance. Lady Eve Balfour who has spent a life time associated with the Soil Association gives in her pamphlet "Soil and Seed" an account of an experiment carried out in the U.S. in which cats were fed on various diets from entirely raw food and milk to diet wholly composed of processed, cooked and pasteurized material. This was carried on for some generations of the cats and those strains which were fed on the raw whole food remained healthy and fertile whereas the others became increasingly sickly and eventually sterile. Moreover, the soil in the pens of the well fed cats was fertile and produced healthy plants whereas the other pens showed various degrees of infertility. This points to the conclusion that health and vitality is a cycle which begins in the soil, goes through plants, animals and man and returns to the soil. See Appendix IV.

sufficient quantities, their presence is indicated by certain signs and abnormal colours on the corresponding areas of the iris. In this way nature makes known by her records in the iris which substances are injurious to the body and which are harmless. Certain mineral elements, such as iron, sodium, lime, magnesium, phosphorus, sulphur etc., which are among the important constituents of the human body, may be taken in the live form in fruits and vegetables or in herb extracts in large amounts, in fact in excess of the actual needs of the body, but they will not show in the iris of the eye because they are easily eliminated from the system. If, however, the same minerals be taken in the inorganic form in considerable quantities, the iris will exhibit certain well defined signs and discolourations in the areas corresponding to those parts of the body in which the mineral substances have accumulated.

Obviously, nature does not intend that these mineral elements should enter the organism in the inorganic form, and therefore, the organs of depuration are not designed to neutralize and eliminate them. Thus, for instance, any amount of iron may be taken in vegetable and herb extracts but will not show in the iris. Whatever is taken in excess of the needs of the body will be promptly eliminated. If, however, similar quantities of iron be taken for the same length of time in the inorganic mineral form, the iron will accumulate in the tissues of stomach and bowels and begin to show in the iris in the form of a rust brown discolouration in the corresponding areas of the digestive organs, directly around the pupil. In similar manner, sodium, which is one of the most important mineral elements in the human body, if taken in the inorganic form such as sodium bicarbonate or sodium salicylate, will show in a heavy white ring near the outer edge of the iris. Sulphur will show in the form of yellowish discolourations in the area of stomach and bowels. Iodine in the inorganic form, prepared from ash or sea weeds, shows in the iris in well defined bright red spots. Phosphorus appears in whitish-yellow streaks and clouds in the areas corresponding to the organs in which it has accumulated.

An interesting exception to this rule is our common table salt (NaCl), sodium chloride), which is an inorganic mineral combination. So far, iridologists have not discovered any sign in the iris indicating that this mineral substance accumulates abnormally in the body. It may be that this salt is more easily eliminated from the system, since it is normally present in large amounts in the blood serum. It is also possible that the salt is split up into sodium and chlorine and that these units enter into new chemical combinations. This might explain why salt is the only mineral substance which is extensively used as food by humanity in general. Advocates of the liberal use of table salt usually argue that animals guided by their natural instinct do not hesitate habitually to visit "salt licks".

Animals will do this when the vegetation on which they subsist is deficient in mineral salts as the result of deficiency of the minerals in the soil. It must, however, be remembered that animals, as well as human beings, may acquire bad habits. Horses will founder on oats when they have free access to grass and hay. In Montana at one time we kept in confinement a splendid elk. He would eat more chewing tobacco in a day than could have been consumed by a dozen cowboys. Though undoubtedly a limited amount of inorganic sodium chloride can be utilized by the body, I do not encourage the excessive use of salt, either in cooking food or at the table. Taken in considerable quantities, it is very injurious to the tissues of the body. The boiling of foods precipitates the salts of sodium, magnesium, potassium, etc. This is the reason why "cooked foods" crave more salt than raw food (The various aspects of the table salt problem are fully discussed in the Nature Cure Cook Book.)

Before the days of canned vegetables and fruits, scorbut or scurvy was a common disease among mariners and others who had to subsist for long periods of time on salted meats and were deprived of vegetables. The disease manifested as a breaking down of the gums and other tissues of the body, accompanied by bleeding and much soreness. As soon as these people partook of fresh fruits and vegetables, the scurvy disappeared. The minerals which occur in organized combinations in these foods furnished the building stones which imparted tensile strength to the tissues and stopped the disintegration of the fleshy structures.

The Nature Cure regimen aims to provide sodium chloride as well as other minerals and salts required by the body in organized form in foods and medicines. When the use of inorganic minerals is discontinued and the proper methods of eliminative treatment are applied, these mineral substances are gradually dislodged and carried out of the system. Simultaneously with their elimination disappear their signs in the iris and the disease symptoms which their presence had created in the organism. In this connection it is significant that those minerals which are congenial to the system, that is, those which in their organized form enter into the composition of the body, are much more easily eliminated, if they have been taken in the inorganic form, than those substances which are naturally foreign and poisonous to the human organism, such as mercury, arsenic, bromide, the different coal tar preparations, etc. This is proved by the fact that the signs of the minerals which are normal constituents of the human body disappear from the iris of the eye much sooner than the signs of those minerals which are foreign and naturally poisonous to the system. The difficulty which we experience in eliminating mineral poisons from the body would seem to indicate that nature never intended them to be used as foods or medicines. The intestines, kidneys, skin, mucous membranes, and other organs of depuration are evidently not constructed or prepared to cope with inorganic poisonous substances and to eliminate them completely. Accordingly these poisons show a tendency to accumulate in certain parts or organs of the body for which they have a special affinity or where the resistance is lowered, there to act as destructive irritants.

The diseases which we find most difficult to cure, even by the most radical application of natural methods, are cases of drug poisoning. Substances which are foreign to the human organism, especially the inorganic mineral poisons, positively destroy tissues and organs and are much harder to eliminate from the system than the encumbrances of morbid materials and waste matter produced in the body by wrong habits of living. The obvious reason for this is that our organs of elimination are intended and constructed to excrete only such waste products as are formed in the organism in the processes of metabolism. Tuberculosis or cancer may be caused in a scrofulous or psoric constitution by overloading the system with meat, coffee, alcohol or tobacco; but as soon as these bad habits are discontinued, and the organs of elimination treated by natural methods, the encumbrances will be eliminated and the much dreaded symptoms will subside and disappear, often with surprising rapidity. On the other hand, mercury, arsenic, quinine, strychnine, iodine, etc., accumulate in the brain, spinal cord, and the cells and tissues of the vital organs, causing actual destruction and disintegration. The tissues affected are not easily rebuilt and it is exceedingly difficult to stir up the destructive mineral poisons and to eliminate them from the system. Therefore it is an indisputable fact that many of the most stubborn, so called "incurable" diseases are drug diseases.

The Importance of Natural Diet

While certain medicinal remedies in organized form may be very useful in supplying quickly a deficiency of mineral elements in the system, we should aim to keep our bodies in a normal healthy condition by proper food selection and combination. A brief description of the scientific basis of "natural dietetics" will be found in a later chapter, but we find that nature has supplied in overabundance all the elements which the human organism needs in natural foods, otherwise she would be a very poor organizer and provider. We should learn, therefore, to select and combine food materials in such a manner as to supply all the needs of the body in the best possible way and thus insure perfect health and strength without the use of medicines. Which is more in harmony with the basic laws of morality and with wise common sense, — to leave people in total ignorance of the principles of natural dietetics, thus allowing them to drift into all sorts of diseases through food and drink poisoning and then to "cure" them with artificial chemical preparations; or, to teach them how to eat and drink in such a way as to establish perfect, natural immunity to disease? Why should we attempt to cure anaemia with inorganic iron, hyperacidity of the stomach with baking soda, swollen glands with iodine, the itch with sulphur, rachitic conditions in infants with lime water, etc., etc., when these mineral elements are contained in abundance and in live, organized form in fruits, vegetables and herbs. Unfortunately, however, a great many individuals, through wrong habits of living and of treating their ailments, have weakened their digestive organs to such a degree that they are incapable of assimilating properly their food and require, at least temporarily, natural stimulative treatment and a supply of the indispensible organic mineral salts through medicinal food preparations. In such cases the mineral elements must be provided in the most easily assimilable form in vegetable extracts which should be prepared fresh every day.

What has been said is sufficient, I believe, to justify the attitude of the Nature Cure school toward medicines in general. It explains why we condemn the use of inorganic minerals and poisonous substances, while we find a wide and useful field for medicinal remedies in the form of blood and tissue foods.[1]

[1]
    Lindlahr does here admit a certain usefulness in the Schuessler tissue salts, but he is not keen on them because of their "inorganic" character. His disciple, Mackinnon, on the other hand, looked on them with much more favour. These salts as originally prepared and advocated by Schuessler do seem to be something of a mystery in that while they appear to be intended as dietary supplements which are given to make up deficiences or to correct imbalances, they are in fact prepared after the manner of homeopathic remedies which normally act in the body in accordance with the law of similars. It would appear very doubtful whether the amount of the minerals contained in them could in fact be sufficient to make up deficiences in the chemical sense. It would seem more likely that the effects which they undoubtedly have are produced rather by causing a change in body metabolism which normalizes that metabolism in specific ways. If this is so, there can be little objection to them on the grounds of their "inorganic" character. More recently there has grown up a school of Biochemic Therapy associated, in England at least, with the name of Dr. Gilbert. This school absolutely denies that there is any essential difference in the case of mineral substances which are required by the body between those derived from animal or vegetable tissue and those derived from inorganic sources. They prepare such minerals from inorganic sources and use them in sufficient quantities to correct deficiencies and imbalances which they believe to exist. Such biochemic food supplements are usually prepared by an elaborate process of trituration but they are not potentized in the same way as homeopathic remedies or the Schuessler salts. It is claimed that not only are they harmless but that they are, in many cases, more easily assimilated and used by the body than the same substances taken in vegetable or flesh foods. There is here a definite conflict of opinion but it may be that there is some element of truth in both points of view though they may at first appear irreconcilable. It does seem that the body is intended to get the mineral substances it needs from food, and Julius Hensel who was the first great exponent of biochemic ideas

believed that health must begin in the soil and that the health of the soil and crops must be maintained not by chemical fertilizers but by putting back into the soil what has been taken from it. This he did largely by the use of ground rocks as well as animal and vegetable residues and manures. Others have done the same thing by the use of seaweed in various forms. On the other hand, it does appear that the body has a certain limited ability to assimilate and use mineral substances more directly either from water or from such substances as common salt and, if Hensel and some of his followers are right, in the form of ground rocks. It is surely not impossible that there is a real difference between minerals derived from vegetable or animal tissues and those derived directly from water or rocks, even though this difference may not be detectable by ordinary chemical analysis. On the other hand, it may be that certain ways of preparing mineral substances by great refinement or grinding may enable them to be used directly by the body in a very effective and rapid manner. Lindlahr may be very right in saying that the ultimate criterion for judging whether a substance is harmful or not is to be found in whether it produces signs or discolourations in the iris.

CHAPTER XXV

HOMOEOPATHY

When I first entered upon the study of medicine I could not believe in the curative power of homoeopathic doses, but experience caused me to change my mind. The well selected remedy administered at the right time often works wonders. True homoeopathic medicines in high potency doses are so highly refined and rarefied that they cannot possibly produce harmful results or suppress nature's cleansing and healing efforts; on the contrary, if employed according to the law of homeopathy: "Like cures like" they assist in producing acute reactions or 'healing crises', thus aiding nature in the work of purification and repair. In order to make clear the minuteness of the high potency doses, I will briefly explain the process of trituration, and it should be noted that the more dilute and refined the dose, the higher the "potency" is said to be. The first potency is prepared by mixing one part of the drug with nine parts of milk sugar. Milk sugar is used because it is a constituent of the human organism and therefore neutral. The mixture is macerated in a mortar for about twenty minutes. The product constitutes the first trituration or "potency" of the drug. The second potency is obtained by mixing one part of the first potency with nine parts of milk sugar and treating the mixture in the same way. The third and subsequent potencies are obtained in the same way and the process can be repeated to obtain potencies up to the hundred thousandth or even higher. In the higher potencies alcohol may be substituted for the milk sugar. It will be seen that, for instance, the fiftieth potency which is not considered a high one represents a dilution of the drug to be written with fifty noughts.

Homoeopathy works with the laws of cure, not against them. "Similia similibus curantur" translated into practice means that a drug capable of producing a certain set of disease symptoms in a healthy body when given in large doses, will relieve or "cure" a similar set of symptoms in the diseased organism, if the drug be given in small homoeopathic doses. For instance, belladonna given in large, poisonous doses to a healthy person will cause a peculiar headache with sharp, stabbing pains in forehead and temples, high fever, violent delirium, dilation of the pupils, dryness and rawness of the throat, scarlet redness of the skin, and extreme sensitiveness to light, jars and noise. It will be observed that this is a fair picture of a typical case of scarlet fever. A homoeopathic physician when called to a scarlet fever patient exhibiting in a marked degree three or more of the above described symptoms would prescribe a trituration of belladonna, say 6 — X. In numberless cases fever has subsided and its symptoms have rapidly disappeared under such treatment. This procedure is altogether different from the allopathic suppression of disease by drugs. The allopathic physician might use belladonna in the same case, but he would use from ten to twenty drops of tincture of belladonna repeated every three or four hours. Such doses are from twenty to forty times heavier than the homoeopathic 3-X or 6-X. The allopathic dose allays the fever symptoms by paralyzing the organism as a whole and the different vital organs and their functions in particular. By such a dosing nature is forcibly interrupted in her efforts of cleansing and healing; the acute reaction is suppressed but not cured. If fever be a healing effort of nature, it may be controlled and modified, but must not be suppressed. A minute dose of homoeopathic belladonna, acting on the innermost cells of the organism and their microzymes, which the coarse allopathic doses would paralyze, stimulates these cells to effort in the right direction. It brings about conditions similar to those produced by healing crises and thus assists nature's purifying effort; it is cooperation instead of counter-operation.

We must now examine how far the laws and theories of homoeopathy agree with and corroborate the laws and principles of Nature Cure philosophy. Hahnemann discovered the law of "similia similibus curantur" accidentally while investigating the effects of quinine on the human organism. Ever since then it has been applied successfully by him and his followers in treating human ailments. However, this law has been used empirically. Neither in the "Organon" nor in any other writings or teachings of Hahnemann and the homoeopathic school can be found a clear and concise explanation of why "Like cures like". This has led to the homoeopathic system being widely ignored or denied. With the aid of the three laws of cure, I believe it is possible to give the reasons and proofs for the workings of the homoeopathic system. The laws to which I refer are:— The Law of Cure, the Law of Dual Effect and the Law of Crises.

"Similia similibus curantur" is only another way of stating the fundamental law of Nature Cure: Every acute disease is the result of a cleansing and healing effort of nature. If a certain set of disease symptoms is the result of a healing effort of nature, and if I give a remedy which produces the same or similar symptoms in the system, am I not aiding nature in her attempt to overcome the abnormal condition? In such a case, the indicated homoeopathic remedy will not suppress the acute reaction, but will help it along, thus accelerating and hastening the curative process. In the last analysis, disease resides in the cell. The well being of the organism as a whole is dependent on the health of the individual cells of which it is composed. In order to cure the man we must free the cell of its encumbrances. Elimination must begin in the cell, not in the organs of depuration. Laxatives and cathartics, by irritating the digestive tract, may cause a forced evacuation of the contents of the intestinal canal but they do not eliminate the poisons which clog the cells and tissues. The eliminating organs do not make waste products; they are elaborated in the tissues. Stimulating the activity of the kidneys or the skin with drugs does not neutralize and oxidize the morbid materials in the cells and tissues. In stubborn chronic diseases, when the cells are too weak to throw off the latent encumbrances of their own accord, a well chosen homoeopathic remedy is often of great service in arousing them to acute reaction.

For instance, if the system is heavily encumbered with scrofulous taints and its vitality is lowered to such an extent that the individual cell cannot of itself throw off the morbid encumbrances by means of vigorous, acute effort, sulphur, if administered in doses sufficiently triturated and refined to affect the minute cells composing the organism and the still more minute microzymes of the cells, will start "disease vibrations" similar to those of acute scrofulosis and thus give the needed impetus to acute eliminative activity on the part of the individual cell. The acute reaction once started may develop into vigorous forms of scrofulous elimination such as skin eruptions, glandular swellings, abscesses, catarrhal discharges, etc.

The efficiency of the high potency homoeopathic doses is often questioned, but we must remember that, in the administration of medicines, the size of the dose should be adjusted to the size of the patient. If half a grain of a certain drug is the normal dose for an adult, the proper dose of the same drug for an infant, say one year old, is one twelfth of a grain. How small, in proportion then, should be the dose given to a cell a billion times as small as an infant? Can we even conceive how infinitely small must be the dose to fit the microzyme? The dose given to an adult would paralyze or perhaps kill an infant. In like manner the minute cell or microzyme would be benumbed and paralyzed by the drug suited to the infant's organism. But this is precisely how allopathy effects its fictitious cures. It suppresses inflammatory processes by paralyzing the cells and organs and their vital activities. Homoeopathy, on the other hand, adapts the smallness of the dose to the smallness of the tiny organism which is to be treated. Herein lies the reasonableness of the high potency dose.

The cell resembles man not only in physical and physiological aspects, but also in regard to the moral law. Elimination must commence in the cell and by virtue of the cell's personal effort. Its work cannot be done vicariously by drugs or the knife. Large allopathic doses of medicine may be given with the idea of doing the work for the cells by violently stimulating or else benumbing the organism as a whole or certain ones of the vital organs, but this is demoralizing and destructive to the cell. The powerful doses calculated to affect the body and its organs as a whole make superfluous or paralyze the individual efforts of the cell, and thus intensify the chronic disease conditions in cells and tissues.

It should also be noted that the late revelations of chemistry, Roentgen rays, X-rays, radioactivity of metals, and other discoveries of science, throw an interesting light upon the seemingly infinite divisibility of matter. A small particle of a given substance may for many years throw off a continuous shower of corpuscles without perceptibly diminishing its volume. For illustration we may take the odiferous musk. A few grains of this substance will fill a room with its penetrating aroma for years. When we smell musk or any other perfume, minute particles of it "bombard" the end filaments of the nerves of smell in the nose. Therefore the musk must be casting off such minute particles continually without apparent loss of substance. With the aid of this recent knowledge of the true nature of matter, of the minuteness and complexity of the atom, we can now understand much better how the highly triturated and refined homoeopathic remedy may still retain the "dynamic force" of the element, as Hahnemann expressed it, and how a remedy so "attenuated" may still be capable of exerting an influence upon the minute cell or the still more minute microzyme. Since chemistry and physiology have acquainted us with the finer forces of nature, demonstrating that they are mightier than the things we can apprehend by weight and measure, the claims of homoeopathy do not appear so absurd as they did a generation ago.

Undoubtedly, the good effect produced by a well-chosen remedy is heightened and strengthened by the mental and magnetic influence of the prescriber. The positive faith of the physician in the efficacy of the remedy, his sympathy and his indomitable will to assist the sufferer affect both the physical substance of the remedy and the mind of the patient. The varying mental and magnetic qualities of prescribers have undoubtedly much to do with the varying degrees of effectiveness of the same remedy when administered by different physicians. The true Hahnemannian homoeopath, who believes in his remedies as in his God, will concentrate his intellectual and spiritual forces on a certain remedy in order to accomplish certain well defined results. The bottle is not allowed to become empty. Whenever the "graft" runs low, it is replenished with distilled water, alcohol, milksugar, or another neutral vehicle. Every time he takes the medicine bottle in his hands these potent thought forms are projected into it: "You are the element sulphur (or whatever it may be), you produce in the human body a certain set of symptoms. You will produce these symptoms in the body of this patient."

If there be any virtue at all in magnetic, mental and psychic healing, the homoeopathic remedy must be also an effective agency for transmitting these healing forces from prescriber to patient. Transmission of these higher and finer forces, whether directly, telepathically, or by means of some physical agent, such as magnetized water, a charm or simile, etc., is the modus operandi in all the different forms of ancient and modern magic, "white" or "black". It is the active principal in mental healing, Christian Science, sympathy healing, voodooism, witchcraft, etc. We may assume, too, that the infinitely minute and sensitive microzymes are even more easily affected by the higher and finer forces and vibrations than the comparatively large and complex cell.

Earlier in this work the Law of Action and Reaction in its application to the treatment of disease was formulated as follows: "Every agent affecting the human organism has two effects; a first, temporary one and a second, lasting one. The second effect is directly opposite to the first." Allopathy, in giving large, toxic doses, takes into consideration only the first effect of the drug, and thereby accomplishes in the long run results directly opposite to those which it desires to bring about. It produces the very conditions which it tries to cure. As an example, note the permanent effects of laxatives, stimulants, and sedatives upon the system. On the other hand, the homoeopathic physician may use the same remedies as the allopath, provided they produce symptoms similar to those of the disease, but he administers the various drugs in such minute doses that their first effect is noticed only as a slight "homoeopathic aggravation", while their second and lasting effect is relied on to relieve and cure the disease. In other words, homoeopathy produces as the first effect a condition "like the disease", and counts on the second and lasting effect of the drug to bring about the opposite, or health, condition. This law of dual effect has been proved by homoeopathy for over a hundred years. An experienced homoeopathic prescriber would no more doubt it than he would doubt the law of gravitation.

If the remedy be well chosen in accordance with the law of "similia similibus curantur", the first homoeopathic aggravation, which corresponds to the Crisis of Nature Cure, will be followed by speedy readjustment. Nature has her way, the disorder runs its course, and the return to normal conditions is quicker and more perfect than if the homoeopathic remedy had not been employed or if nature's healing processes had been forcibly interrupted and suppressed by large, poisonous allopathic doses. Homoeopathy assists nature in removing the old encumbrances, whereas allopathy changes the acute, inflammatory healing effort into chronic destructive disease.

The law of "like cures like" is also of great practical importance from another point of view, that of economics. The best engineer is he who accomplishes the maximum result with the minimum expenditure of force and with the least friction. The same is true of the physician and his remedies. We have learned that drugs given in coarse allopathic doses attack and affect the organism as a whole. If, for instance, there is a catarrhal affection of the mucous membranes of the respiratory tract accompanied by fever, the allopath will give quinine in large doses to change this condition. He may accomplish his aim; but if so, he does it by paralyzing the heart, the respiratory centres, the red blood corpuscles and the excreting cells of the mucous membranes. The body as a whole and certain parts in particular are saturated with the drug poison and correspondingly weakened. As allopathy itself states it: "Quinine reduces fever by depressing the metabolism". On the other hand homoeopathic materia medica teaches that bryonia has a special affinity for the mucous membranes of the respiratory tract, and that its symptomatic effects correspond closely with those described in the preceding paragraph. If, in accordance with the law of "similia similibus curantur", a homoeopathic dose of bryonia be given to a patient exhibiting these symptoms, the remedy will assist nature in her work of cure. In doing this it will not attack and affect the entire organism, but only those mucous tissues for which it has a special affinity and which are most seriously affected. In other words, the large allopathic dose paralyzes the whole organism in order to produce its fictitious cure. The small homoeopathic dose, on the other hand, goes right to the spot where it is needed, and by mild harmless stimulation of the affected parts assists and supports the cells in their acute eliminative efforts. Thus homoeopathic medication is not only curative but also conservative and in the highest degree economic.

Finally, having become convinced of the truth of Hahnemann's law of similars and having occasion daily to observe its practical results in the treatment of acute and chronic diseases, we should not be justified in omitting homoeopathy from our system of treatment. The triturated homoeopathic doses of certain drugs may be of great service in bringing about the acute reactions which we so earnestly desire, especially in the treatment of chronic diseases of long standing. I am aware of the fact that in severe and obstinate conditions homoeopathy is often apparently

185

of no avail. But when the system has been strengthened by our natural methods — a rational vegetarian diet, hydrotherapy, neurotherapy, massage, corrective exercise, air and sun baths, normal suggestion, etc. — the homoeopathic remedies will work with much greater promptitude and efficiency. It is the combination of all the various healing factors which constitutes the perfect system of treatment. No disease conditions, even when apparently hopeless, can be pronounced incurable unless all these different healing factors, properly combined and applied, have been given a thorough trial. It is no charlatanic boast, but the simple truth, that the various natural methods of treatment properly applied, can and do cure so called incurable diseases, such as tuberculosis, cancer, locomotor ataxia, epilepsy, eczema, neurasthenia, insanity, and the worst forms of chronic dyspepsia and constipation — always providing that the patients possess sufficient vitality to react to the treatment and that destruction of vital parts and organs has not advanced too far. Hence our claim that while there are incurable patients, there are no incurable diseases.(1)

[1]
   The following additional explanation of the modus operandi of homoeopathic remedies has been given by an experienced homoeopathic physician:- "In nature it would seem that the higher the division of a particle, the very much greater is its proportional surface area and the very much more active is its power of chemical combination. For instance, a block of aluminium placed in a jar of oxygen shows no reaction when brought into daylight; whereas the same aluminium in the form of very fine filings will be stimulated by the daylight to a violent reaction with the oxygen so that the flask will be blown to pieces. Hence the finer the particle the quicker the reaction. The finer the division (that is the higher the potency) of the drug in the homoeopathic pill the quicker is its chemical reaction with the cell elements of the nerve endings in the mucosa and the greater the stimulus to the body to antidote the substance in the pill. Also, in the physiology laboratory it is well known that an electrical stimulus to a nerve below a certain threshold produces no reaction whereas an additional stimulus added to this to bring the total stimulus above the reactive threshold will produce a reactive contraction of the muscle supplied by the nerve." It is clear that in the administration of homoeopathic remedies we are not concerned with putting measurable quantities of any chemical substance into the body. We are dealing rather with energies and this is particularly so when we use high potencies. These remedies appear in the first instance to give a powerful stimulus to the nerve endings in the mucosa which causes the body to react in a particular way. Only if low potencies and tinctures are used could any of the substance get into the blood stream or tissues or exercise a direct influence on body chemistry. Another interesting point is that the symptom pictures on which homoeopathic prescribing is based lay as great emphasis on emotional and psycho-somatic states as on purely physical symptoms. This is even more so in the case of the Bach remedies which must be regarded as closely allied to conventional homoeopathy. This could point to the possibility that high potency homoeopathic remedies may be acting on the spiritual body or on a different plane to the purely physical and that the effects on the physical body are secondary to this as appears to be the case in some forms of "miraculous" or spiritual healing. While it is still difficult to give an entire explanation of the workings of homoeopathy in terms of conventional science, it would seem to be much less so than it used to be. There are two respects in which homoeopathy can be said to be highly scientific. (1) The remedies are administered in accordance with an universal principle or law, the law of similars, and (2) the provings of the various substances which are used in the remedies have been carried out over the years since the

time of Hahnemann in a most elaborate and scientific manner and are based on a profound knowledge of toxicology and of the effects produced by the administration of the various substances to healthy persons in ordinary dosages. Also the tendency of modern science has for some time now been towards a greater study and manipulation of energies and towards a realization of what can be achieved by the study of the infinitely small. This is already beginning to have an effect on medical practices and concepts and can be expected to do so increasingly in future. This should lead to an increased understanding in scientific terms of the modus operandi of homoeopathic procedures.

CHAPTER XXVI

NATURAL DIETETICS

The chemical composition of blood and lymph depends upon the chemical composition of food and drink and upon the normal or abnormal condition of the digestive organs. The purer food and drink, the less it contains of morbid matter and poison producing materials and the more it contains of the elements necessary for the proper execution of the manifold functions of the organism, for the building and repair of tissues and for the neutralization and elimination of waste and systemic poisons, the more normal and the more natural will be the diet.

The system of dietetics of the Nature Cure school is based upon the composition of milk, which is the only perfect natural food composition in existence. In its composition milk corresponds very closely to red, arterial blood and contains all the elements which the new born and growing organism needs in exactly the right proportions, providing, of course, that the human or animal body which produces the milk is in good health and lives on pure and normal foods. Therefore, if any food combination or diet is to be normal or natural it must approach in its chemical composition the chemical composition of milk or of red, arterial blood. This furnishes a strictly scientific basis for an exact science of dietetics and proves true not only in the chemical aspect of the diet problem but also in every other aspect and in its practical application.

The orthodox school of medicine pays little or no attention to rational food regulation. In fact, it knows nothing about it, because the subject of natural dietetics is as yet not taught in medical schools. As a result, the dietary advice given by the majority of old school practitioners is something as follows: "Eat what agrees with you: plenty of good nourishing food. There is nothing in dietetic fads. What is one man's meat is another man's poison, etc., etc." However, if we study dietetics from a strictly scientific point of view we cannot help finding that certain foods — among these especially the highly valued fleshfoods, eggs, pulses and cereals — create in the system large quantities of morbid, poisonous substances; while fruits and vegetables which are rich in organic salts, tend to neutralize and to eliminate from the system the waste materials and poisons created in the processes of protein and starch digestion. The accumulations of waste and systemic poisons are the cause of the majority of diseases arising within the human organism. Therefore it is imperative that the neutralizing and eliminating foods be provided in sufficient quantities. Around this revolves the entire problem of natural dietetics. While the old school of medicine looks upon starches, fats and proteins as the only elements of nutrition worthy of consideration, Nature-Cure aims to reduce these foods in the natural dietary and to increase the purifying and eliminating fruits and vegetables.

In this volume we cannot go into the details of the diet question; this will be done in another volume. I will mention here in a general way that in the treatment of chronic diseases, with few exceptions, I favour a strict vegetarian diet for the reason that most chronic diseases are created by the accumulation of the fæces of the cells in the system, as before stated. Every piece of animal flesh is saturated with the excrement of the cells in the form of uric and many other kinds of acids, alkaloids of putrefaction, xanthins, ptomaines, etc. The organism of the meat eater must dispose not only of its own impurities produced in the processes of digestion and of cell metabolism, but also of the morbid substances which are already contained in the animal flesh. Since the curing of chronic diseases consists largely in purifying the body of morbid materials, it stands to reason that a chronic must cease taking these in his food and drink. To do otherwise would be like sweeping the dirt out of a house through the back door and throwing it in again through the front door. Whether one approves of strict vegetarianism as a continuous mode of living or not it will be admitted that the change from meat diet to a non meat diet must be of great benefit in the treatment of chronic diseases. The cure of chronic conditions depends upon radical changes in the cells and tissues of the body. The old, abnormal, faulty diet will continue to build the same abnormal and disease encumbered tissues. The more thorough and radical the change in diet toward normality and purity, the sooner the cells and tissues of the body will change towards the normal and thus bring about the complete regeneration of the organism. Anything short of this may be palliative treatment, but is not worthy of the name of "cure".

CHAPTER XXVII

FASTING

Next in importance to building up the blood on a natural basis is the elimination of waste, morbid matter and poisons from the system. This depends to a large extent upon the right diet; but it must be promoted by the various methods of eliminative treatment: fasting, hydrotherapy, massage, physical exercise, air and sun baths, and, in the way of medicinal treatment, homœopathic remedies.

Foremost among the methods of purification stands fasting, which of late years has become quite popular and is regarded by many people as a panacea for all human ailments. However, it is a two-edged sword. According to circumstances it may do a great deal of good or a great deal of harm. Kuhne, the German pioneer of Nature Cure, claimed that "disease is a unit", that it consists in the accumulation of waste and morbid matter in the system. Since his time many "naturists" claim that fasting offers the best and quickest means of eliminating systemic poisons and other encumbrances. To "fast it out" seems simple and plausible but it does not always prove to be successful in practice. Fasting enthusiasts overlook the fact that in many cases lowered vitality and weakened powers of resistance precede and make possible the accumulation of morbid matter in the organism. If the encumbrances consist merely of superfluous flesh or fat or of accumulated waste materials, fasting may be sufficient to break up the accumulations and to eliminate the impurities. If however, the disease has its origin in other causes or if it is due to a weakened, negative constitution and lowered powers of resistance, fasting may aggravate the abnormal conditions instead of improving them. We hear frequently of long fasts extending over many weeks, recklessly undertaken without the prescription and guidance of a competent dietetic adviser, without proper preparation of the system and the right subsequent treatment. Many a good constitution has thus been permanently injured and wrecked.

When Fasting is Indicated

Persons of sanguine, vital temperament, with the animal qualities strongly developed, enslaved by bad habits and evil passions, will be greatly benefited by occasional short fasts. In such cases the experience, aside from promoting morbid elimination, affords a fine drill in self discipline, strengthening of self control and conquest of the appetites. Vigorous, fleshy people, positive physically and mentally, especially those who do not take sufficient physical exercise, should take frequent fasts of one, two or three days' duration for the reduction of superfluous flesh and fat and for the elimination of systemic waste and other morbid materials. Such people should never eat more than two meals a day and many get along best on one meal.

However, different temperaments and constitutions require different treatment and management. People of a nervous emotional temperament, especially those who are below normal in weight and physically and mentally "negative", may be seriously and permanently injured by fasting. They should never fast except in acute diseases and during eliminative healing crises, when nature calls for the fast as a means of cure. People of this type are usually thin, with weak and flabby muscles. Their vital activities are at a low ebb and their magnetic envelopes (aura) are wasted and attenuated like their physical bodies. The red aura, which is created by the action of the purely animal functions and forces, is more or less deficient or entirely lacking. Such people have a tendency to become abnormally sensitive to conditions in the magnetic field (the astral plane). Next to the hypnotic or mediumistic process, there is nothing that induces abnormal psychism as readily as fasting. During a prolonged fast the purely animal functions of digestion, assimilation, etc. are almost completely at a standstill. The depression of the physical functions arouses and increases the psychic functions and may produce intense emotionalism and abnormal activity of the senses of the spiritual material body, the individual thus becoming abnormally clairvoyant, clairaudient and otherwise sensitive to conditions on the spiritual planes of life. This explains the spiritual exaltation, visions of "heavenly" scenes and beings or the fights with demons which are frequently, indeed uniformly reported by hermits, ascetics, saints, yogi, fakirs and dervishes.

Fasting facilitates hypnotic control of the sensitive by positive intelligences either on the physical or on the spiritual plane of being. In the one case we speak of hypnotism, in the other of mediumship, obsession or possession. These conditions are usually diagnosed by the medical practitioner as nervousness, nervous prostration, hysteria, paranoia, delusional insanity, double personality, mania, etc. (The various forms of abnormal psychism are fully described in "Nature Cure Eugenics".)([1]) The destructive effects of fasting are intensified by solitude, grief, worry, introspection, religious exaltation or any other form of depressive or destructive mental and emotional activity. Spirit "controls" often force their subjects to abstain from foods thus rendering them still more negative and submissive. Psychic patients when controlled or obsessed will frequently not eat unless they are forced or fed like an infant. When asked why they do not eat, these patients reply: "I mustn't. They will not let me." When we say, "Who?" the answer is, "These people. Don't you see them?" pointing to a void and becoming impatient when told that no one is there. The allopathic school says "delusion", we call it abnormal clairvoyance. In other instances the control tells the subject that his food and drink are poisoned or unclean. To the obsessed victim these suggestions are absolute reality. To place persons of the negative sensitive type on prolonged fasts and thus to expose them to the dangers just described is little short of criminal. Such patients need an abundance of the positive dairy products and vegetable foods in order to build up and strengthen their physical bodies and their magnetic envelopes which form the dividing and protecting wall between the terrestrial and astral planes.

A negative vegetarian diet, consisting principally of nuts, cereals and pulses but deficient in animal foods (the dairy products, eggs, honey) and in vegetables growing in or near the ground, may result in conditions similar to those which accompany prolonged fasting. Animal foods are elaborated under the influence of a higher life element than that controlling the vegetable kingdom and foods from the animal kingdom are useful to develop and stimulate the positive qualities in man. In the case of the psychic who is already deficient in the physical (animal) and over developed in the spiritual qualities, it is especially important in order to restore and maintain lost equilibrium to build up in him the animal qualities.

At all times some of our patients may be found to be fasting, but they do not begin until the right physiological and psychological moment has arrived — until the fast is indicated. When the organism, or rather the individual cell, is ready to begin the work of elimination, then assimilation should cease for the time being because it interferes with the excretory processes going on in the system. To fast before the system is ready for it, means mineral starvation and defective elimination. Given a vigorous, positive constitution, encumbered with too much flesh and with a tendency to chronic constipation, rheumatism, gout, apoplexy and other diseases due to food poisoning, a fast may be indicated from the beginning. But

([1])
As stated previously the volume entitled 'Nature Cure Eugenics' did not appear, but Lindlahr does give considerable information on the treatment of psychological and mental disorders both in this volume and in the 'Practice of Nature Cure'.

it is different with persons of the weak negative type.

Ordinarily the organism resembles a huge sponge which absorbs the elements of nutrition from the digestive tract. During a fast the process is reversed, the sponge is being squeezed and gives off the impurities contained in it. However, this is a purely mechanical process of flushing and deals only with the mechanical aspect of disease — with the presence of waste matter in the system. It does not take into consideration the chemical aspect of disease. We have learned that most of the morbid matter in the system has its origin in the acid end products of protein and starch metabolism. In rheumatism and gout the colloid and earthy deposits collect in the joints and muscular tissues; in arteriosclerosis, in the arteries and veins; in paralysis, epilepsy and kindred diseases, in brain and nerve tissues. The accumulation of these waste products is due, in turn, to a deficiency in the system of the alkaline, acid binding and acid eliminating mineral elements. In point of fact, almost every form of disease is characterized by a lack of these organic mineral salts in blood and tissues. Stones, gravel (calculi), etc. grow only in blood surcharged with acid elements and they must be eliminated by rendering the blood alkaline. This is accomplished by the absorption of alkaline salts contained most abundantly in the juicy fruits, leafy and juicy vegetables, the husks of cereals and in milk.

How are these all important solvents and eliminators to be supplied to the organism by total abstinence from food? Prolonged fasting undoubtedly lowers the patient's vitality and powers of resistance. But natural elimination of waste products and systemic poisons (a healing crisis) depends upon increased vitality and activity of the organism and the individual cells which compose it. For these reasons we find in most cases that proper adjustment of the diet, both as to quality and quantity, together with the various forms of natural treatment, must precede fasting. The great majority of chronic patients have become chronics because their skin, kidneys, intestines and other organs of elimination are in a sluggish condition. As a result the system is overloaded with morbid matter which must be promptly eliminated to prevent reabsorption. Even normal organs, unless properly prepared, eliminate waste with difficulty. This may explain why patients frequently suffer severely without any demonstrable lesion in the iris. The atrophic condition of the organs of depuration makes prompt elimination impossible and there are not enough alkaline mineral elements to neutralize the destructive acids. Therefore the impurities remain and accumulate in the system and may cause serious aggravation and complications. Therefore before fasting is enforced it is wiser first to build up the blood on a normal basis by natural diet and to put the organs of elimination in good working order by natural methods of treatment. This is, indeed, the only rational procedure and will always be followed by the best results.

When under the influence of a rational diet the blood has regained a more normal composition; when mechanical obstructions have been removed by manipulative treatment; when skin, kidneys, bowels, nerves and nerve centres, in fact every cell in the body has been vitalized into vigorous activity by the various methods of natural treatment — then the cells themselves begin to eliminate their morbid encumbrances. The waste materials are carried in the blood stream to the organs of elimination and incite them to acute reactions or healing crises in the form of diarrhoeas, catarrhal discharges, fevers, inflammations, skin eruptions, boils, abscesses, etc. Now the sponge is being squeezed and cleansed of its impurities in a natural manner. The mucous membranes of stomach and bowels are called upon to assist in the work of house cleaning; hence the coated tongue, lack of appetite, digestive disturbances, nausea, biliousness, sour stomach, fermentation, flatulency, and occasionally vomiting and purging. These digestive disturbances are always accompanied by mental depression, "the blues", homesickness, irritability, fear, hopelessness, etc. With the advent of these cleansing and healing crises the physiological and psychological moment for fasting has arrived. All the processes of assimilation are at a standstill. The entire organism is eliminating. We have learned that these healing crises usually arrive during the sixth week of natural treatment. To take food now would mean to force assimilation and perchance to interfere with or check a beneficial healing crisis. Therefore we regard it as absolutely essential for the patient to stop eating as soon as any form of acute elimination makes its appearance and we do not give any food except acid fruit juices diluted with water until all signs of acute eliminative activity have subsided whether this requires a few days, a few weeks, or a few months. Some time ago we treated a severe case of typhoid malaria. No food except water mixed with a little orange or lemon juice passed the lips of the patient for seven weeks. When all disease symptoms had disappeared we allowed a few days for the rebuilding of the intestinal mucous membranes. Thereafter food was administered with the usual precautions. The patient gained rapidly and within six weeks weighed more than before the fever. A thorough discussion of the technique of fasting will be found in a later volume.

The majority of those who undergo their first long fast are most pleasantly surprised to find that the terrors of "starvation" exist only in people's minds. It has happened that people stranded on barren islands or lost in desert places or entombed in mines, even where they had water, have died apparently from starvation in the course of a week or two.

It is now fully proved by thousands who have fasted for long periods ranging from forty to ninety days that death in such cases is not due to actual starvation. The real cause must be fear and apprehension, showing again that we tend to materialize the things we fear. It cannot be too much emphasized that fear is a perversion of the great law of faith; it is faith in evil. By submitting to it we give evil power over us. The most necessary requirement therefore for a successful fast is. the profound conviction that it cannot harm us in any way but that, on the contrary, it will prove of great benefit, physically, mentally and morally, because it will not only purify the body but will strengthen will power and self control. Self control is the master key to high attainment. There is no other practice that has so desirable an effect upon the highest and finest qualities of the soul as fasting under the right conditions. It subdues the animal cravings, appetites and passions. It proves to us that we can master the most primitive instincts of our animal and human natures. To attain such control is the very purpose of being, for self mastery is the key to all higher development, mentally, morally and spiritually. It is the only key to mastership. This is the gist of the teachings of all the saviours of mankind and of the wise men of all ages. It is the sum and substance of science, philosophy and religion.

Nature Cure philosophy of natural living in strict accord with nature's laws is for this reason the only true and safe foundation for all higher development. While he who has not mastered completely his physical habits of living may claim high mental and spiritual development, these great attainments will not save him from physical and consequent mental shipwreck if he persists in violating nature's laws on the physical plane. Time and again I have seen people of high attainment who had become spiritual giants and a source of inspiration to thousands of hungering souls suffer mental and moral shipwreck before their work was finished, thus cutting short the most brilliant careers and consigning to oblivion great constructive movements which might have blessed humanity for ages to come; all because they attempted to master spiritual and psychical conditions before they had learned to conquer the physical. The most brilliant woman I have ever known, a woman whose writings were epoch making in the realms of science and philosophy, had many a friendly tilt with me over my "radical ideas". She contended that a little meat and coffee did not hurt anybody but were necessary in order to maintain a positive condition of body and mind, and that allopathic drugs had their good as well as bad effects. The result of her "positive" diet and of the poisonous heart tonics which she was in the habit of taking in order to suppress symptoms of uric acid poisoning, brought about a total collapse at a time of life when her work had just attained its highest degree of usefulness to humanity. Through pathogenic clogging and the benumbing effects of long continued drug poisoning her system failed to react to further stimulation and she passed away after a few days coma. There was no reason why, under natural living and treatment, her life should not have been doubled in years.

Strict compliance with the natural laws of living means much more than the curing of physical pains or frazzled nerves. It is the foundation for all higher development on the mental, moral and spiritual planes. He who has not learned to control his physical habits will never attain mastership on the intellectual, moral and spiritual planes of being. Those who have attained perfect control of the physical plane will however find the way clear and easy to higher attainment. It is a fact we see continually verified in every day experience that most people find it more easy to exert necessary self control in moral matters than in their common, every day habits of life.(1)

[1] Lindlahr's attitude towards fasting as a therapeutic procedure is broadly speaking that it should not be used except in acute feverish diseases or when the body has clearly undertaken a strong elimination by way of skin, bowels or mucous membranes. It is no doubt true that this is a sound rule but there seem to be circumstances in which a more or less prolonged fast may be beneficial and time saving at the beginning of an effort to cope with a chronic condition or to bring about a general cleansing and rejuvenation of the body, It has the effect of giving the digestive organs a complete rest and of knocking the body out of a rut of inertia. On the other hand there is reason to think that in most cases if not in all better results may be obtained by doing the 'Grape Cure' than by absolute fasting. It appears that grapes and grape juice throw so little strain on the digestive system and are so non-toxic and assimilible that their use makes an exception to the general rule that the body cannot assimilate and eliminate, tear down and build up at the same time. The successful use of the Grape Cure in cases in which the body was too weak to sustain a long fast or to benefit by it is discussed in the books on the Grape Cure by Brandt and Shackleton.

CHAPTER XXVIII

WHAT IS POSITIVE, WHAT IS NEGATIVE?

Everywhere in the literature of the day and in general conversation we meet with the expressions "positive" and "negative". Science speaks of positive and negative substances, forces and energies. We hear of positive and negative personalities and traits of character. Nature Cure philosophy claims that all disease — physical, mental, moral, spiritual and physical — is originally negative, and that health on all planes of being is positive. We must, then, seek to define what constitutes positivity and negativity.

As regards substances, science divides the atoms of matter and their corresponding elements into positive and negative, according to their electromagnetic qualities. In lectures I have frequently been asked the question: "How do you know whether a substance is positive or negative?" It is a relative proposition, very much as with heat and cold. Nobody can fix the dividing line where cold ceases and heat begins. The scales of heat and cold on the various kinds of thermometers are based on arbitrary starting points and standards. So, also, is the positivity and negativity of atoms a relative proposition. For instance, if we arrange the elements of matter found in animal and human bodies and in the foods which they require in such a manner that the negative elements, carbon, oxygen, hydrogen, nitrogen, phosphorus, sulphur, fluorine, chlorine, and iodine are placed to the left of hydrogen, and the positive elements, iron, lime, sodium, potassium, manganese, magnesium and lithium, on the right of hydrogen, then we find that hydrogen is positive to the negative elements on its left but negative to the positive alkaline mineral elements on the right. For, while hydrogen is the positive and dominating element in negative substances like acids, ptomaines, alkaloids, xanthins, etc., it has to relinquish its dominating position at the approach of a positive alkaline mineral element. The latter will take its place and change the negative acid or xanthin into a new substance, a neutral salt. Both kinds of elements display varying degrees of positivity and negativity among themselves. However, there are certain tests by which positive and negative polarity can be determined. The positive pole of a magnet attracts negative elements and repels the positive. In similar manner can the polarity of substances be determined by electrolysis. Positive substances will gravitate towards the negative pole, and vice versa.

The law of polarity is one of the fundamental laws, if not the fundamental, of nature. On it are based the constitution and vital activities of this universe. According to this basic law of nature every entity seeks vibratory correspondence or union in or with another like entity of opposite polarity. In harmony with this law, electromagnetically positive atoms are attracted to and seek vibratory union with negative atoms, and vice versa. This attraction which manifests in the mineral kingdom as electromagnetic affinity, appears in the vegetable kingdom in the rudiments of sex life. Separation of the sexes becomes physically complete in the animal kingdom. On the human plane, sex influence manifests in and modifies the mental, ethical, moral and spiritual qualities as well as the purely physical characteristics. Thus the law of polarity or the law of sex runs all through nature, from the affinities and repulsions of atoms to the subtle sympathies and antipathies, affinities or "Wahlverwandtschaften" of the most highly developed and cultured human beings.

The question, "What are electricity and magnetism?" could be answered by saying, "Everything is electricity". One modern scientist never tires of saying, "There is nothing but electrons" — and electrons are negative particles or charges of electricity. A few thousand years ago Pythagoras and many other wise men and mystics of antiquity claimed that "all matter is made up of three elements, substance (the one primordial substance), motion and numbers". Now advanced modern science seems to verify the teachings of the ancient wise men. The discovery and the study of the X-rays, of radium and radioactivity has revealed the fact that atoms of all the different kinds of matter are made up of negative charges or particles of electricity, called electrons or corpuscles, which revolve around one another without ever touching as the planets in the starry heavens swing around their central suns. These electrical whirls or vortices tear through the ether (primordial substance) like the centripetal force of the eddy tears through the water.

Furthermore, it has been found that the number of the particles of negative electricity (electrons) vibrating in the atom determines the physical qualities of the atom or element. In other words, whether an atom or element impresses our sensory organs with the physical properties of iron, carbon, hydrogen, oxygen, or any one of the other elements of matter depends on the number of electrons in the atom and their modes of vibration. It has been found that the number of electrons or corpuscles in the atom determines its atomic weight. Science has gone so far as to be able to count approximately the number of electrons in the atoms. The electrons, or negative charges of electricity in the atom, are accompanied by or surround spheres of positive electricity. Thus again we find the teachings of the ancients and mystics verified by the discoveries of modern science. The "primordial substance" of Pythagoras is the ether in various stages of refinement. "Motion" is the oscillation or vibration of the electrons in the atom, and "numbers" is the number of electrons or corpuscles which make up the atom of matter.

Science teaches that the electromagnetically negative atom has more (negative) corpuscles than are necessary to balance its positive electricity, and that the electromagnetically positive atom has fewer negative corpuscles than are needed to balance its positive sphere of electricity. It is this deficiency or superfluity of negative corpuscles which constitutes positive and negative magnetism or polarity, which causes the desire of the negative atom to equalize its polarity by union with a positive atom. This is what constitutes the chemical affinity or valency — combining power — of the various atoms or elements of matter. The greater the surplus of negative corpuscles in an atom, the greater will be its desire or chemical affinity for atoms having a deficiency of negative electrons or which are, in other words, surcharged with positive electricity. Therefore, according to the predominance of the positive or negative qualities in a force, matter or entity, we speak of them as positive or negative. We learn from the foregoing that the law of polarity is fundamental in nature. On the activities which it provokes and regulates are built the entire structure of the universe. The cessation of these activities for the fraction of a second would cause the universe to disappear into nothingness in a flash.

From the foregoing it becomes apparent that a substance is positive or negative according to the electromagnetic quality of the elements of which it is composed. Thus we speak of wheat as being a negative food because it contains very large amounts of negative food elements in the forms of starch, dextrin, sugar, fat and protein, while it ranks exceedingly low in positive mineral elements. On the other hand we speak of spinach as being a positive food because it contains only negligible amounts of starch, protein and sugar, but large amounts of positive mineral elements.

However, the positivity or negativity of substances as well as of forces and energies is influenced by another factor of equal importance. This second factor is the life element which dominates the substance, force or energy in question. In every higher sphere matter is made to vibrate to higher velocities and is moulded into compounds of greater refinement and of increasing complexity. The higher the degree of complexity, refinement and vibratory activity of a compound or substance, the greater its potential energy. Four distinct life elements or ranges of vibratory activity control the four great kingdoms of nature. The lowest plane is under the domination of the electromagnetic life element; the next higher, or vegetable kingdom is controlled by the vitochemical life element; the still higher animal kingdom is animated by the spiritual or animal life element, and the highest, or human plane, by the soul life element. On the lowest plane the electromagnetic life element binds together the elements into the simple inorganic compounds of the mineral plane. The vibrations of this plane are the slowest and its substances are the coarsest in our planetary universe. In the vegetable kingdom the vitochemical life element by the aid of sun energy builds up the elements of air, water and minerals into the refined and complex living molecules of organic vegetable matter. While the compounds of the mineral kingdom are crystalloid in structure, the substances of the vegetable kingdom are colloid or amorphous (without form) in structure. It is well to remember this distinction in order to be able to judge whether foods or medicines belong to the mineral or to the vegetable kingdom. For instance, water belongs to the mineral kingdom as proved by the fact that it crystallizes in the form of ice and snow. However, here a vital distinction becomes necessary. Most chemists look upon carbon compounds as organic and alive and as belonging to the vegetable kingdom. Professor Béchamp, the discoverer of microzymes, has pointed out the error of this by showing that carbon compounds should not be regarded as alive or belonging to the vegetable kingdom unless they contain living microzymes. This constituted the difference between ordinary calcareous rocks unable to produce fermentation and the calcareous rock of the "chalk of Sens" capable of producing fermentation. The term "organic" for carbon compounds belonging to the mineral kingdom is therefore inappropriate. The term should be applied only to substances that are alive, have organs and are capable of using organs. All such things are alive by virtue of their microzymes. In these discussions I have not deviated from common usage in the employment of the term "organic" but truly living beings I have called organized or alive in distinction from the lifeless carbon compounds of the mineral kingdom. As, for instance, white sugar may be called by chemists "organic" but it is no longer alive, while the natural product of the maple, cane and beet, is live food in the true sense of the word. The dead product of the refineries is crystalloid in form, while live, unrefined sugar is amorphous.(1)

[1]
    Béchamp drew a very careful distinction between what he called "proximate principles" (principes immédiats) which were non-living substances of organic origin such as sugar and starch and "natural organic substances" (matières organiques naturelles) such as meat which had once been actual parts of living plant or animal tissue.

The spiritual life element governing the animal kingdom seizes upon the living matter of the vegetable plane and refines, organizes and vivifies it to still higher potencies of vital force and creative energy. The life principle governing the animal kingdom has been called the spiritual life element because it manifests in the phenomena of consciousness, animal intelligence and volition. The life element dominating the human kingdom has been called the soul life element because it manifests in the human entity as self consciousness which differs from animal consciousness in that it is capable of reasoning and philosophizing upon its own nature, origin and destiny, of which the animal is incapable. The intellectual and volitional capacity of the animal is limited and circumscribed by heredity and instinct. Materialistic science would make us believe that animal instinct is altogether the product of adventitious influences, of the struggle for nutrition in a hostile environment, of the struggle for reproduction, etc. This, however, is unthinkable on the face of it. If that were true, then the various individuals of the same species or family of animals would not display the marvellous uniformity and identity of structure and of instinctive impulse. There would be as many different shades and degrees of physical, intellectual and volitional qualities and tendencies as there are individuals according to the varying conditions of hostile environment, of struggle for nutrition, reproduction, etc. We find, however, that marvellous as is the instinctive recognition and application of social, mathematical and geometrical principles revealed in the doings of the bee and the ant, their intellectual and social activities are the same today as they were thousands of years ago. They must be fixed and regulated by something more stable than the struggle for existence, for nutrition and reproduction in an hostile environment, and this something is the spiritual life element which manifests in animal intelligence and instinct. On the other hand we find that human intelligence is not hampered by heredity and instinct but is capable of infinite development and expansion until it has assimilated all there is to be learned and experienced in the sidereal universe. We cannot imagine limitations of the possibilities of growth and expansion of the human mind and soul anywhere this side of the Godhead itself.

To recapitulate: The four great kingdoms of earth life are animated and governed by four distinct life elements which are equivalent to progressively higher, more refined and more potent ranges of vibratory activity. Increase of vibratory activity means increase of potential and kinetic or working energy. The building of atoms into molecules involved the absorption of the energy which builds into that which it is building; therefore every additional atom in the molecule means additional inherent potential energy. Every higher kingdom of nature in addition to

201

its own life elements is animated by the qualities of the life elements governing the lower kingdom. Thus the vegetable kingdom in addition to the vitochemical life element is animated by the electromagnetic life element of the mineral kingdom, etc. While as yet on this earth we have become acquainted with only four kingdoms of nature and their corresponding life elements, I do not believe these constitute the entire range of vibratory planes or of life and action. It seems very probable that, in accordance with the septimal law, there are three higher kingdoms which will become manifest.

The ascending life elements, or progressive manifestations of vital force, resemble the power of steam at different degrees of tension. Steam at ten pounds of pressure may be sufficient to run a churn or grindstone but it would not be powerful enough to run a harvester or a traction engine. Steam at one hundred pounds' pressure can perform a much greater amount and variety of work than steam at fifty pounds' pressure. In similar manner, each higher expression of vital force exhibits more powerful potential and kinetic energy and produces substances of greater refinement and complexity than a lower one. The greater the tension of steam, the greater its capacity for work; the higher the vibratory tension of the life element, the more potent, complex and refined its manifestations and products. This is illustrated in the formation of ice. The "cold" which solidifies the molecules of water is absorbed and becomes latent in the icy crystals which it builds. When the particles of ice disintegrate under the influence of "heat", cold is liberated. In a similar manner the "heat" which gives warmth and comfort to our homes is sun warmth which was absorbed in the formation of vegetable cells in the growing plants and trees of primeval jungles and forests. Coal, though classed among the minerals, possesses infinitely greater heat producing qualities than other minerals because originally its elements were elaborated under the vibratory influence of the vitochemical vegetable life element. The latter element ranges much higher in the scale of vibratory activities than does the electromagnetic life element which elaborates and controls the simple compounds and crystals of the mineral kingdom.

The animal cell being synthetised under the operation of the spiritual or animal life element, is alive with still higher potencies of vital force than those in the vegetable cell. It is for this reason that animal food substances contain something that is not present in the vegetable protoplasm, namely, the animal life element or animal magnetism. This aspect of the food question is overlooked by our friends, the simon pure vegetarians or advocates of raw food diet who exclude from their dietary the dairy products. However, in order to receive the benefits of the animal life element or animal magnetism in our diet, we do not need to consume animal flesh with its systemic poisons and alkaloids of putrefaction. This subtle but potent life principle which is absent in the products of the vegetable kingdom is presented to us in the most refined form, unimpaired by cooking, in the dairy products because nature has refined milk, eggs and honey and charged them with the highest potencies of animal magnetism to serve as food for the newborn animal and human.

It is interesting to note that the "newly" discovered vitamins of orthodox medical science are identical with the life elements of Nature Cure philosophy. In fact the word "vitamin" is a literal translation of "life element". I predict that one of the next great "new" discoveries of medical science will be the fact that the positive mineral elements are the carriers of the life elements in the lower kingdoms of nature. The life elements in the mineral and vegetable kingdoms are vital force transformed into electromagnetic and vitochemical or physiochemical energies. Positive mineral elements are good conductors; negative elements are poor conductors for these electromagnetic energies. We cannot conduct electricity over ropes made of starchy or protein matter; this requires wires made of metals. Science now admits that nervous energy is a form of electromagnetic energy. This explains the great importance of the mineral elements as carriers and conductors of the vital or nervous energies in animal and human bodies.

As already explained, the principles of positivity and negativity affect sexual, mental, emotional and psychical activities as well as the qualities of so called inanimate substances, forces and energies. In sex life, the positive male qualities manifest as creative power, initiative, self reliance, aggressiveness and love of material and intellectual domination. The corresponding faults are coarseness, self indulgence, obstinacy and intellectual vanity. The predominating negative qualities of the female sex nature are intuitional, emotional, passive, conservative and pacific. The corresponding faults are excessive emotionalism, deceitfulness and personal vanity.

In the mental and emotional sphere one can compare the positive characteristics such as will power, self-control, self reliance, courage, aggressiveness, initiative, confidence, faith, cheerfulness, creativeness, happiness, love, helpfulness, altruism with the negative characteristics of indecision, vacillation, self-indulgence, diffidence, laziness, fear, worry, anxiety, apprehension, hatred, jealousy, selfishness, depression, melancholy, self-pity. Considered from the psychical viewpoint, positivity means predominance of reason, will power and self-control over the emotions, appetites and passions — independence and poise of character. These positive qualities are the best safeguards against psychical negativity or subjectivity which may lead to hypnotic subjection, mediumship, obsession and possession and their various manifestations of abnormal psychism.

CHAPTER XXIX

HEALTH IS POSITIVE, DISEASE NEGATIVE

To prove the truth of the proposition that health is positive and disease negative one must study the law of polarity in the lower kingdoms, insofar as these are concerned in the production of wholesome foods and medicines and of harmful substances and destructive poisons. Chemical science so far has discovered in animal and human bodies and likewise in the foods which sustain them, seventeen elements in appreciable quantities. These seventeen elements must be present in animal and human bodies and consequently in their food supplies in well balanced and sufficient quantities to fill all their requirements and thus to insure healthy tissue and normal function. If some of these elements are present in over-abundance and if others are deficient or entirely lacking in food and drink, then the chemical balance of the organism and its functions will be disturbed and abnormal function or disease will, sooner or later, be the inevitable result.(1)

Let us now study more closely the chemical processes which determine health or disease. Practically all diseases arising in animal and human bodies, always barring accidents and surroundings uncongenial to life and health, are caused ultimately by the deleterious and destructive action of certain acids, ptomaines, alkaloids, xanthins or other pathogenic substances and toxins. These disease producing chemical substances to which we refer collectively as pathogens are made up of hydrogen in combination with negative elements. If food and drink consist almost entirely of these negative, pathogen producing elements, then in time abnormal or diseased conditions must develop.

The foods most highly valued by the medical profession and the laity for their "nourishing" qualities, namely proteins, dextrins, starches, fats

---

(1)
The number of elements normally present in human, animal and plant tissue and required by living things for their health and well being is now believed to be greatly in excess of seventeen. Also, the recent researches of the French scientist, C. L. Kervran, would appear to imply that biological transmutations can take place which bring about changes of one element into another in the soil and in animal tissues to a limited degree in certain circumstances.

and sugars are, when chemically pure, made up of hydrogen, nitrogen, phosphorus and sulphur. Hydrogen is the basic element in all acids. Oxygen is found in practically all acids, ptomaines, xanthins and colloids. These two basic elements are reinforced in pathogenic (disease producing) substances by more or less of carbon, nitrogen, phosphorus, sulphur, chlorine, fluorine, iodine and other negative elements found in foods, medicines and tonics. Carbon, hydrogen and nitrogen are the basic elements in all toxic substances in the body. This explains why the customary American meat-white-bread-potato-pie-and-coffee diet, unbalanced by organic mineral salt foods, must in time produce abnormal conditions in the tissues and functions of the human body. In the "Nature Cure Cook Book and ABC of Natural Dietetics" I have quoted a selection of disease producing acids, ptomaines, xanthins, colloids and toxins. It will be seen that not one of these contains a single positive element. Nor have I been able to find one in any other of these negative, pathogenic substances.

Naturally the question arises, how can we prevent the formation of these negative, disease producing substances? The simple answer to this is: by providing in foods and medicines sufficient amounts of positive, alkaline, mineral elements in the live organic form. If this is taken into consideration and properly attended to then the positive mineral elements will, through chemical affinity, unite with the negative atoms and molecules and thus produce chemically balanced combinations which are not injurious but rather beneficial in the vital economy of the body. Physiological science now admits that all cell waste is chemically acid and that it must be neutralized by alkaline elements as quickly as it is formed in order to prevent the accumulation of morbid waste products. Thus the salts eliminated through kidneys and skin are neutralized acids. When through the excessive intake of negative foods and the subsequent excessive production and neutralization of acids, more salts are formed than can be eliminated by the organs of depuration, then those salts also form morbid deposits and become pathogenic substances in rheumatic joints, in calculi, "hardened" arteries and obstructed capillaries.

The diagram illustrates the chemical changes involved in cell nutrition and in the neutralization and elimination of cell waste. Column I which shows the three principal classes of cell foods; Carbohydrates (starches, dextrins and sugars), Hydro-carbons (fats and oils), Proteins. The first two, when chemically pure, consist of carbon, oxygen and hydrogen, the third contains also nitrogen, phosphorus and sulphur. Column II shows, in schematic outline, the nature of the cell substances or protoplasm. Column III gives the common forms of cell waste into which the cell protoplasm and its food materials are broken down in the metabolic processes of cell life (digestion, nutrition and elimination). All this cell

CELL NUTRITION	CELL SUBSTANCE PROTOPLASM	ACID WASTE PRODUCTS	POSITIVE ALKALINE MINERAL ELEMENTS	NEUTRALIZED WASTE PRODUCTS	PTOMAINS AND LUKOMAINS
Carbohydrates~COH (Starches, dextrines and sugars)	C	Carbonic—$H(CO_3)$		Sodium carbonate-$NaH(CO_3)$	Cadaverin—$C_5H_{14}N_2$
	O	Lactic—$C_3H_6O_3$	Iron——Fe	Urea——$CO(NH_2)_2$	Cholin — $C_5H_{15}NO_2$
	H	Oxalic—$C_2H_2O_4$		Calcium oxalate-$Ca(C_2HO_4)$	Amylamin—$C_5H_{13}N$
	N	Diacetic—$C_4H_6O_3$		Potassium acetate—$K(C_2H_3O_2)$	Gadinin—$C_7H_{17}NO_2$
Hydrocarbons-COH (fats and oils)		Butyric—$C_4H_8O_2$	Lime——Ca	Magnesium butyrate-$Mg(C_4H_7O_2)$	Betain $C_5H_{11}NO_2$
		Nitric—HNO_3		Sodium nitrate— $Na(NO_3)$	Hydrocollidin-$C_8H_{15}N$
		Nitrous—HNO_2	Sodium——Na	Sodium nitrite—— $Na(NO_2)$	Putrescin~ $C_4H_{12}N_2$
	P	Uric—$C_5H_4N_4O_3$		Sodium urate-$Na(C_5H_3N_4O_3)$	Neurin — $C_5H_{13}NO$
	S	Glycoholic-$C_{26}H_{43}NO_6$	Potassium—K	Iron glycoholate-$Fe(C_{26}H_{41}NO_6)$	Mydatoxin-$C_6H_{13}NO_2$
		Bilivirdinic—$C_{16}H_{18}N_2O_4$		Iron bilivirdinate-$Fe(C_{16}H_{18}N_2O_4)$	Guanidin—CH_5N_3
Proteids COHNPS (Meat, fish, fowl, eggs, cheese, nuts, beans, peas, lentils, mushrooms, etc.)		Indol & Skatol—C_8H_7N	Lithium— Li	Indican salt—— $K(C_6H_4NSO_4)$	Gerontin—$C_5H_{14}N_2$
		Phosphoric—$H_3(PO_4)$		Sodium phosphate-$Na_3H(PO_4)$	Paraxanthin-$C_7H_8N_4O_2$
		Phosphorous-$H_3(PO_3)$	Magnesium-Mg	Sodium phosphite-$Na_3H(PO_3)$	Xanthin-$C_5H_4N_4O_2$
		Sulphuric—$H_2(SO_4)$		Calcium sulphate——$Ca_2(SO_4)$	Xanthocreatnin-$C_5H_{10}N_4O$
		Sulphurous—$H_2(SO_3)$	Manganese-Mn	Calcium sulphite—$Ca_2(SO_3)$	Reducin-$C_6H_{13}N_4O$
		Hydrochloric—HCl		Sodium chloride——NaCl	

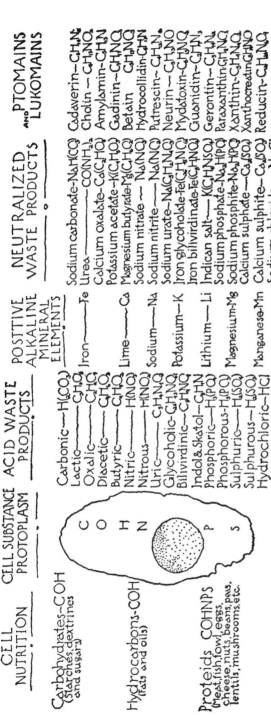

A Ptomaine is a toxic amine derived from intestinal (large intestine) putrefaction by bacteria e.g. Escherichia coli. This involves decarboxylation of amino-acids; intestinal bacteria appear to possess a decarboxylase enzyme for most amino acids. Ptomaines can be absorbed by the colon into the portal circulation and are metabolized and removed by the liver if this organ is intact. Bacterial fermentation can yield methane, hydrogen sulphide and ammonia. Ammonia intoxication can arise in patients on a high protein diet with liver dysfunction.

The following are ptomaines: Cadaverine (from lysine), neurine (from lecithin), choline (from lecithin), putrescine (from ornithine).

Others present include: agmatine, tyramine, histamine, spermine, spermidine and ethanolamine.

Betaine is derived from methylation of glycine. Xanthine is a purine base present as caffeine, theophylline and theobromine in tea, coffee and cocoa and derived from purine bases of DNA and synthesised from glycine and aspartic acid. Guanidine is present mainly in invertebrates and is of little significance in humans. Xanthocreatinine does not appear to exist as such, though creatinine derived from creatine phosphate is present. Xanthine may be used instead of paraxanthine. Collidine exists though not necessarily in the body.

The following either do not exist or they are old names; at least they are never mentioned in modern texts: Amylamine, Gadinin, Mydatoxin, Gerontin and Reducin.

Bases are anions and any acid buffering capacity resides in these e.g. Citrate anion, Malate anion and bicarbonate anion. Sodium is freely ionized, as is potassium and magnesium. Many cations are complexed. However, they do not participate in neutralisation of acid waste products.

F. I. WHITEHOUSE

waste is acid as it as made up of atoms of hydrogen and four or five other negative forming acid elements. The acid cell waste products given in this Column III are convertible into neutral salts, by combination with positive alkaline mineral elements, shown in Column IV. These alkaline elements neutralize the acids and change them into harmless neutral salts. A number of these salts are given in Column V. Column VI contains morbid products of abnormal cell and food metabolism which are constituents of what we designate as pathogen. These substances when they accumulate in the system in excessive quantities may cause (in the form of leucocytes and colloid matter) capillary obstruction, followed by inflammation and exudation of the pathogenic materials into the neighbouring tissues, resulting in putrefactive changes as described in the chapters dealing with inflammation. These morbid processes favour the development of normal as well as abnormal microzymes into bacteria. The bacteria feed on and decompose the pathogenic materials (leucocytes and colloids) into simple compounds, suitable for neutralization by alkaline elements and for elimination through the natural channels. When the pathogenic materials have been decomposed the bacteria are either eliminated from the system or the microzymes consume the protoplasm of their own bacteria, leaving nothing but the microzymes themselves. These under favourable conditions, that is, in a congenial morbid soil in their own or other bodies, may again develop into scavengers, or bacteria, as called upon. That this process under certain circumstances actually takes place is admitted by orthodox science. The name "spores" is given to what Béchamp called microzymes. The foregoing explains why healing crises become necessary when the pathogenic encumbrances in the body of a "chronic" contain excessive amounts of morbid encumbrances classified in Column VI.([1])

The human body is made up of acid and alkaline constituents; in order to have normal conditions and functions of tissues and organs both must be present in the right proportions. If either the acid or the alkaline elements are present in excessive or insufficient quantities, then abnormal conditions and functions, that is Disease, will be the result. Acidity and alkalinity undoubtedly play an important part in the generation of electricity and magnetism in the human organism. Every electric cell and battery contains acid and alkaline elements; and the human body is a dynamo made up of innumerable minute electric cells and batteries in

---

[1] The author here gives a long quotation from the "Principles of Bacteriology" by A. C. Abbott, a standard work of the time. This puts forward an explanation of the behaviour of cells under adverse conditions almost identical with that of Béchamp.

the forms of living, protoplasmic cells and organs. It has been claimed that what we call "vital force" is electricity and magnetism and that these forms of energy are manufactured in the human body. This, however, is but a partial statement of the truth. It is true that vital force manifests in the body as electricity and magnetism, but vital force is not itself generated in the system. Life is a primary force. It is the source of all activity animating the universe. From this primary force other, secondary forces are derived, such as electricity, magnetism, mental, emotional and nervous energy. These secondary derived forces and energies cannot be changed back into vital force in the human organism. Nothing can give Life but Life itself. When the physical body is dead, as we call it, the life which left it is active in the spiritual body. It is independent of the physical organism just as electricity is independent of the incandescent bulb in which it manifests as light.

If we continue to consider the cause and development of acid diseases, we see that nearly every disease originating in the human body is due to or accompanied by the excessive formation of different kinds of acids or other pathogenic substances in the system. These are formed during the processes of protein and starch digestion and in the waste products of cells and tissues. Of these waste products uric acid probably causes the most trouble in the organism. The majority of diseases arising within the human body are due to its erratic behaviour. Together with oxalic acid and oxylates it is responsible for arteriosclerosis, arthritic rheumatism and the formation of calculi. Their presence in excessive quantities aggravates all other forms of disease.

Dr. Haig of London has done excellent work in the investigation of uric acid poisoning, but he becomes onesided when he makes it the scapegoat for all disease conditions originating in the organism. In his philosophy of disease he fails to take into consideration the effects of other acids and systemic poisons. For instance, he does not mention the fact that carbonic acid is produced in the system somewhat similarly to the formation of coal gas in the furnace; and that its accumulation prevents the entrance of oxygen into the cells and tissues, thus causing asphyxiation or oxygen starvation, which manifests in the symptoms of anaemia and tuberculosis. Neither does Dr. Haig explain the effects of other destructive byproducts formed during the digestion of starches and proteins. Sulphurous acid and sulphuric acid (vitriol) as well as phosphorus and phosphoric acids actually burn up the tissues of the body. They destroy the cellulose membranes which form the protecting skins or envelopes of the cells, dissolve the protoplasm, and allow the latter to escape into the circulation. This, together with pathogen obstruction, accounts for the symptoms of Bright's disease — the breaking down of the cells and the presence of albumen (cell protoplasm) in blood and urine, the clogging of the circulation, the consequent stagnation and the accumulation of blood serum (dropsy) and the final breaking down of the tissues (necrosis) resulting in open sores and ulcers. Excess of phosphorus and the acids derived from it overstimulate the brain and the nervous system, causing nervousness, irritability, hysteria and different forms of mania. An example of this is the "distemper" of a horse when given too much oats and not enough grass or hay. The excess of phosphorus and phosphoric acids formed from the protein minerals of the grain, if not neutralized by alkaline minerals contained in grasses, hay or straw, will overstimulate and irritate the nervous system of the animal and cause it to become nervous, irritable and vicious. These symptoms disappear when the ration of oats is decreased and when more fresh grass or hay is fed in place of the grain. Hard working horses develop distemper when their food contains over five per cent total protein. What about inactive humans consuming much larger proportions of protein and starch foods? Similar effects to those produced upon the horse by an excess of grains are caused in the human organism, especially in the sensitive nervous system of the child, by a surplus of protein foods, of meat, eggs, grains and pulses. Still, when patients suffering from overstimulation of the brain and nervous system consult the doctor, his advice in almost every instance is: "Your nerves are weak and over-wrought. You need plenty of good nourishing food (broths, meat and eggs), a good tonic and rest". The remedies prescribed by the doctor are the very things which caused the trouble in the first place.

As stated before, uric acid is undoubtedly one of the most common causes of disease and therefore deserves especial attention. Through the study of its peculiar behaviour under different circumstances and influences the cause, nature and development of all acid diseases will become clearer. Like urea, uric acid is one of the end products of protein digestion. It is formed in much smaller quantities than urea, in proportion of about one to fifty, but the latter being more soluble is more easily eliminated from the system. The principal ingredient in the formation of uric acid is nitrogen, one of the six elements which enter into all protein or albuminous food materials, also called nitrogenous foods. Uric acid, as one of the byproducts of metabolism, is therefore always present in the blood and in moderate quantities serves useful purposes in the economy of the human and animal organism as do other waste materials. It becomes a source of irritation and cause of disease only when it is present in the circulation or in the tissues in excessive amounts.

How Uric Acid is Precipitated

The potentially alkaline blood takes up uric acid, dissolves it and holds it in solution until it is neutralized, its salts carried to the organs of depuration and eliminated in perspiration and urine. If, however, through the excessive use of nitrogenous foods or through defective elimination, the amount of uric acid and other waste products in the system is increased beyond a certain limit, the blood loses its power to dissolve and neutralize these substances and they form a sticky, gluelike "colloid" substance which occludes or blocks up the minute blood vessels (capillaries) so that the blood cannot pass readily from the arterial system into the venous circulation. This interference with the free passing of the blood increases in proportion to the distance from the heart, because the farther from the heart the less force behind the circulation. Therefore we find that slowing up of the blood currents, whether due to uric acid occlusion or to any other cause, is more pronounced in the surface of the body and in the extremities than in the interior parts and organs. The occlusion of the surface circulation can be easily observed and even estimated by a simple test. Press the tip of the forefinger of one hand firmly on the back of the other and release it. A white spot will be formed where the blood has receded from the surface because of the pressure. Now observe how quickly or how slowly the blood returns into this white patch. Dr. Haig states that if the reflux of the blood takes place within two or three seconds the circulation is normal and not obstructed by uric acid. If, however, the blood does not return for four or more seconds it is a sign that the capillary circulation is obstructed by colloid occlusion. When this occlusion of the circulation by uric acid or other pathogenic substances prevails through the body, the blood pressure is too high in the arterial blood vessels and in the interior organs, such as heart, lungs, brain, etc., and too low in the surface, the extremities and in the venous circulation. This gives rise to the much dreaded high blood pressure. The return flow of the blood to the heart through the veins is sluggish and stagnant because the force from behind, that is, the arterial blood pressure, is obstructed by pathogen which clogs the minute capillaries that form the connection or bridge between the arterial and the venous systems.

Because of interference with the normal circulation and distribution of the blood, uric acid produces many annoying and deleterious effects. It irritates the nerves, the mucous membranes and other tissues of the body, thus giving rise to headaches, rheumatic pains in joints and muscles, congestion of blood in the head, flushes, dizziness, depression, fainting and even epilepsy. Other results are inflammatory and catarrhal con-

211

ditions of the bronchi, lungs, stomach, intestines, genito-urinary organs; also rapid pulse, palpitation of the heart, angina pectoris, etc. These colloid substances occlude the minute ducts and capillaries in liver, kidneys and other organs, interfering with their normal functions and causing the retention of morbid matter in the system. All these troublesome and destructive effects of uric acid poisoning may be greatly augmented by excessive accumulation of sulphuric, phosphoric and other acids and by the formation of ptomainas, leukomains, and poisonous alkaloids incidental to the metabolism of protein substances.

The entire group of symptoms caused by the excess of uric acid or pathogen in the system and the resulting occlusion of the capillary blood vessels by colloid substances is called "collemia". If in such a condition of collemia the amount of uric acid or pathogen in the system is still further increased by the taking of uric acid producing food and drink and the saturation point of the blood is reached, that is, if the blood becomes overcharged with acid materials, a curious phenomenon may be observed; the collemic symptoms suddenly disappear as if by magic, giving way to a feeling of physical and mental buoyancy and strength. This wonderful change has been wrought because the blood has lost its capacity for dissolving uric acid and holding it in solution and the acid has been precipitated, thrown out of the circulation and deposited in the tissues of the body. After a period of rest, that is, when no uric acid and xanthin producing foods have been taken for some time, say over night, the blood regains its alkalinity and its capacity for dissolving and carrying uric acid and begins to reabsorb it from the tissues. As a consequence the blood again becomes saturated with uric acid and the collemic symptoms reappear. This explains why the hilariousness and exaltation of spirits at the banquet is followed by "Katzenjammer" in the morning. It also explains why many people do not feel "fit for their day's work" unless they take a stimulant of some kind, "a hair of the dog that bit them", on arising. Their blood is filled with pathogen to the point of saturation and the extra amount of xanthins contained in the meat, coffee or alcohol causes uric acid precipitation, giving temporary stimulation and relief. Every time this precipitation of uric acid from the circulation is repeated some of the morbid materials remain and accumulate in different parts and organs. If these irritating substances become lodged in the joints and muscles, arthritic or muscular rheumatism is the result. If acids, xanthins and oxalates of lime form earthy deposits along the walls of arteries and veins, these vessels harden and become inelastic and their diameter is diminished. This obstructs the free circulation of the blood and causes malnutrition of the brain and other vital organs. Furthermore, the blood vessels become brittle and break easily, and there is danger of haemorrhages.

This explains the origin and development of arteriosclerosis, high blood pressure and apoplexy. Apoplexy may also be caused by other acids and drug poisons which soften, corrode and destroy the walls of the blood vessels in the brain. In individuals of certain constitutions accumulations of uric acid, xanthins, oxalates of lime and various other earthy substances form stones, gravel or sandy deposits in the kidneys, the gall bladder and in other parts and organs.

Haig distinguishes two distinct stages of uric acid diseases: the collemic stage, marked by an excess of uric acid or pathogen in the circulation and resulting in occlusion of the capillary blood vessels and in local irritation; and the arthritic stage, marked by permanent deposit of uric acid and other earthy substances in the tissues of the body. During the prevalence of the collemic symptoms, that is when the circulation is saturated with uric acid, the urine is also highly acid. When precipitation of the acid materials from the blood into the tissues has taken place the amount of acid in the urine materially decreases. Xanthins have the same effect upon the system as uric acid. Caffein and theobromin, the narcotic principles of coffee and tea, are xanthins and so is the nicotine contained in tobacco. Peas, beans, lentils, mushrooms and peanuts, besides being very rich in uric acid producing proteins, carry also large percentages of xanthins which are chemically almost identical with uric acid and have a similar effect upon the organism and its functions.

From what has been said it becomes clear why the meat eater craves alcohol and xanthins in the form of coffee, tea, etc. When by the taking of flesh foods the blood has become saturated with uric acid and the annoying symptoms of collemia make their appearance in the forms of lassitude, headache, and nervous depression, then alcohol and the xanthins contained in coffee, tea and tobacco will cause the precipitation of the acids from the circulation into the tissues of the body and thus temporarily relieve the collemic symptoms and create a feeling of well being and stimulation. Gradually, however, the blood regains its alkalinity and its acid dissolving power and enough of the acid deposits are reabsorbed by the circulation to cause a return of the symptoms of collemia. Then arises a craving for more alcohol, coffee, tea, nicotine, or xanthin producing foods in order to gain temporary relief and stimulation, and so on, ad infinitum. The person addicted to the use of stimulants is never himself. His mental, moral and emotional equilibrium is always unbalanced. His brain is muddled with poisons and he lacks the self-control, clear vision and steady hand necessary for the achievement of success in any line of endeavour. We can now understand why one stimulant creates a craving for another, why it is almost impossible to give up one stimulant without giving up all the others as well.

From the foregoing it is clear that the stimulating effect of alcohol and of many so-called tonics depends upon their power to clear the circulation temporarily of uric acid or pathogen. This effect is, however, deceptive and temporary and is followed by a return of the collemic symptoms in aggravated form leading eventually to chronic pathogenic conditions. Not understanding the deceptive effects of artificial stimulation and acid precipitation, people will say "Why not take a cup of tea (a toddy or a cigar, as the case may be) when you know it does you good?" This sounds reasonable enough, but the position is really somewhat as follows: A man may carry a burden of fifty pounds on his shoulders without difficulty or serious discomfort. Let this correspond to the normal solving power and carrying capacity of the blood for uric acid. Suppose you add gradually to the burden on the man's back until its weight has reached 150 pounds. He may still be able to carry the burden, but as the weight increases he will begin to show signs of distress. The increase of weight and the attendant discomfort correspond to the increase of uric acid in the blood and the accompanying symptoms of collemia. If you increase the burden on the man's shoulders still further, beyond his individual carrying capacity, a point will be reached when he can no longer support its weight and he will throw it off entirely. This climax corresponds to the saturation point of the blood when the limit of its acid carrying capacity is exceeded and its acid contents are precipitated into the tissues.

The treatment of acid diseases is the same as of all other diseases which are due to violation of nature's laws, namely, purification of blood and tissues from within, and building up of the vital fluids (blood and lymph) on a natural basis through normal habits of eating, dressing, bathing, breathing, working, resting and thinking as outlined in these volumes. In severe cases which have reached the chronic stage, the treatment must be supplemented by more aggressive methods of strict diet, hydrotherapy, curative gymnastics, massage, neurotherapy and homoeopathic medication. The only permanent preventive for acid diseases is not to take in excessive amounts of pathogen making food and drink. If, indeed, we substitute the terms pathogen and pathogenic for Dr. Haig's "uric acid", we have a still better picture and a clearer understanding of the condition prevailing in a human body saturated with colloid or mucoid matter in the form of uric acid and other waste and morbid materials (proteins, starches and fats) and of normal cell and tissue waste. The accumulation of these morbid byproducts of digestion and of the metabolic changes in the system is further increased through defective elimination. The mucoid detritus clogs the capillaries and forms morbid deposits in the system, especially in those parts and organs whose vitality and resistance are

214

already lowered. Nature attempts to rid the system of these pathogenic encumbrances through the mucous membranes of the internal tracts and cavities, thus giving rise to all kinds of catarrhal troubles, but orthodox medical science with its suppressive treatment of catarrhal conditions forces the disease matter again into the system. If through the chilling of the skin or for any other reason an excessive amount of this mucoid matter is concentrated into a weakened organ the tiny capillaries become clogged so that the blood cannot pass through. This distends the capillaries, the pressure from behind forces the mucoid matter and leucocytes from the blood vessels into the neighbouring tissues, thus developing inflammation and fever wherever the mucoid obstruction occurs.

The statements made in the preceding pages concerning the disease producing effects of high acidity on the system have been repeatedly verified in our institutional practice and through special laboratory experiments conducted by a member of our staff. Before proceeding to explain the nature of these experiments, let us consider briefly the role performed by acids, alkalines and salts in the human body.

During the chemical changes which occur in the cells of the body and in the food while it is being digested or metabolized, acid compounds are formed in considerable quantities. The more the foods contain of negative elements, the greater the production of acids, ptomaines, xanthins, etc. However, from the following it will become evident that the system is strongly fortified against the accumulation of these negative pathogenic substances. The blood and lymph contain from two-tenths to three-tenths per cent of potential alkalies; hence all acids tend to be neutralized into salts immediately upon their formation. These chemical reactions take place in conformity with the following laws: When an acid combines with a base (one or more alkaline elements) the positive alkaline element neutralizes the acid and changes it into a salt. These salts are easily eliminated through the kidneys and skin. Should the potential alkalinity of the blood be insufficient to neutralize all the acids and other pathogenic substances, then kidneys and skin eliminate the acid products in order to maintain a slight predominance of the basic (alkaline) elements over the acids and other negative substances in the blood stream. The amount of acid found in the urine during the twenty-four hour period, therefore, furnishes a reliable clue as to the amount of acid which the system is unable to neutralize. The amount of salts in the urine, on the other hand, indicates the amount of acids which the system has succeeded in neutralizing. Physicians, students and nurses employed in our institutions have submitted at different times to dietetic experiments in order practically to demonstrate the foregoing statements. When their urine showed a low state of acidity as the result of a vegetarian low protein diet they were given three meals rich in negative acid forming proteins, starches and fats, such as eggs, legumes, bread, potatoes, butter, etc., with no additions of fruit and leafy vegetables. In every case the acidity of the urine increased considerably during the next twenty-four hours. The ordinary mixed diet or a vegetarian diet like the above, persisted in for a considerable length of time, inevitably results in hyperacidity and this causes irritation and in time destruction of cells and tissues. Nerve cells being especially sensitive, are more readily affected than other cells. This is the reason why hyperacidity causes nervousness, neurasthenia, neuritis and neuralgia.

Further experiments and observations have confirmed and extended these findings. It was found if, as in the above experiments, the high protein diet was accompanied by fresh fruit and green vegetables, the increase in acidity was reduced by about half. Other experiments have shown that the neutralizing action of sodium bicarbonate had only very temporary effects on the urine by comparison to alkalising substances in true organic form. It was also shown that it is not satisfactory to try to balance excessive quantities of such things as meat, white bread, eggs and pastry by large quantities of fruits and vegetables. Where the acidity was thus neutralized, it was found that the amount of solid waste products was raised dangerously high. Vigorous, healthy, eliminating organs may be able to cope with this extra work for some time. Sooner or later, however, they are bound to give way under the strain and will then fail to eliminate even the regular daily amount. The urine, in such cases, shows a percentage of solids less than normal, indicating the retention of these waste products in the system. The autopsy of a well known Chicago physician and surgeon who died in middle life when he should have been at his best as far as professional efficiency is concerned, showed deposits of urates and carbonates of sodium in the heart muscles. We see this further verified in the composition of stones, gravel and earthy deposits in various parts of the body. For instance, kidney and bladder stones are composed of the following constituents, mentioned in the order of their frequency: (1) uric acid and urates of sodium, potassium and calcium; (2) phosphates of sodium and calcium; (3) oxides of calcium; (4) carbonates of calcium; (5) xanthins, cystin, indican, etc. Of these nos. 1, 2 and 5 result from excessive protein food; nos. 3 and 4 from excess of starches, sugars and fats. This means that these calculi are made up largely of salts which are neutralized acids. The only safe rule, therefore, as regards diet, is to limit the consumption of starches, proteins and fats — the pathogen or mucous forming elements — to the proportions and amounts which science and experience has taught us to be the normal.

Further light is thrown on the nature of acid diseases by what happens during healing crises. During the first five weeks of natural living and treatment the acidity is greatly reduced. As a rule, from the beginning of the sixth week on, acute eliminative crises develop in the form of purgings, skin eruptions, boils, acute catarrhal discharges, inflammations, fevers, haemorrhoids, haemorrhages, etc. With the onset of these acute reactions we usually find a considerable increase in the acidity of the urine. Frequently it rises to 110 degrees and even as high as 150. Since these patients for many weeks have lived on a low protein diet, in other words have not consumed acid forming materials, there is but one explanation for the sudden rise in acidity and other waste products in the urine. That is, they must have come from the pathogenic deposits in the tissues of the body. This sudden increase in the urine and other excretions of the body during healing crises also confirms our claim that these acute reactions are indeed purifying, healing efforts of nature.

It frequently happens that patients come to us whose urine registers 100 to 150 degrees acidity. Such abnormally high acidity is usually accompanied by high blood pressure. As explained in the previous pages, there is a direct relationship between the two. Hyperacidity means excessive amounts of colloid or mucoid matter in the circulation. These obstruct the capillary circulation, especially in the surface. This in turn makes the blood surge back into the internal large blood vessels of the heart, lungs and brain. During the last few years high blood pressure has become the bugbear of the medical profession and of life insurance companies. Many years ago in my lectures and writings I called attention to the prevalence of colloid obstruction and its causes, and also explained the natural treatment. Life insurance companies are losing many millions of dollars of new business annually because they reject people on account of high blood pressure. Thereby they admit that their eminent medical advisers are unable to cope with the simple problem. Under natural living and treatment hyperacidity and high blood pressure decrease with wonderful rapidity. Many patients have come to us because examiners of life insurance companies had rejected them on account of arteriosclerosis, high blood pressure and heart disease. This, together with fear of apoplexy, induced them to give natural methods a fair trial. We have taken many such patients who registered a blood pressure of 250 degrees or more and reduced it to normal or near normal within three to nine months time. They were then able to secure life insurance without further difficulty.

One of the stock arguments met with in talking natural dietetics to our friends and patients is that many men and women have lived to the age of seventy, eighty or more on the ordinary meat diet and have used tea, coffee, tobacco and whisky and have remained in good health. The answer to this is that these fortunate people were born with excellent constitutions and good vitality. Their organs of elimination were strong enough to throw off the food and drink poisons so that they did not endanger life and health. Few of us, however, are endowed with such excellent constitutions and active organs of depuration; therefore we cannot indulge in reckless habits of living without suffering the penalty. Because my neighbour can drink a quart of whisky every day and consume a dozen cigars without showing any immediate ill effects, it is not to be assumed that I can do likewise with impunity. Another common argument met with is that of the Christian or Mental Scientist: "Why should I pay attention to rules of diet, since nature in her great wisdom transmutes foods in the system into the substances most needed and best adapted to the body?" Anyone can see that this is very superficial reasoning. Nature will indeed do the best she can to maintain the integrity of the human organism to the very limit of her resources. Nature Cure philosophy teaches and emphasizes this over and over again. Yet there is a limit to nature's ability to neutralize injurious and toxic substances and she certainly does not change her immutable laws of chemical affinity to please the fancies of Mental or Christian Scientists. Moreover, if the reasoning of these "Scientists" be sound it should hold good in the animal creation which is truly under the guidance and control of Mother Nature. It is now positively proved that the terrible beri-beri disease results from the prevalence of polished rice or white flour products in the diet. Pigeons or other test animals fed for a few months on white flour or polished rice develop symptoms of the disease and die unless they are given in time small quantities of the husks of the grain or polishings of rice which contain the positive mineral elements (and together with these the vitamins) which neutralize the poisonous acids and ptomaines responsible for the development of beri-beri, scurvy, rachitic diseases, etc. A striking example of the disease producing effect of a one sided starchy diet occurred a few years ago when the Kronprinz Frederick, a German raider, surrendered to the United States authorities at Newport News because ninety per cent of the crew were ill with a disease resembling beri-beri. The explanation was that during the many months of chasing and being chased on the high seas, they were unable to make port anywhere and had been thereby limited to a daily diet of potatoes, rice, cereals, meat, coffee, and cakes and bread made from white flour. After medical treatment had utterly failed to bring about any improvement in the condition of the men, a dietary of fruits and vegetables brought speedy recovery. As long as forty years ago scientists of the Nature Cure school proved by actual experimentation that animals fed on nothing but white sugar or pure starch (organic but not live food) died sooner than those who received no food at all. If Christian Scientists by concentration on metaphysical formulae could change the results of such experiments on animals or human beings, the truth of their theories might be accepted.

CHAPTER XXX

CONSERVATION OF VITALITY

In Chapter V I named as the first of the primary manifestations of disease, lowered vitality. What can be done to increase vitality? Old school physicians and the public in general seem to think that this can be done by consuming large quantities of "nourishing" food and drink and by the use of stimulants and tonics. We often hear the cry: "Oh, doctor, if you could only prescribe for me some nourishing food or tonic to give me more strength, then I would be all right." Through all the ages alchemists, doctors and scientists have been searching in vain for the wonderful elixir which will rejuvenate the body, cure all human ills and prolong human life indefinitely.

Ever since I began to study the problems of health, disease and cure I have been convinced that we would be able to cure all disease instantaneously if we could increase the activity of vital energy sufficiently. All disease is caused by something which interferes with, diminishes or disturbs the normal inflow and distribution of vital energy throughout the system. Acute disease represents a temporary increase in activity of the vital force in order to overcome obstructions in the system caused by pathogenic conditions. Chronic disease is permanent obstruction to the activity of vital energy. In chronic disease the cells and tissues are so heavily encumbered with waste, morbid matter and poisons that they cannot rouse themselves to acute healing efforts in the form of acute disease or healing crises. In other words, acute disease is the battle between the healing forces and the diseased condition. Cure means the victory of the vital energies over the pathogenic obstruction. Vitality, physical and mental energy, power of resistance and capacity for the enjoyment of life are various forms and manifestations of vital energy, and these are transmutations of vital force. The problem, then, before us in the healing of disease as well as in maintaining the highest possible efficiency and capacity for the enjoyment of life, is to increase the inflow and distribution of life force, which means "life more abundant". This glorious consummation has been and always will be doomed to failure as long as the medical profession and the laity look for the source of vital energy in "nourishing foods, strengthening tonics and stimulants". These substances cannot give life because they are secondary manifestations of life. Secondary derived energies cannot be transmuted back into life force — the primary source of all force. If this were possible we could, indeed, prolong life indefinitely. The relation of the life force and its derivatives, vitality, strength and recuperative power, to foods, medicines, drugs and stimulants has been described as follows in my book on dietetics: "This life force which flows into us from the one great source of all life in this universe — from that which we call God, Nature, Creative Force, or Universal Intelligence — is the primary source of all energy, from which all other forms and kinds of energy are derived. It is as independent of the body and of food and drink as the electric current is independent of the glass bulb and the carbon thread through which it manifests as heat and light. The breaking of the glass bulb, though it extinguishes the light, does not in any way diminish the amount of electricity back of it. In a similar manner, if the physical body should "fall dead" as we call it, the vital energy would keep on acting with undiminished force through the spiritual material body, which is the exact duplicate of the physical body but whose material atoms and molecules are infinitely more refined and vibrate at infinitely greater velocities than do those of the latter.

This is not merely a matter of faith and of speculative reasoning, but a demonstrated fact of natural science. When St. Paul said (I Cor 15:44) "If there is a natural body there is also a spiritual body" he stated an actual fact in nature. Indeed, it would be impossible to conceive of the survival of the individual after death without a material body which serves as the vehicle of consciousness, memory and of the reasoning faculties and as an instrument for physical functions. Without a body it would be impossible for the soul to manifest itself to other souls or to communicate with them. Therefore, if survival of the individual after death be a fact in nature, and if the achievement of immortality be a possibility, a spiritual material body is a necessity. Someone may say, "If the life force is independent of the physical body and of food and drink, why do we have to eat and drink to keep alive?" The answer is: Food and drink are necessary to keep the organism in the right condition, so that vital force can manifest and operate through it to the best advantage. To this end food is needed to build up and repair the tissues of the body. It also serves to a certain extent as fuel material, which is transmuted into animal heat and vital energy. Furthermore, just as coal has to come in touch with fire before it can be transmuted into heat, so the life force is needed to "burn up" or to "explode" the fuel materials. When "life" has departed even large amounts of sugars, fats, proteins, tonics and stimu-

221

lants are not able to produce one spark of vital energy in the body. On the contrary, digestion and assimilation of food and drink and elimination of waste materials require the expenditure of considerable amounts of vital energy. Therefore all food taken in excess of the actual needs of the body wastes vital force instead of giving it. If these facts were more generally known and appreciated people would not habitually overeat under the mistaken idea that their vitality increases in proportion to the amount of food they consume; neither would they believe that they can derive strength from poisonous stimulants and tonics. They would not be so much afraid of fasting. They would better understand the necessity of fasting in acute diseases and healing crises and would avail themselves more frequently of this most effective means of purification. They would no longer believe themselves in danger of dying if they were to miss a few meals. Briefly stated, all that food and drink can do is to keep the body in normal, healthy condition. On this depends the flow of life force into the body and its free distribution by way of the nervous system to the various organs and to every individual cell.

Anything and everything in natural methods of living and treatment that will help to build up the blood on a normal basis, that will purify the system of waste and morbid matter, that will correct mechanical lesions and harmonize mental and emotional conditions will insure a greater supply of life force and its derivatives, strength, vitality, resisting and recuperative power. In other words, the more normal, healthy, and perfect the organism, the more copious will be the inflow of vital energy. Never before in any writings dealing with dietetics or food chemistry has there been revealed the true relationship between the life force and food, medicines, tonics and stimulants. All the different schools, systems and cults of healing deal only in a partial way with the problem of vital force. Some confine their efforts to dietetic measures, others to the administration of drugs and to surgical treatment. The hydropath stimulates the flow of vital fluids and nerve currents through hot and cold water applications. Manipulative schools of healing endeavour to facilitate the distribution of vital energy through the system by correcting mechanical lesions in the bony structures, ligaments, muscles and connective tissues. Mental scientists, Christian Scientists and spiritual healers confine their efforts to establishing the right mental and spiritual attitudes. All these and other systems of treating human ailments deal only with one or several phases of the problem. The only system so far devised that endeavours to combine and apply all that is good in natural healing methods is Natural Therapeutics. It draws the line only at the employment of destructive methods such as the use of poisonous drugs, promiscuous, uncalled for surgical operations, hypnotism and mental therapeutics based on erroneous and misleading premises.

Ignorance of the simple truths outlined above leads to the most serious mistakes. Physicians and people in general do not stop to think that excessive eating and drinking tend to rob the body of vitality instead of supplying it. The Romans had a proverb: "Plenus venter non studet libenter" — "a full stomach does not like to study". The most wholesome food if taken in excess will clog the system with waste matter just as too much coal will dampen down and exstinguish the fire in the furnace. Furthermore, the morbid materials and systemic poisons produced by impure, unsuitable or improperly combined food clogs the cells and tissues of the body, cause unnecessary friction and obstruct the inflow and the operations of the vital energies, just as dust in a watch clogs and impedes the movements of its mechanism. The greatest artist living cannot draw harmonious sounds from the strings of the finest Stradivarius if the body of the violin be filled with dust and rubbish. Likewise, the life force cannot act perfectly in a body filled with morbid encumbrances. The human organism is capable of liberating and manifesting daily a limited quantity of vital force, just as a certain amount of capital in the bank will yield a specified sum of interest in a given time. If more than the available interest be withdrawn the capital in the bank will be decreased and gradually exhausted. Similarly, if we spend more than our daily allowance of vital force, "nervous bankruptcy", that is nervous prostration or neurasthenia, will be the result. It is the duty of the physician to regulate the expenditure of vital force according to the income. He must stop all leaks and guard against wastefulness.

Much stimulation which is now done is, in effect, stimulation by paralysis. Stimulants are poison to the system. Few people realize that their exhilarating and apparently tonic effects are produced by the paralysis of an important part of the nervous system. As we have learned, wholesome food and drink in themselves do not contain and therefore cannot convey life force to the human body. Much less can this be accomplished by stimulants. The human body has many points of correspondence with a watch. Each has a motor or driving mechanism and an inhibitory or restraining apparatus. If it were not for the inhibiting balance, the wound watchspring would run off and spend its force in a few moments. The expenditure of the latent force in the wound spring must be regulated by the inhibitory and balancing mechanism of the timepiece. Similarly, the nervous system in the animal and human organism consists of two main divisions: the "motor" or driving and the "inhibitory" or restraining mechanism. The driving power is furnished by the sympathetic nerves and the motor nerves. They convey the vital energies and nerve impulses to the cells and organs of the body, thus initiating and regulating their activities. We have found that the human body is capable of liberating in a given time, say twenty four hours, only a certain limited amount of vital energy, just as the wound spring of a watch is capable of liberating in a given time only a certain amount of kinetic energy. As in the watch the force of the spring is controlled by the regulating balance (the anchor), so in the body the expenditure of vital energy must be regulated in such a manner that it is evenly distributed over the entire running time. This is accomplished by the inhibitory nervous system. Every motor nerve must be balanced by an inhibitory nerve. The one furnishes driving force, the other applies the brake. For instance, the heart muscle is supplied with motor force through the spinal nerves from the upper dorsal region, while the pneumogastric nerve (vagus) retards the action of the heart and in that way acts as a brake.

Another brake is supplied by the waste products of metabolism in the system, the uric acid, carbonic acid, oxalic acid, etc. and the many forms of xanthins, alkaloids and ptomaines which make pathogen. As these accumulate in the organism during the hours of wakeful activities they gradually clog the capillary circulation, benumb brain and nerves, and thus produce a feeling of exhaustion and weariness and a craving for rest and sleep. In this way, by means of the inhibitory nervous system and the accumulation of fatigue products in the body, nature forces the organism to rest and to recuperate when the available supply of vital force runs low. The lower the level of vital force, the more powerful the inhibitory influences.

Stimulants have the effect of benumbing and paralyzing temporarily the inhibitory nervous system and the inhibitory mechanism generally. In other words they "lift the brakes" from the motor nervous system and allow the driving powers to run wild when nature wanted them to stop. To illustrate: A man has been working hard all day. Toward the night his available supply of vitality has run low, his system is filled with uric acid, carbonic acid and other benumbing fatigue products and he feels tired and sleepy. At this juncture he receives word that he must sit up all night with a sick relative. In order to brace himself for the extraordinary demand on his vitality, our friend takes a cup of strong coffee or a drink of whisky or whatever his favourite stimulant may be. The effect is marvellous; the tired feeling disappears and he feels as though he could remain awake all night without effort. What has produced this apparent renewal and increase of vital energy? Has the stimulant added to his system one iota of vitality? This cannot be, because stimulants do not contain anything that could impart vital force to the organism. What, then, has produced the seemingly strengthening effect? The caffein, alcohol or whatever the stimulating poison may have been has precipitated the fatigue products from the blood and deposited them in the tissues and organs of the body. Furthermore, the stimulant has benumbed the inhibitory nerves, it has lifted the brakes from the driving part of the organism so that the wheels are running wild. By this means we draw upon the reserve supplies of vital energy which nature wants to save for extraordinary demands upon the system in times of illness or extreme exertion. Therefore this procedure is contrary to nature's intent. Nature tried to force the tired body to rest and sleep so that it could store up a new supply of vital force. Under the paralyzing influence of the stimulants upon the inhibitory nerves the organism now draws upon the reserve stores of nerve fats and vital energies for the necessary strength to accomplish the extra night work. At the same time remaining awake and active during the night prevents the storing up of a reserve supply of vital energy for the next day's work, which means that the latter also has to be done at the expense of the reserve supply of life force.

Only during sleep do we replenish our reserve stores of vitality. The expenditure of vital energy ceases, but its liberation in the system continues. Therefore sleep is the great restorer. Nothing can take its place. No amount of food and drink, no tonics or stimulants can make up for the loss of sleep. Continued complete deprivation of sleep is bound to end in a short time in physical and mental exhaustion, in insanity and death. That the body during sleep acts as a storage battery for the vital energy is proved by the fact that in deep, sound sleep the aura disappears entirely from around the body. The aura is to the organism what the exhaust steam is to the engine. It is formed by the electromagnetic fluids which have performed their work in the body and then escape from it, giving the appearance of a many coloured halo. With the first awakening of conscious mental activity after sleep the aura appears, indicating that the expenditure of vital energy has recommenced. The return of the aura is more fully described in the chapter entitled "Magnetic Treatment".[1]

[1] In spite of what is here said there do seem to be some well authenticated cases of people who could not sleep and who went for very long periods or even permanently without sleep, suffering no serious effects and leading normal lives. Such persons would seem to have acquired the ability to relax the body very completely and so restore their vitality and get rid of fatigue. Usually, however, persons who relax thoroughly go to sleep without trying to and indeed most people who have insomnia can overcome it by learning to relax instead of trying to go to sleep. We should, in fact, relax in order to go to sleep rather than go to sleep in order to relax. The physiology of sleep would not seem to be at all well understood and it is doubtful if it can be understood except on the basis that it is a mechanism by which the normal relationship between the physical body and the energies which are working on it and through it are changed. This gives the body a chance to store up energy and repair wear and tear. There is little doubt that the healthier a person is and the more integrated his personality is the better the quality of his sleep will be and the less quantity of it he will require. A conclusion to which we can come is that it is very doubtful whether sleep which is induced by drugs is of as much value as rest and relaxation without sleep.

225

The truth of the matter is that the person who resorts to stimulants to keep up his strength or to increase it, is never normal, never "on the level", never at his best. He is either overstimulated or abnormally depressed; his efforts are bound to be fitful and his work uneven in quality. Furthermore, it is only a matter of time until he exhausts his reserve supply of vital energy and then suffers nervous bankruptcy in the form of nervous prostration, neurasthenia or insanity. The same principles hold true with regard to stimulants given at the sick-bed. One of the arguments I constantly hear from students and physicians of the old school of medicine is: "What would you do at the sickbed of a patient who is so weak and low that he may die at any moment? Would you just let him die? Would you not give him something to keep him alive?" I certainly would if I could, but I do not believe that poisons can give life. If there is enough vitality in that dying body to react to the poisonous stimulant, then that same amount of vitality will keep the heart beating and the respiration going a little longer at the slower pace. Nature regulates the heart beat and other functions according to the amount and availability of vital force. If the heart beats slow it is because nature is trying to economise vitality. In the inevitable depression following the artificial "whipping up" of the vital energies, many times the flame is snuffed out entirely when otherwise it might have continued to burn at the slower rate for some time longer. However, I do not deny the advisability of administering stimulants in cases of shock. When a shock has caused stopping of the wheels of life, another shock by a stimulant may set them in motion again.(1)

The mental and emotional exhilaration accompanying the indulgence in alcohol or other poisonous stimulants is produced in a manner similar to the apparent increase in physical strength under the influence of these agents. Here, also, the temporary stimulation and seeming increase in power are effected by paralysis of the governing and restraining faculties of mind and soul: of reason, modesty, reserve, reverence, etc. The moral, mental and emotional capacities and powers of the human entity are governed by the same principle of dual action that controls physical activity. We have on the one hand the motor or driving impulses and on the other hand the restraining and inhibiting influences. In these higher realms appetite, passion, imagination and desire correspond to the motor

(1)
    It is not very clear in what circumstances stimulants should be administered or what kind of stimulants should be used. It does, however, seem that a distinction is here being drawn between cases in which the patient is in extremis as the result of shock and cases of severe illness. Homoeopathy of course has an important contribution to make to the treatment of shock.

system in the physical organism and the power of the will and reasoning faculties represent the inhibitory nervous system. The exhilarating and stimulating influence of alcohol and narcotics such as opiates, "hashish", etc. upon the animal spirits and the emotional and imaginative faculties is caused by the benumbing and paralyzing effect of these stimulants upon the powers of will, reason and self control, which are the brakes on the lower appetites, passions and desires. However, what is gained in emotionalism and imagination is lost in judgement and logic.

Alcohol, nicotine, theo-bromin, luppulin (the bitter principle of hops), opium, cocaine, morphine, etc., when given in certain doses, all affect the human organism in a similar manner. In small quantities they seemingly stimulate and animate; in larger amounts they depress and stupefy. In reality, they are paralyzers from the beginning and in every instance and their apparent, temporary tonic effect is deceptive. They benumb and paralyze not only the physical organism but also the higher and highest mental and moral qualities, capacities and powers. These higher and finer qualities are located in the front part of the brain. In the evolution of the species from lower to higher, the brain gradually developed and enlarged in a forward direction. Thus we find in the lowest order of fishes that all they possess of brain matter is a small protuberance at the upper extremity of the spinal cord. As the species and families rose in the scale of evolution, the brain developed proportionately from behind forward and became differentiated into three distinct divisions — the medulla oblongata, the cerebellum, and the cerebrum. The medulla oblongata, situated at the base of the brain where it joins the spinal cord, contains those brain centres which control the purely vegetative, vital functions, the circulation of the blood, respiration, regulation of animal heat, etc. The cerebellum, in front of and above the medulla, is the seat of the centres for the co-ordination of muscular activities and for maintaining the equilibrium of the body. The frontal brain, or cerebrum, contains the centres for the sensory organs, also the motor centres which supply the driving impulses for the muscular activities of the body and in the occipital and frontal lobes the centres for the higher qualities of mind and soul, which constitute the governing and restraining faculties on which depend the powers of self control. Thus we see that the development of the brain has been in a forward direction, from the upper extremity of the spinal cord to the frontal lobes of the cerebrum, from the low, vegetative qualities of the animal and the savage to the complex and refined activities of the highly civilized and trained mind. It is an interesting and most significant fact that paralysis of brain centres caused by alcohol and other stimulants, or by hypnotics and narcotics, proceeds reversely to the order of their development during the processes of evolution. The first to succumb are the brain centres in the frontal lobes of the cerebrum which control the latest developed and most refined human attributes. These are modesty, caution, reserve, reverence, altruism. Then follow in the order given, memory, reason, logic, intelligence, will power, self control, the control of muscular coordination and equilibrium and, finally, consciousness and the vital activities of heart action and respiration. When the conscious activities of the soul have been put to sleep paralysis extends to the subconscious activities of the Life or Vital Force. Respiration and heart action become weak and laboured and may finally cease entirely.

In order to verify this let us study the effects of alcohol, the best known and most used of stimulants. Many people believe that alcohol increases not only physical strength but mental energy also. Medical science considers it a valuable tonic in all cases of physical and mental depression. It is often administered after surgical operations and in accidents with the idea of prolonging life. I have frequently found the whisky or brandy bottle at the bedside of infants and on it the directions of the attending physician. Watch the effect of this tonic on a group of convivial spirits at a banquet. Full honour is done to the art of the chef and the wine flows freely. The flow of animal spirits increases proportionately — conviviality, wit and humour rise by leaps and bounds. But the apparent joy and happiness are in reality nothing but the play of the lower animal impulses unrestrained by the higher powers of mind and soul. The words of the after dinner speaker, who when sober is a sedate and earnest gentleman, flow with unusual ease. The close and unprejudiced observer notices, however, that what the speaker has gained in eloquence, loquacity and exuberance of style and expression, he has lost in logic, clearness and good sense. As alcohol tightens its grasp on the merry company, the toasters and speakers lose more and more their control over speech and action. What was at first mischievous abandon and merry jest gradually degenerates into loquaciousness, coarseness and querulous brawls. Here and there one of the maudlin crowd drops off in the stupor of drunkenness. If the liquor be strong enough, and the debauch continued long enough it may end in complete paralysis of the vital functions or in death.

Again we find the seeming paradox of "stimulation by paralysis" exemplified in the phenomena of hypnotism and obsession. The abnormally exaggerated sensation, feeling and imagination of the subject under hypnotic control are made possible because the higher, critical and restraining faculties and powers of will, reason and self control are temporarily or permanently benumbed and paralyzed by the stronger will of the hypnotist or of the obsessing intelligence. There is the most interesting resemblance between the effects of stimulants, narcotics or hypnotic control and blind, unreasoning faith. The latter also benumbs and paralyzes judgement and reason. It gives full sway to the powers of imagination and thus may produce seemingly miraculous results. This explains the modus operandi of faith cures as well as the fitful strength of the intoxicated and the insane, or the beautiful dreams and "delusions of grandeur" of the drug fiend. The close resemblance and relationship between hypnotic control and faith became vitally apparent to me while witnessing the performance of a professional hypnotist. His subject on the stage was a young woman who under his control performed extraordinary feats of strength and resistance. Several strong men could not lift or move her in any way. What was the reason? In the ordinary waking condition her judgement and common sense would tell her: "I cannot resist the combined strength of these men. Of course they can lift me and pull me here and there." As a result of this doubting state of mind she would not have the strength to resist. However, the control of the hypnotist had paralyzed her reasoning faculties and therewith her capacity for judging, doubting and "not believing." Her subconscious mind accepted without question the suggestion of the hypnotist that she did possess the strength to resist the combined efforts of the men and as a result she actually manifested the necessary powers of resistance. It is an established fact that the impressions (records) made upon the subconscious mind under certain conditions, as for instance under hypnotic influence, absolutely control the activities of the physical body.

Does not this throw an interesting light on the power of absolute faith, on the saying: "Everything is possible to him who believeth"? Blind, unreasoning faith benumbs and paralyzes judgement and reason in similar manner as do hypnotic control or stimulants, and in that way gives free and full sway to the powers of imagination and autosuggestion for good or ill, for "white magic" or "black magic" according to the purpose for which faith is exerted. It also becomes apparent that such blind, unreasoning faith cannot be constructive in its influence upon the higher mental, moral and spiritual faculties. These can be developed only by the conscious and voluntary exercise of will, reason and self control. These subjects will be more fully considered in another volume entitled "Nature Cure Eugenics."

From the foregoing it will have become evident that we cannot increase vital force in the body through any artificial means or methods from without, by food, drink or stimulant. What we can and should do, however, is to put the organism into the best possible condition for the liberation and manifestation of life force or vital energy. The more normal the chemical composition of the blood and the more free the tissues from clogging impurities, poisons and mechanical obstructions such as lesions of the spinal column, the more abundant will be the available supply of vital energy, and the freer its liberation. Therefore perfect, buoyant health which ensures the greatest possible efficiency and enjoyment of life, can be attained and maintained only by strict adherence to natural ways of living and, when necessary, by natural treatment of disease.

CHAPTER XXXI

ONANISM OR MASTURBATION

Undoubtedly one of the most serious leaks of vital force is created through onanism or masturbation. This destructive habit is exceedingly common among those who can least afford it, namely young people and children who need their vital energies for the upbuilding of their physical organism and for the development of their mental, imaginative and creative faculties, capacities and powers. There is a close relationship between genius and virility. Therefore the wasteful expenditure of sex fluid and sex life stunts growth and development in all directions. It lowers resistance to physical disease and creates negative conditions on the mental, moral and spiritual planes of being which may lead to serious mental and psychical disorders.

The main reason why this body and soul destroying habit is so common among those of tender age is because the subject, like that of venereal diseases, is too much avoided in discussions and instruction in the school, church and home. The topic is taboo especially among those who pride themselves on their education and refinement. In view of the untold harm done by this foolish avoidance and concealment of a vital problem, religious instructors, teachers, parents and physicians should learn how to deal properly with this delicate but vital phase of child life. Therefore the free discussion of the subject should be encouraged among those most deeply concerned and in health culture literature.

First let us examine some of the causes of this disease, for disease it truly is. The causes of it are not well enough understood. The seed of this weakening indulgence is frequently sown during the prenatal period. Abnormally strong sexuality in one or both parents may be transmitted hereditarily, and especially so if intercourse takes place during pregnancy. This is a real crime against the pregnant mother and the unborn child. In the animal world the female is never sexually active during the period of gestation, and so it should be with man. It is a sad commentary on our system of education, scholastic as well as religious, that our young people are not instructed in these all important laws of nature. We all know how the slightest prenatal characteristics are repeated in the offspring; how the unborn infant is apt to be "marked" by transitory impressions, especially by sudden fright and other strong emotions. Is it any wonder that the most powerful of human emotions should leave its impress upon the growing sex centres in the brain and nervous system of the child, causing abnormal and precocious development? Truly in such cases perversion is born and bred in the flesh and bone before the child sees the light of day. The mother cannot be blamed for this if she has not been instructed on the subject. Also, being in a dependent position, she feels bound to submit to the demands of her husband at these times in order to maintain her hold upon him. Much of the fault therefore lies with the men and with those of the medical profession who teach them that the free indulgence of sexual passion is not only legitimate but necessary to manly vigour. If our young men were taught that greater happiness is attained by the exchange of tender affection than by the frequent indulgence of the appetites and that the creative forces thus preserved develop and strengthen their finest capacities of body, mind and soul they would be wise as well as chivalrous in protecting mother and child. Many a man whom we have thus advised has become a lifelong friend in consequence. Young men should be made aware that in this regard as well as in other habits desire grows with indulgence, and that through such indulgence he who should be the master becomes the abject slave. This is true of overeating, drinking, gambling and drugging as well as of the habits under discussion. This places the responsibility not so much with the "defective" child as with the ignorant or inconsiderate parents.

In connection with this subject I must mention that, in the course of my professional work, a woman will sometimes confide to me that the real cause of her physical, nervous or mental ailments lies in excessive intercourse; that this produces loathing and revulsion which she dares not reveal to her husband, being afraid that she might disappoint and offend him. On occasion I have taken it upon myself, without the knowledge of the patient, to have a confidential talk with the husband and to apprise him of the situation. In every instance the man expressed great surprise and regret for having in his ignorance caused such suffering and anguish of mind. His reply would be somewhat as follows: "I was under the impression that her desire was as strong as mine and often thought it necessary to her. I will cheerfully exercise self control for her sake as well as my own." In several instances understanding and confidence established in this way between husband and wife have transformed a very unhappy relationship into perfect and affectionate harmony.

There is something very wrong with a system which permits people to enter upon a relationship of such vital importance as marriage in total ignorance of its fundamental laws. Ignorance as well as excessive delicacy and hypersensitiveness prevent many well-intentioned people from establishing a thorough understanding concerning this intimate relationship. This leads to much unnecessary suffering, unhappiness and anguish of spirit which might easily be avoided by a freer and more sympathetic exchange of conjugal confidence. Among the animals copulation does not take place except for reproduction. While I am not prepared to take the extreme stand that this should be the ironclad rule in the human family, still continence is certainly to be desired, and self mastery will enhance true conjugal affection and love instead of diminishing or destroying it. Few men are aware of the fact that the normally constituted woman craves affection and kindly consideration rather than sexual indulgence. Many men, afraid of real or imaginary weakness, remain single because they have a false idea of the sexual demands of woman. A free and confidential understanding in regard to these matters between those who contemplate matrimony would frequently prevent marital unhappiness.

Next in importance to prenatal influence comes the diet after weaning and during early childhood and adolescence. Most of the poisonous acids and alkaloids contained in the flesh of dead animals are powerful stimulants. I have frequently noticed that people who have long abstained from meat on first partaking of it again experience symptoms resembling those of intoxication. We have already seen that those stimulating principles of meat are similar to alcohol, caffein, thein and nicotine and that meat eating invariably fosters an appetite and craving for these and other stimulants. The legumes or pulses, peas, beans and lentils, are close seconds to meat in pathogen producing qualities. Eggs also contain considerable ready made uric acid and a great deal of phosphorus and sulphur which form many nerve stimulating acids, alkaloids and ptomaines. For these reasons meat, pulses and eggs are always danger foods to the child. The most serious aspect of this question lies in the stimulating influence of these food poisons on the sex centres in the brain and nervous system. It is a well known fact, verified by close observation, that flesh foods stimulate the sexual passions to a marked degree. This tendency is greatly influenced by the use of tea, coffee and alcoholic stimulants in the form of wines, liquors and medicines. If the sensitive nervous organism of the child is overwrought by these powerful irritants there can be but one result, precocious sexual awakening.

Next to prenatal influence and stimulating food and drink, ignorance is the main cause of sexual perversion. If religious instructors, teachers and parents do not early enough give the child the necessary information concerning the sex functions and their legitimate use and abuse, the child may learn concerning these things from unscrupulous and vicious servants and playmates in a way not at all conducive to health and morality. This subject, instead of being something to be shunned as unclean by refined and sensitive people, is worthy of confidential discussion between parent and child. The marvels of creative life and its modes of manifestation in the vegetable, animal and human kingdom can be introduced to the mind of the child. The workings of the procreative principle may be traced through the ascending kingdoms of nature without any offence to the sensibilities.

We must now consider the weakening and destructive effects of masturbation. I have become thoroughly convinced through much experience in dealing with such cases that the destructive effects of onanism are in many instances more of a mental and psychical than of a physical nature. Too weak to resist the almost uncontrollable desire, the victim of the disease struggles vainly in loneliness and silence with no one to confide in and no one to go to for advice and encouragement. The vague allusions to the terrible consequences of the habit which he hears and reads about here and there, the terrifying literature of quack doctors and unscrupulous medical publicists who prey upon the fears of these unfortunates, fill their minds and souls with remorse, dread of the future and expectancy of impotency and early decline. As is always the case, fear materializes that which it fears. Fear is faith in evil, and faith has creative power for evil as well as for good. Deep down in his soul the victim of morbid imagination sees himself weak, diseased, impotent, prematurely old and in an early grave, and "as he thinketh in his heart so he is." Much experience in an extensive practice has taught me that the physical effects of the habit can be overcome easily by natural methods of living and treatment as soon as the patient ceases to violate the laws of his being. Sympathetic advice and the right kind of suggestive treatment will greatly aid him in doing this. But also his self confidence must be aroused, his faith renewed and his will power strengthened. I find this as a rule more difficult than the regeneration of the physical organism. He must be made to realize that his consciousness is part of the universal intelligence, that his will is an expression of divine creative force, that these are superior to the weakness and the animal desires and propensities of the lower self. The best way to awaken and to strengthen this constructive faith is to practice the formulas given in the last chapter of this book. This auto suggestive treatment may be practised at any time during the day when there is an opportunity for concentration, even though it may be only for a few minutes. The best time in the twenty-four hours is, however, just before going to sleep. If this is done faithfully and persistently, with fervent desire of the spirit and uncompromising determination of the soul, the patient cannot possibly fail in his resolve. This mental attitude was what Jesus had in mind when he said, "What things soever ye desire, when ye pray, believe that ye receive them and ye shall have them". Simple as these methods may seem, there is no better way to strengthen the weakened will, or to overcome bad habits and establish better ones.

In a general way, the natural ways of living and treatment are the simplest and most efficient remedies for overcoming physical and nervous debility. A well balanced vegetarian diet will nourish the body abundantly, while it does not overstimulate the sex centres in the brain and spinal cord as is done by meats and eggs, coffee, tea, alcoholic liquors and tobacco. Nothing on earth stimulates a sluggish circulation and tones up a debilitated nervous system like a brisk cold rub in the morning and a cold sitz bath in the evening. The morning cold rub should be followed by deep breathing and other exercises in the nude. Corrective gymnastics, especially internal massage and exercises while lying on the back will strengthen and vivify the flabby muscles and debilitated nerves of the abdominal and genital organs. Overeating and the use of meat, eggs, coffee, tea, alcoholic liquors and tobacco should be strictly avoided. Faithful adherence to this natural regimen will overcome indigestion, malnutrition, constipation and sluggish circulation, which usually accompany sexual weakness and nervous debility and help to produce them.

Doctors almost universally treat involuntary emissions too lightly. They say that such discharges are an indication that the sex organs are generating an excess of sex fluids, and that these might just as well be got rid of through nocturnal emissions. Some doctors, and many habitual masturbators apply similar sophistry to the practice of onanism. Such opinions, however, are based upon grave error. It is a fact that, as a rule, the sexually strongest individuals are not subject to involuntary emissions, while those so afflicted are most often weakly, sickly and of the nervous debilitated type. The true explanation is that any excess of sex fluids is normally absorbed into the system through the lymphatic structures of the inguinal glands, and serves to stimulate and invigorate all the vital functions and the creative capacity of mind and soul. But if these glands are engorged with pathogenic materials the sex fluids are not absorbed into the system; they stagnate in the sex organs and cause abnormal sex stimulation, neurotic dreams, unnatural craving for intercourse or masturbation, or, as an alternative, involuntary emissions. Such pathogenic obstruction in the absorbent glandular structures we overcome by natural diet and treatment, particularly by manipulative treatment of the lymphatic glands themselves, for the purpose of relieving them of pathogenic engorgement. In hundreds of the most stubborn cases we have proved the wonderful efficacy of these natural methods in combination with constructive mental, moral and psychical influences.

In order to correct actual impotence, doubt and nervous impatience must be overcome. Perfect confidence and serenity must be established. The treatment should be undertaken not in a spirit of doubt and anxiety, but in the "I-do-not-care-whether-I-succeed-or-not" attitude of mind, exactly the same attitude with which one must meet insomnia or the performance of difficult tasks in any line of effort; as, for instance, passing a difficult examination or giving a public performance. While in all effort there must be strong resolve to succeed and the concentration of mind to do so, this must be accompanied by the "care-less" attitude of mind.

In conclusion, it may be said that it is the duty of all parents to warn their growing children of the pitfalls and vices which lie in their path and threaten their welfare. Too often this duty is shirked or postponed until boys and girls learn from undesirable sources what they should have learned quietly, and without undue emphasis from their fathers and mothers. Fathers have not fulfilled their duty to their sons until they have counselled them along right lines.(1)

[1]
This chapter contains a number of important points. It is to be noted that a very definite distinction is here drawn between genuine virility with sexual and reproductive power and efficiency on the one hand and abnormal sexuality and sexual excitability on the other. It is contended that when the latter is present it can be a great source of loss of vitality and that it can be due to a number of causes among which are prenatal influences, wrong dietary habits and an unhealthy congestion of the pelvic organs. Dr. Lindlahr is here dealing mainly with the question of masturbation and he has more to say about other sexual problems in a later volume. However, it would appear that certain criticisms might be made of what he here says or omits to say. He would seem to imply that sexual activity has little real justification except for purposes of reproduction and that the more continence there is the better it is for the health and development of all concerned. It may be argued that while it is true that celibacy as a way of life is perfectly possible and compatible with good health it should be a genuine sublimation of the physical and emotional energies of the personality deliberately undertaken for the love and service of God or mankind and that in a general way suppression or denial of all sexuality can be harmful both on the physical and the emotional planes. Points which should be considered are (1) that physical love seems to be something of an art and an art cannot flourish unless it is sometimes practised, (2) that both men and women who have been life long celibates do frequently seem to be in a way uncompleted and immature both physically and emotionally. (3) that while sexuality may be coarsening and weakening and an hindrance to the intellectual and spiritual life if it is excessive or indulged entirely from habit or for physical pleasure or release, it yet may be beneficial physically and emotionally for both parties if it is the expression of a genuine relationship and it may then be a help and not a hindrance to high development in intellectual, artistic and moral spheres. Also that it is important that people should learn to love one another and that there are many who do not love at all unless they are allowed at least to start by loving with their bodies. And (4) that the close connection of the endocrine balance and health is a very important matter and is a necessary basis for the good life whether this good life be envisaged as one of celibacy or of controlled sexual activity. Also (5) that masturbation and excessive sexual activity, in so far as its physical effects are concerned, would appear to be more damaging to males than to females since they are on the giving rather than the receiving end of sexual activity, though excessive child bearing can obviously be very harmful to the female.

CHAPTER XXXII

SPINAL MANIPULATION AND ADJUSTMENT

by Jean du Plessis M.D.

History

In many European countries "bone-setters" have, in a crude way, been treating strains and sprains of the spinal column since time immemmorial. These bone-setters usually belong to the peasantry and the art has been transmitted from father to son for many generations. Incidentally, these simple people observed that their treatment relieved not only sprained, tired and painful backs — the result primarily aimed at — but frequently exerted a favourable influence upon disease processes in remote organs and parts. This empirical discovery led to a wider application of this method of treatment.

The various modern systems of spinal manipulation, namely, osteopathy, chiropractic, naprapathy, neuropathy, spondylotherapy and our own neurotherapy are all of distinctly American origin. During the last quarter of a century millions of Americans through personal experience have become staunch adherents to one or more of these systems of treatment. This fact has been instrumental in directing the attention of numerous sincere and scientific investigators to the spinal column with its associated structures as a mechanism through which to apply therapeutic measures. Something therefore must be said about the theories and methods of the various schools of manual and manipulative therapy, all of which differ somewhat from each other both in their theoretical basis and in their technique, though all of them have behind them the idea that there is a close relationship between structure and function and that health and disease in the body are conditioned by its structural, mechanical and postural state.

Osteopathy, which was initiated by Dr. A. T. Still in 1874, was based on the idea that "lesions" of the skeletal structure of the body were the main cause or maintaining factor of disease conditions. The way in which these lesions produced their effects was, in Dr. Still's view, by creating a disturbance of circulation. The form of treatment which

Dr. Still devised consisted in work upon and around joints, particularly those of the spine, with a view to normalizing joints and repositioning bones. Chiropractic which was initiated somewhat later by Dr. D. D. Palmer who tended to regard the ill-effects of "lesions" or "subluxations" as being due to their interference with nerve impulses rather than with circulation. The type of technique of the chiropractors was also somewhat different and laid emphasis on the use of "thrusts" of a particular kind for moving individual spinal joints. The chiropractors also showed much less interest at first in joints other than spinal joints than was shown by the osteopaths. It is undoubtedly true to say that in recent times osteopaths and chiropractors have tended to draw closer together both in their theories and in their technique. It must also be admitted that any controversy as to whether blood supply or nerve supply is the more important is largely academic. The circulatory and nervous systems are in very close association both anatomically and functionally, the circulatory system being largely under nervous control and the nervous system being dependent on the circulatory system for nutrition and drainage. It is a hard matter to say which is of primary importance and which of secondary.

While the osteopaths and the chiropractors have been and still are the most numerous of those engaged in manual and manipulative treatment (except in so far as this type of work is done by masseurs and physiotherapists) there have been and are other schools of manual therapy which have contributed both theories and techniques of great value to all who seek to become experts in manual methods of healing. In the early years of this century a certain Dr. Oakley Smith proclaimed the "connective tissue doctrine of disease." According to this theory vertebrae do not become displaced without being fractured or dislocated. What is called a bony lesion by the osteopath and a subluxation by the chiropractor is something which is due to what Dr. Smith called a "ligatight", that is a shrunken condition of the connective tissue forming the ligaments that bind the vertebrae together. Dr. Smith gave the name of Naprapathy to his theory and technique, which consisted in certain "directos" designed to stretch shrunken connective tissues. In more recent times various systems of manual treatment have been developed or discovered which are somewhat different from manipulation of the framework of the body of the kind which we have been describing. These systems make use of nerve reflexes to obtain their results. Thus osteopaths from early times made use of stimulation and inhibition of spinal nerve centres in treatment, especially of acute conditions. In his method of treatment known as "Spondylotherapy" Dr. Albert Abrams used the stimulation of spinal nerve centres by concussion, pressure or electricity. The system of treatment called "Neuropathy" advocated by Drs. Arnold and Walter was based on a somewhat similar idea. They found that where a certain organ or part of the body was disturbed or diseased there were corresponding changes, as well as tenderness, in the spinal tissues associated neurologically with such organs or parts. By manipulation and thermal applications to these spinal tissues they found that a corresponding effect could be produced on the organs or parts concerned. They also laid great stress on stimulation of the lymphatic system.(1)

We of the Nature Cure school have endeavoured in the manual and manipulative treatment which we use to combine all that is useful in the methods of all schools, provided that they harmonize with the fundamental laws of cure. The resulting system which we have evolved has been named "Neurotherapy". This system and method will be more fully discussed in a later chapter.

If we survey the spinal column and its associated structures we find that the spinal column is made up of a series of separate bony segments called vertebrae. These are placed one on top of another thus forming a pillar or column. Throughout the length of this runs a hollow cylindrical canal which lodges and protects the spinal cord. Between the vertebrae of human beings are found pads of tough, resilient fibro-cartilage which form the main bonds of union and serve as shock absorbers. To the vertebrae are attached strong bands of tough fibrous tissue called ligaments which serve to restrict the motions of the spine. These motions are regulated by the spinal muscles which are responsible for actively holding the vertebrae in alignment. Between the adjacent vertebrae on either side are found oval openings called intervertebral foramina, which communicate with the spinal canal and each of which contains the following structures:—

(a) The spinal nerve, composed of fibres from the various parts of the body to the cord, as well as fibres which convey instructions from the cord to the outlying organs and parts. The spinal cord therefore, is the

---

(1)
    Mention should here be made of a method and theory which is of more recent origin than those here discussed. Dr. Ida Rolf's system of Structural Release and Integration lays stress on the condition of muscles and fasciae as being the basic factor in the creation and development of structural, postural and mechanical faults in the body and of "spinal lesions". It is accordingly to muscles and fasciae that treatment should be mainly directed. If the work of releasing and balancing up the musculature and fascial structures of the body is thoroughly and properly performed the various parts of the body will be brought into proper relationship to one another and to the gravity line and individual lesions or groups of lesions will disappear. The particular technique which is used in this work is highly original and is applied in accordance with a definite plan or sequence. My own feeling is that the contributions of Dr. Rolf both in theory and technique represent a very great advance in manipulative therapy and should be studied by all who wish to undertake this kind of work, although it would be rash to contend that they entirely supercede in all cases the methods and ideas of other schools in this field.

switchboard, as it were, of the nervous system controlled by the brain.

(b) A few small arteries which carry nourishment to the corresponding segment of the spinal cord.

(c) A few small veins and lymph vessels which drain waste products away from the corresponding segment of the cord. The nerve cells in each segment of the cord are, therefore, supplied on both sides by arteries and drained by veins and lymphatics.

(d) A small amount of fibrous connective tissue which surrounds all these structures and forms a cobweb-like arrangement the meshes of which are filled with:—

(e) Semifluid compressible fat tissue which is the most abundant substance present and fills all space not occupied by other structures.

A careful study of the skeletons of all backboned animals reveals the significant fact that the spine comprises the central sustaining shaft which supports all the rest of the framework. For instance, the skull is attached to it in front, the ribs and forelimbs to the sides, the hip bones, hindlimbs and tail in the rear. Broadly speaking, the various parts of the skeleton are mere offshoots from this central pivot, the spine. In the field of biology this is perhaps best illustrated in the gradual development of the complete skeleton of a frog from the "lineshaft" of a tadpole.

Another important fact is that all backboned animals walk on all fours. The suspension of the spine in a horizontal direction makes possible a perfect interlocking of the articular processes of the vertebrae. The human spine, however, has to perform its function in the erect position. This not only prevents the proper interlocking of the vertebrae but also brings the weight of the head and chest outside the centre line of the body, thus necessitating the development of the normal curves of the spine maintained by powerful supportive muscles along the back. In the erect position the weight of the body, sustained by the spinal column, rests upon the pelvic girdle or platform. This, in turn, is supported from underneath by the two thigh bones. Since these are placed in sockets which are placed well toward the front, the body weight resting upon the rear of this platform actually falls far behind these two points of support, the thigh bones. From an engineer's standpoint, therefore, the biped man indulges in a constant struggle to maintain the erect position thereby rendering his weight-bearing column more susceptible to strains and sprains of all kinds.(1)

(¹)
    There can be little doubt that the physical body of man is evolved or developed from some form of four-legged vertebrate. It may however be doubted whether the life of man needs to be a constant struggle against gravity, though there is always a danger of its becoming so. If the musculature of the body is properly balanced the spinal column will be maintained in the erect position without strain much as a tent pole is supported by

The term "lesion" in its broadest sense signifies any departure from the normal. Spinal lesions may be defined as those deviations from the normal of the bones, ligaments or muscles concerned with the spine, which lead to or result from disease in corresponding organs and parts. Since the spine is the weightbearing shaft which supports the entire framework all external force, no matter where or how applied, is transmitted to this central axis. From time to time the infant falls out of its cradle, through the rough and tumble life of childhood, all the way through youth and maturity to old age, the human spine is constantly subjected to falls, jars, blows, twists, over-exertion, fatigue, etc. These mishaps, however, the individual promptly dismisses from his mind; hence he rarely sees the relation between a past accident and his present ailment. The above mentioned strains and sprains, unless severe enough to produce an actual dislocation, result in a wrenched or overstrained condition of the ligaments of the injured joint. Since the body manifests a constant tendency to return to normal this strain is frequently repaired during sleep when all muscles are relaxed and the spine is in a recumbent position with no weight to support. In more severe cases, however, the proliferation and subsequent shrinkage of the connective tissue of the injured ligaments decrease the motility of the affected intervertebral joint or series of such joints. The function of a stiffened region of the spine is readily compensated for by an increased motility of the spinal joints above and below it. Being thus allowed to remain inactive, it becomes fixed to a varying degree. This process is greatly assisted by the presence of an excessive amount of waste products in the system. A process of stiffening tends to follow also sprains of such joints as the ankle, the wrist, the knee, etc. However, since it is hardly possible for these joints to shift their function, slight adhesions which form here are more readily broken up.

In view of all the foregoing facts, is it any wonder that osteopaths, chiropractors and naprapaths would have us believe that as long as human beings are unfortunate enough to possess spinal columns these will persist in getting out of order? It should be remembered, however, that the spine is immune against most such injuries unless they are severe enough or prolonged enough to overcome the resistance of the supporting muscles and ligaments. In other words, the degree of force required to produce a lesion is determined by the degree of strength of the body framework. Injuries, therefore, constitute merely the exciting cause of

guy ropes. It cannot, however, be denied that man, by reason of his erect posture and the enormous variety of ways in which he uses his body, is more prone to postural and spinal derangement than other animals and that such derangement is less likely to be spontaneously corrected.

lesions. The predisposing factor is a weak spine, which in turn is the result of insufficient exercise, malnutrition, faulty posture in standing, sitting or lying and other debilitating factors.

Another important cause of spinal lesion, from the standpoint of Natural Therapeutics, is the following: Nerve impulses coming to the spinal cord from inflammatory processes are promptly reflected to the supporting structures of that region of the spine. Here these abnormal impulses subsequently bring about sufficient irritation to produce lesions such as will be described presently. Since abuse of function causes disease even in an individual with a perfectly normal spine, it is evident that many spinal lesions are the effects and not the primary causes of disease. These secondary lesions in turn tend to perpetuate the original disturbance, thereby establishing a vicious circle.

Different people at different times have held different theories as to what spinal lesions actually are and just how they produce the harmful effects for which they are held responsible. Some of these theories and claims would appear to be confirmed by spinal dissection and some not. Suffice it to say that a lesion is invariably associated with an increase in and a shrunken condition of the connective tissue comprising the ligaments of the affected joint. Most noticeable is a decrease in the thickness and the resiliency of the intervertebral disc — either in part or as a whole (author's note). In major lesions dissection reveals, in addition to the above, a slight shifting of the adjacent articular processes upon each other. Either a bony or a ligamentous lesion alters both the size and the shape of the adjacent intervertebral foramen. This tends to interfere with the function of the structures passing through it. Within each foramen the spinal nerve is comparatively well protected. It occupies on an average only one fifth of the total area, is situated in the largest part of the foramen, is free from all bony contact and is embedded in semifluid compressible fat tissue. The functions of the blood and lymph vessels, however, are more readily disturbed by changes in the size and shape of the foramen. As the nerves and vessels leave the foramen, the fat surrounding them gradually decreases while the connective tissue increases in amount, until finally they are entirely clothed in fibrous connective tissue. Shrinkage of this connective tissue, brought about as previously described, is bound to have an untoward effect, if not on the nerves and vessels within the foramen then surely on their branches immediately outside the foramen. Irritation to the nerve, according to a law in neuro-

(author's note)
  As a result of wrong living it is usual for the discs to become compressed and less resilient with advancing years. Finally the adjacent vertebrae may become entirely ankylosed.

logy, first increases and later decreases the intensity of the nerve impulses conveyed to the corresponding organs or parts, thus giving rise first to acute and later to chronic disturbances.

The motility of a joint in which a lesion occurs is invariably decreased. This is due partly to the shrunken connective tissue already described and partly to tension or infiltration of the muscles governing that joint. The degree of normal activity in any joint determines the amount of blood supply to that joint and to its adjacent structures. Restricted motion of an invertebral joint, therefore, will impair the nutrition of the corresponding segment of the spinal cord. This will naturally pervert the functions of the nerve cells from which originate the nerve fibres coming through the affected foramen. Interference with the nerve supply to any part of the body predisposes that part to the secondary causes of disease, thereby leading first to functional and later to organic derangement.

It should be borne in mind that lesions occurring in other joints of the body give rise to disturbances also. This is especially true of the joints uniting the hip bones and the ribs to the spine. The so called "innominate" lesions are far more frequent than is generally suspected. During pregnancy all the joints of the pelvis become more supple. Even after pregnancy these joints frequently remain in a relaxed condition due to improper food and irrational living before, during and after this important period. Again, in order to compensate for rigidity in the small of the back, the joints between the hip bones and the sacrum almost invariably become abnormally relaxed. As already explained, the erect position places the pelvis at a mechanical disadvantage, thereby subjecting these joints to a considerable strain. Should they be weakened from any cause, then falls, twists, false steps, over exertion, etc. frequently result in lesions which give rise to sciatica, urinary and menstrual disturbances and other pelvic disorders. Lesions at the junction between the ribs and the vertebrae, between the coccyx and the sacrum and in other joints of the framework are of great importance also. Lack of space, however, excludes the discussion of their causes, nature and effects.(1)

[1]
The importance of innominate or sacro-iliac lesions can hardly be overemphasized. The pelvic girdle is a sort of pivot on which the posture and mechanics of the whole body is based and when its integrity is impaired, as it is when sacro-iliac subluxations take place, the effects are very fundamental and far-reaching. The sacro-iliac joints appear to be shock-absorbers rather than moveable joints of the ordinary kind and if they become deranged the effects appear to be both mechanical and neurological. The mechanical effects are mostly due to the fact that the relative length of the two extremities is altered so that the sacral base on which the spine rests is tilted and the relationship of the lower extremities to the spine is upset. The neurological effects can be extremely varied, producing symptoms in various organs and parts of the body. Daniel Mackinnon in his book "The Conquest of Pain" lists a number of symptoms which are almost invariably due to innominate lesions in whole or in part.

In diagnosing any given abnormal manifestation, a careful analysis of the corresponding region of the spine furnishes indispensible information as to the role played by structural lesions in causing or perpetuating the trouble in question. The most elaborate examination, therefore, is incomplete without a painstaking analysis of the spine and those parts of the framework attached to it. The most important steps in this procedure consist in noting peculiarities of gait and posture, the absence or presence of the normal spinal curves, the relative tone of the spinal tissues, the absence or presence of tender spots along the spine, the alignment of the vertebrae, ribs and hip bones; but, above all, the degree of motility of each joint of the spine and its attached structures. The above procedure necessitates the viewing of the bodily mechanism through the eyes of an engineer. It also requires a sense of touch sufficiently keen to detect the least variation in the density and motility of the various parts of the spine and framework; it literally means "seeing" with the finger tips. Every vertebrae apparently out of line does not necessarily indicate the presence of a lesion. It may merely signify a deformed spinous process. On the other hand, where inspection and palpation of the spine suggest no apparent abnormalities, tests for motility reveal obscure lesions in the form of more or less fixed joints. This impaired mobility is usually compensated for by increased pliability of the joints above and below it. Briefly stated, a spinal lesion manifests, among other characteristics, varying degrees of tenderness and muscular rigidity during its acute stage and tension in the joint during its chronic stage. In puzzling cases an X-ray examination may be of great assistance.

Structural analysis constitutes only one of several procedures to be employed in arriving at a definite diagnosis. It must be supplemented by physical examination, iridiagnosis, urine, gastric and faecal analysis, blood count, sputum examination, basic diagnosis and every other method of examination that will throw light on the past and present condition of the patient. Often not until after the findings from all these sources have been compared and correlated can there be established a diagnosis that will reveal not only the nature of the abnormal process but also its underlying causes, both primary and secondary.

Dealing with acute and chronic lesions in the best way requires skill and experience and may vary from case to case, but certain general rules and principles can be indicated. Acute lesions tend to require rest of the parts affected, careful inhibition over the tender areas and, in severe cases, cold packs. Graded massage and passive movements are to be given at an early date. Thrusts and directos during this period are generally not only uncalled for but likely to prove positively detrimental. Chronic lesions, as above stated, imply joints which have become stiffened to a varying degree. Treatment, therefore, should aim at re-establishing normal motility. We caution against the manipulation of tubercular joints in the spine or elsewhere and also against indiscriminate attempts at the breaking up of long standing ankyloses.

Although the application of neurotherapy differs with each individual case, the procedure in general consists of the following steps. These are not necessarily administered in this sequence nor are they all employed at the same time.

(a) The muscles governing the affected joints are deeply kneaded if infiltrated, and stretched if contracted.

(b) The spine as a whole is put on a good general stretch in every direction. The ligaments of the stiffened joints naturally are the first to feel this force because those of the normal joints are slack.

(c) To the tensed joints are applied such osteopathic moves as tend to re-establish normal motility in every direction. These enhance the metabolism of the joints and neighbouring structures including the spinal cord.

(d) To the bony lesions, careful chiropractic thrusts are given. These tend to readjust the shifted articular processes by stretching those bands of shrunken connective tissue which are responsible for maintaining the bony lesions.

(e) The ligamentous lesions are corrected by means of naprapathic directos. These aim at stretching the definite strands of shrunken connective tissue in the ligaments of the affected joints.

(f) Spondylotherapy concussion is given whenever indicated.

(g) At the end of each treatment the flabby areas of the spine are stimulated and the overactive areas and tender spots are carefully inhibited by neuropathic manipulations.

This last process is of the utmost importance because in addition to correcting structural lesions, every osteopathic spinal twist, stretch or pressure, every chiropractic thrust, every naprapathic directo, will and does originate nerve reflexes. These reflexes exert either a beneficial or a detrimental influence on some other abnormality from which the patient may be suffering at the time.

In recent years chiropractors have been teaching that during and after the removal of a lesion the disease process caused by the lesion gradually reverses itself. It begins to pass from the abnormal back to the normal. The symptoms which manifest themselves as a result are spoken of as "retracing" symptoms. These are looked upon by the medical profession as "aggravations" if they occur in the diseased part itself. Should they appear elsewhere they are dealt with as "complications". Naprapaths have been referring to such symptoms as "repair changes". The school of Nature Cure for more than half a century has recognized these apparently alarming symptoms as attempts at reconstruction or healing crises. These crises tend to develop during each and every disease process, whatever its cause, no matter whether it is being treated correctly or wrongly or not at all. This whole matter of crises and the laws governing them has been dealt with in an earlier chapter.

For the purpose of restoring the normal curves of the spine, active movements (curative gymnastics) are devised. These aim at developing those groups of muscles which are responsible for maintaining the normal spinal curves, thereby keeping the weight of the head and chest within the centre-line or gravity line of the body. Other active and stretching movements are devised for promoting suppleness and for strengthening the spine as a whole. These exercises are specific for each case and are not prescribed until the more severe lesions have been corrected. Physical culturists in general devote entirely too much time and effort to those exercises which bring into play mainly the upper and lower extremities. If they realized that man is as young as his spine is limber and strong, they would pay more attention to developing the spine and to limbering up each of its joints. By so doing they will derive twice the benefit in one-half the time and will prevent the harmful effects resulting from indiscriminate exercises which do not take into consideration the normal curves or the presence of lesions.([1])

According to the teachings of Doctors Still, Palmer and Smith, the human organism is self-regulating — health is automatic. Disease is merely a process during which health is labouring under difficulties — it is health handicapped. Since the body is also a self-repairing organism, treatment calls for nothing more nor less than the removal of handicaps. Spinal lesions and their correction, therefore, constitute all there is to the cause and cure of disease. In this relation we may note the following which appears in naprapathic literature: "If a puddle of water is produced by a small leak in the roof, find, treat and cure the leak. The naprapath, instead of treating the organic or functional disturbance (the puddle), finds, treats and cures the diseased ligament (the leak)." If a puddle of

[1]
It is undoubtedly true that many forms of "physical jerks" and physical exercises which are prescribed for people or which they prescribe for themselves leave much to be desired and are often useless or positively harmful. However, we have in yoga a method of reconstructing and maintaining the framework of the body which has stood the test of time and which would, if more widely followed, render unnecessary much of the work which is now done by the various schools of manipulative therapy. Yoga may also be used in combination with manual and manipulative methods with very good results. There are, however, some cases in which even simple yogic postures and routines should only be attempted under expert guidance and instruction and with an intelligent appreciation of the requirements and capabilities of the patient, and the more advanced forms of yoga should in any case not be undertaken without the guidance of a competent teacher.

water is on your floor as a result of a leak in your roof, would you leave the puddle to spoil your floor and merely patch up the leak, leaving your roof in such a condition that it is liable to spring other leaks? That is what the naprapath, chiropractor or osteopath does when he merely adjusts the spine. Would you not carefully wipe up the puddle, repair the leak and so reinforce your whole roof that it will be able to withstand future rain storms? That is what Natural Therapeutics does when it promotes the elimination of morbid matter from the system (wiping up), readjusts the spine (the repairing), and makes it lesion proof by means of corrective exercises (the reinforcing). It is encouraging to note that osteopaths in general have already detected the inadequacy of their slogan, "Find the lesion and remove it." The fact, however, that they are gradually adopting also the allopathic maxim, "Find the germ and kill it", proves that they are not as yet familiar with the fundamental laws of cure. As evidence of this, osteopaths are today advocating the use of germicides, antitoxins, serums and vaccines. In addition, they practice major surgery and allow advertisements of patent medicines in their journals. Let it be understood that in order to manifest perfect health the body cells demand not only unimpaired nerve and blood supply, but also the proper amount and kind of nourishment, as well as the prompt elimination of their waste products. Given an unimpaired nerve supply under natural surroundings, health would be automatic. It is essential, however, to "adjust" not only the patient's spine but also his food supply, his mental attitude, his environment and his habits of living in general.(1)

(1) The criticisms of Osteopathic theory and practice made by Dr. du Plessis, the writer of this chapter, and by Dr. Lindlahr himself are to some extent justified, but it is doubtful if they are entirely fair to the profession as a whole. Dr. Still himself was not a very highly educated or articulate person but he was a practical genius with a great idea, a very profound knowledge of anatomy and an understanding of its relationship to body functioning. Some of his early disciples were, however, scholars and thinkers of distinction who very much developed and widened osteopathic theory and correlated it to sciences such as physiology, pathology, endocrinology and biochemistry. The most outstanding among these pioneers were, perhaps, Drs. Hulett, Lane and Martin Littlejohn, the founder both of the Chicago College and of the British School of Osteopathy. These men retained the belief that Osteopathy in its widest sense was a complete system of therapeutics but they were far from regarding all disease as being due to "a bone out of place" which only had to be "fixed" to bring about cure. Dr. Littlejohn conceived of Osteopathy as a method of healing by adjustment and this included not only anatomical adjustment but physiological adjustment and a proper adjustment as between the patient and his environment, including diet. His basic philosophy of health and disease was actually not very far removed from that of Dr. Lindlahr in that he firmly believed in the tendency of the body to be healthy and in its ability to overcome disease provided that it was properly adjusted so that its own resources were fully liberated and rightly directed. This was to be done mainly by manual techniques on the framework and nerve pathways of the body but in other ways too when this was indicated. He rejected the use of inorganic drugs and of serums and vaccines for much the same reasons as Dr. Lindlahr. In treatment the differences between the two appear mainly to be of emphasis. Littlejohn placed greater reliance on manual procedures and not so much on dietetics, hydrotherapy and homeopathy. He was also prepared to allow a larger role to surgery than was acceptable to Lindlahr.

CHAPTER XXXIII

NEUROTHERAPY

Osteopathy, chiropractic, naprapathy, neurotherapy and spondylo-therapy are various systems of manipulative treatment which have been devised mainly to correct spinal and other bony lesions, shrinkage and contracture of muscles, ligaments and other connective tissues. In the previous chapter a detailed explanation was given of the philosophy and practice of these various systems. I shall now only throw on them a few sidelights from the viewpoint of Natural Therapeutics. Important as these methods are in the treatment of acute and chronic diseases, by themselves they are not all sufficient because they deal only with the mechanical causes of disease, not with the chemical, thermal, nor with the mental and psychical. The most efficient spinal treatment cannot make good for the bad effects of an unbalanced diet which contains an excessive amount of poison producing materials and is deficient in all the important mineral elements or organic salts. Just as surely as mental therapeutics and a natural diet cannot correct bony lesions produced by external violence, just so surely is it impossible to cure monomania or obsession, or to supply iron, lime, sodium, etc., to the system by correcting spinal lesions.

The trouble with the manipulative schools and their graduates is that they adhere too closely to the mechanical theory and treatment of disease; that they reject practically all natural methods of treatment aside from the manipulative, and that so far as the osteopathic school is concerned its practitioners show a strong tendency to fall back upon the old school methods of drugging and of surgical treatment. This is due to the fact that in many types of disease manipulative treatment by itself has proved insufficient to produce satisfactory results.

In order to do justice to our patients and not to neglect our respon-sibilities towards them we must use in the treatment of disease all that is good in all the natural methods of healing. In serious chronic cases any single one of these methods, whether it be pure food diet, hydrotherapy, massage, spinal treatment, mental therapeutics or homoeopathy, is not by itself sufficient to achieve satisfactory results or to produce them fast

248

enough. To use an illustration: "Suppose a wagon full of freight requires the combined strength of six horses to move it and suppose that number of horses is available. Would it not be foolish to try to move the load with one, two, three, four, or even five horses? Would not common sense suggest the saving of time and effort by working all six horses at once?

In Natural Therapeutics every one of the various methods of treatment is supplemented and assisted by all the others. The manipulative schools of healing maintain that practically all disease is caused by mechanical abnormalities of the spinal column or of muscles, ligaments and other connective tissues, due to injury or impingement. The philosophy of Natural Therapeutics, on the other hand, points out that a large proportion of such spinal and other mechanical lesions are secondary manifestations of disease, not primary causes; that acute or sub-acute inflammatory conditions in the interior of the body may cause nervous irritation and thereby contraction of muscles and ligaments and, as a result of these, luxations of vertebrae or of other bony structures.

The naprapathic theory of disease postulates that it is the shrinkage and contraction of the connective tissues, which serve as a support and protection for the nerve matter contained in the nerve trunks and filaments, that causes interference with the normal nerve supply of cells and tissues and thereby abnormal function and disease. The philosophy of Natural Therapeutics points out that this shrinkage and contraction of the connective tissues surrounding and permeating the nerve trunks and filaments is caused by certain acids and other pathogenic materials which are produced by faulty diet and defective elimination, and that the same causes produce accumulation of waste and morbid matter in the tissues of the body which, all through the system, interfere just as effectually with nutrition, drainage and innervation of the cells and tissues as do spinal lesions and ligatights. While the other systems of manipulative treatment confine themselves almost entirely to the correction of bony and other connective tissue lesions, to "pressing the button" as it is called, neurotherapy, besides this, aims at other very important results. In disease the tissues are either in an abnormally tense and contracted or in a weak, relaxed condition. The functional activities are either hyper-active as in acute inflammation, or sluggish and inactive as in chronic atonic and atrophic conditions. These extremes can be powerfully influenced and equalized by manipulative inhibition, relaxation or stimulation. During an acute attack of gastritis, for instance, the neurotherapist would exert strong inhibition on the nerves which supply the stomach. This is accomplished by deep and persistent pressure on the nerves where they emerge from the spinal openings (foramina). This diminishes the rush of blood and nerve currents to the inflamed organ, and thereby eases but does not suppress the inflammatory process and the attending congestion and pain. In case of extreme tension in any part of the system, relaxation of the shrunken tissues can be brought about by gentle but persistent stretching of the nerves and adjacent muscles and ligaments, in a manner similar to that of the naprapathic directos. When the vital organs and their functions are weak and inactive or when nerves, muscles, ligaments and other connective tissues are in a relaxed, atonic or atrophic condition, certain stimulating movements applied to the nerves where they emerge from the spinal column will energize the vital functions all through the system. Many patients imagine that such manipulative treatment is superficial. To them it is just "rubbing" and seems all alike. They do not realize that manipulative stimulation applied to the nerves near the surface of the body travels all along the branches and filaments like electricity along a complicated system of copper wires, and thus reaches the innermost cells and organs of the body, making them more alive and active. This internal stimulation of vital activities is attained also by good massage through energizing the nerve endings all over the surface of the body.

Some of my readers may entertain the idea that the chiropractic, naprapathic and osteopathic schools have practically the same conception of acute diseases and healing crises as the school of Natural Therapeutics. This, however, is not the case. On the contrary, osteopaths, naprapaths and chiropractors on the whole adhere to the allopathic idea of acute disease as being in itself harmful and dangerous to health and life, something which therefore ought to be checked as quickly as possible. If anyone should doubt this, the following extracts from an article in the International Chiropractic Journal, entitled "Fevers", will convince him to the contrary. Similar criticisms of the Nature Cure conception of acute disease and healing crises have also appeared in osteopathic journals:—

"The Chiropractic theory (of fever), which I affirm, is briefly this: The primary cause of every fever is vertebral subluxation impinging nerves so as to disturb the heat regulating mechanism of the body. The subluxation operates chiefly by controlling the calibre of the blood vessels and thus the amount of blood in a given part of the body at a given time. Fever is a process, instituted through the co-operation of primary cause (subluxation) and secondary cause (poison, germ, etc.) which is destructive to the body and tends to destroy life unless checked. It is a malign process which nature strives to prevent and correct when once in operation.

"The Nature Cure theory, which I deny, is in brief: Fever is a process resulting from a house-cleaning effort on the part of nature, who seeks to remove from the body the filth accumulated there through faulty habits of living. It is a beneficient process which should not be checked lest its arrest harm the organism and leave it in its state of filth. The primary cause of fever is error of diet, lack of exercise, etc.

"Let us contrast the two theories. A recent discussion brought out the fact that Chiropractors seek suddenly to check, or abort a fever by adjustment and that all believe that less damage is done to the body, that there is less liability of unpleasant sequels when fever is checked as soon as possible. If the Nature Cure theory is correct, then every Chiropractor should avoid 'breaking up' a fever. Logically, he should aid elimination and do as much as possible to give vitality to the patient, but the fever should run until the body is thoroughly 'cleansed'.

"Here are some facts of common experience. The most frequent reduction of temperature in pneumonia is two degrees in from five to ten minutes following the adjustment. It is a rule that all acute fevers disappear in from a few minutes to two days after adjustment is commenced ... If the Chiropractic theory is correct, we check the fever by reversing the process of its causation."

I shall not comment at length upon the above extracts. This entire volume constitutes my answer to this and other criticisms of Nature Cure. However, I can say that, in the first place, I do not believe acute disease of a serious character such as scarlet fever, diphtheria, typhoid fever, pneumonia, cerebro-spinal meningitis, etc., after they once have a good and well defined start, can be suppressed by osteopathic, chiropractic, naprapathic or manipulative treatment. In the second place, if such suppression were possible it should not be permitted because it would surely result in serious harmful after effects and pave the way to chronic disease as do other forms of suppression of nature's acute reactions. I am justified in expressing an opinion in this matter because for over fifteen years graduates of the best osteopathic, chiropractic and naprapathic schools have been working and teaching in our institutions. Suppose a person should develop a good healing crisis in the form of a diarrhoea, acute catarrhal inflammation, skin eruption, boils, carbuncles or some other inflammatory feverish form of elimination. What would happen to such a purifying, healing effort of nature under purely chiropractic care aimed at its immediate arrest by manipulative adjustments? Undoubtedly the patient would be thrown back into the chronic condition if the manipulative measures were such that they did suddenly abort the acute crisis. This does not mean that manipulation, properly applied, may not be very helpful in the treatment of acute diseases. But I do insist that inflammatory processes, after they have once started, must not be checked or suppressed — that the most essential part of the natural treatment in such cases consists in fasting and hydrotherapy. These promote the elimination of morbid matter more thoroughly than does any other method of treatment. The underlying causes of disease must be removed before we can bring about a normal condition of the organism. Suppose the chiropractor, osteopath or naprapath should succeed in suddenly stopping a fever. The patient would continue to "load up" with more morbid materials (especially as these schools tend not to teach the importance of natural dietetics), and it would only be a matter of time until the morbid accumulations in the body would excite new acute reactions, necessitating more adjustments. In the long run this can have but one result, and that is chronic disease.

Massage has very much the same effects upon the system as cold water treatment. It accelerates the circulation, draws blood to the surface, relaxes and opens the pores of the skin, promotes the elimination of morbid matter and stimulates the electromagnetic energies of the body. We have learned that one of the primary causes of chronic disease is the accumulation of waste matter and systemic poisons in the tissues of the body. These morbid encumbrances obstruct the circulation, interfere with osmosis and prevent the normal activity of the organs of elimination, especially the skin. The deep going massage, the squeezing, kneading, rolling and stroking, actually squeezes the stagnant blood and morbid accumulations out of the tissues into the venous and lymphatic circulation, speeds this return circulation, charged with waste products and poisons, on its way to the lungs and other organs of elimination and enables the arterial blood with its freight of oxygen and nourishing elements to flow more freely into the less obstructed tissues. Thorough manipulation of the deeper tissues draws the blood to the surface of the body, and in this way greatly facilitates the elimination of morbid matter through the relaxed and opened pores of the skin. Very important too are electromagnetic effects of good massage upon the system. The positive magnetism of the masseur stirs up and intensifies the latent electromagnetic energies in the body of the patient, very much as a piece of iron or steel is magnetised by rubbing it with a magnet. The more normal and positive, morally and mentally as well as physically, the masseur, the more marked will be the good effects of the treatment upon the weak and negative patient.

CHAPTER XXXIV

MAGNETIC TREATMENT

During the first years of my work as a practitioner of Natural Thera-peutics I administered magnetic treatment in addition to the regular manipulative movements and corrections. The ordinary magnetic treatment is administered by laying the hands on the affected parts or by making passes over the body while at the same time exerting the power of therapeutic faith, will and sympathy. I soon discovered, however, that by some patients the nature and meaning of the treatment was misunder-stood, that they looked upon it with suspicion and fear as a sort of witch-craft or hypnotic process. Such apprehension is unfounded. Hypnotic and magnetic treatments differ decidedly in method and effect. Through the hypnotic process the operator or hypnotist benumbs and paralyses temporarily, or in extreme cases, permanently the highest powers and faculties of his subject, namely, reason, will and self-control. While these higher attributes of the soul are temporarily benumbed and paralyzed the hypnotist, through the concentrated exertion of his imagination and will power, dominates the subconscious mind and by suggestion controls and directs the physical, mental and emotional activities of his subject. This process is, indeed, to be feared because it is destructive in its effects upon both operator and subject. It involves the usurpation of the highest functions of mind and soul. It results in a kind of soul murder and has been called the great psychological crime.(1)

The magnetic healer does not attempt to subdue and control the will power and mental and emotional faculties of his patient. The latter

(1)
Lindlahr loses no opportunity of expressing his disapproval of hypnotism and emphasizing the difference between it and mesmerism (with which it is often confused) and techniques of deep relaxation with suggestion. He is undoubtedly right that techniques which reduce a patient to a state in which he is not normally conscious and in which his reason, will and subconscious mind are subordinated to another are gener-ally speaking evil and dangerous and ultimately harmful even when honestly used for therapeutic purposes. However, it can be argued that there are circumstances in which hypnotic techniques can be used usefully and constructively in emergencies to produce sleep or anaesthesia and in the treatment of some forms of mental illness or obsession. These matters are very interestingly discussed in the works of Mr. Max Freedom Long.

remains during the treatment fully conscious and self possessed. The magnetic treatment affects only the purely vital conditions of the subject. It arouses, strengthens and harmonizes his weakened, negative and discordant vibrations. As has been demonstrated in other chapters disease is negative, health positive. The one is discordant the other harmonious vibration of the parts and particles composing the human entity on the physical, mental and psychical planes of being. As the life force enters the human organism it is transmuted on the lower planes into electromagnetic and vitochemical energies. The ordinary electric cell contains two plates of opposite polarity immersed in acidulated water. For instance, one of the plates may be zinc which is positive, the other copper which is negative. The vessel is partly filled with a weak solution of sulphuric acid. The plates of zinc and copper are connected by copper wires at the top. The current flows from the zinc to the copper within the fluid and from the copper to the zinc through the wire connecting the upper ends of the plates above the fluid, thus making a complete voltaic circle. The positive electricity of the zinc traverses the liquid to the copper over which it flows through the copper wire to the zinc. The effect is that the part of the wire attached to the copper is positive (+) and is called the positive pole or electrode, while the end attached to the zinc is negative (—) and is called the negative pole or electrode. The generation of this current is accompanied by chemical action in the cell. Experiment shows that the mere contact of dissimilar materials such as copper and zinc electrifies them, zinc being positive and copper negative; but contact alone does not yield a continuous current of electricity. When we plunge the two metals, still in contact either directly or indirectly through a wire, into water, preferably acidulated, a chemical action is set up, the water is decomposed and the zinc is consumed. Water, as is well known, consists of oxygen and hydrogen. The water combines with the zinc to form oxide of zinc and the hydrogen is set free as gas on the surface of the copper plate. So long as this process continues, that is to say so long as there is zinc and water left, we get an electric current in the circuit. The existence of such a current may be proved by a very simple experiment. Place a penny above and a dime below the tip of the tongue, then bring the edges into contact and you will feel an acid taste in the mouth.

A living body is a great electric battery for the production of electromagnetic and vitochemical energies. Every minute cell in the body is an electric cell. Cell substance or protoplasm, as we have learned, is made up of hydrogen plus negative substances. Protoplasm is, therefore, negative in character. Under the microscope the cells appear like tiny islands surrounded by moving streams of blood and lymph. The blood is highly charged with positive mineral elements and also contains small amounts of acids. Here, then, we have all the constituents present in an electric cell or battery, the negative elements in the protoplasm in contact with the positive mineral elements in the blood, and the acid constituents of blood and lymph corresponding to the acid fluid in the electric cell. Acting through these cells and batteries in living bodies, the life force is transmuted into electromagnetic and vitochemical energies. All the tissues and organs of the body are electromagnetic batteries made up of innumerable minute electric cells. The internal and external membranes of the various organs and tissues, like the two elements in an electric cell, are of opposite polarity. In some organs the inner membranes are electromagnetically positive while the outer membranes are negative. In other organs, the electromagnetic conditions are reversed. The secretions of these membranes, also of opposite polarity, mingle and promote the liberation of electromagnetic and vitochemical energies. I use the word "liberation" advisedly because these energies cannot be permanently produced by the physical material elements of the body. Vital force is transmuted through the electric cells and batteries which make up the living body into electromagnetic and vitochemical energies. When vital force leaves the body at death the production of vital energy ceases, although the physical material alkaline and acid elements are still present in the rapidly disintegrating body. For these reasons we should not say that the body produces but rather that the body liberates vital energy. According to the ancient vedic teachings, vital force enters the body through the pituitary bodies and is distributed through the sympathetic and central nervous systems. Modern physiology affirms that the involuntary functions and activities of the body are controlled through the sympathetic nervous system. The brain is the most powerful and active electromagnetic battery in the body. In its infinite multitude of glandular structures and minute cells and batteries, vital force is transmuted into nervous, intellectual and emotional energy. The brain and nervous system are the central power stations whose batteries and dynamos supply all the organs with the various forms of vital energy. The nerves and their ramifications are the wires which conduct and transmit vital energy.

Health, which is the normal activity of the vital functions, depends upon the perfect balance of the positive and negative elements and energies, and this, in turn, depends largely upon the correct combination of food elements. Electricity and magnetism produced by inanimate objects such as electric batteries or machinery belong to the mineral kingdom. These forms of electromagnetic energy are three kingdoms removed from the human. Their vibratory activities are, therefore, too slow and coarse for human bodies and not suitable for the treatment of disease. In each higher kingdom of nature, under the influence of the life elements, all forms of matter and energy undergo constant refinement and assume higher velocity of vibration and greater complexity of structure and function. It is for the foregoing reasons that in our work we have discarded electromagnetic treatment by means of electric contrivances. Several years of experimentation convinced me that this kind of treatment in the long run did more harm than good. In place of these dangerous agencies we apply through the various forms of manipulative and magnetic treatment the healing and harmonizing influences of the vital energies of the human plane. As these vital energies are expended in the organism in the forms of physical, nervous, mental and emotional energy, they are thrown off and form around the body the multi-coloured aura which corresponds somewhat to the exhaust of an engine. The aura is visible only during the hours of wakeful activity. It disappears entirely during sound sleep and reappears on awakening with the beginning of physical and mental activity. The weaker and more negative a person is, the weaker the aura; the healthier and stronger and more active mentally, the more voluminous the aura. It varies from dark and muddy colours to the most beautiful tints of the rainbow. The more harmonious the vibratory conditions on the ascending planes of being, the brighter and more beautiful the colour effects of the aura.

The vital energies manifest in higher or lower ranges of colour according to their higher or lower degree of vibratory velocity and refinement. Thus purely vital energy, that which has been called "animal magnetism", appears close to the body as a vivid red, the colour of blood. Red represents the lowest vibratory range in the colour scale. The higher the degree of velocity and refinement of the vital activity, the higher it manifests in the vibratory range of the colour scale. The finer shades of red express activity of sex passion; the higher love nature produces beautiful effects in pink and lavender; emotions of a religious character appear in shades of blue; intellectual activity, in shades of yellow. Violet and purple indicate intellectual and moral development of a high degree. They are the badge of mastership and royalty. We are told that on the spiritual planes of life angelic beings of a high order of spiritual development appear surrounded by a golden aura. This is the significance of the golden halo with which painters surround the heads of saints and angelic beings.

It is the vibratory quality of the aura of a person which affects us pleasantly or otherwise. This constitutes attraction or repulsion, sympathy or antipathy. Likewise the vibratory quality of the aura determines the therapeutic effect of magnetic and manipulative treatment. The purer and more powerful the magnetic vibrations, the greater the healing power. The more passive and sensitive the vibratory condition of a person, the more amenable he is to the tonic and harmonizing influences of a pure and powerful aura. This explains why certain persons have a soothing effect upon children and sick people, while others have a disturbing effect. It is a problem with which we have to deal in the selection of our operators.

The belief in a healing power emanating from spiritual or celestial planes of life may not be as superstitious as it appears to the worldly wise. Since we understand the possibilities of the wireless telephone, why should it be impossible for the powerful auras of angelic or divine beings to affect those who open themselves to their healing influence? Why should it not be possible for the emanations of the highest spiritual and celestial spheres, filled with beings of godlike nature and divine power, to penetrate into the lower planes of this planetary universe? As we connect our mental and emotional wireless with the higher spiritual and celestial planes of life or with the hells and purgatories, so will be the character of the influx — harmonizing or discordant, constructive or destructive. Since spiritual love is the highest possible vibratory activity of the human soul, it is therefore the most powerful element in magnetic, mental and spiritual healing. The sympathy healers among the peasantry in European countries rightfully name sympathy as one of the basic elements in occult healing, the other two being absolute faith and the positive will. To these I would add a vivid imagination. The secret of the healing power of Jesus undoubtedly lay in his great love for and sympathy with suffering humanity. Those who give manipulative and magnetic treatment shoulder a great responsibility. On the purity and power of their own physical, mental and moral vibrations depends the therapeutic effect of their treatment.

I am often asked the question, "Is there danger of losing my vitality and becoming negative by giving manipulative and magnetic treatment?" It is true that manipulative and magnetic work, like everything else, can be overdone and that thereby it may produce harmful effects upon the operator. But within reasonable limits, massage and magnetic treatments will not deplete the power of the person giving them, provided he keeps his system in good condition. His own vibrations must be harmonious on all planes of being — the physical, mental, moral and spiritual. He must be inspired and actuated by the faith that he can heal, by the positive will to heal and by sympathy with the one he is trying to heal. Such an operator makes himself an instrument for the transmission of the life force, which is healing force, from the source of all life. As he gives, so he receives, for this is the basic law of the universe, the law of compensation. If he gives the treatments in the right spirit he will gain vital force instead of losing it. He will actually feel his own intensified life vibrations and after treating he will experience a feeling of buoyancy and elation which nothing else can impart to him. The magnetic healer who tunes up and harmonizes the weakened and discordant vibrations of his patient may be likened to a musician who tunes up and harmonizes the relaxed strings of his instrument. In so doing he puts himself in harmony with the basic law of compensation. "Give and ye shall receive" and "With what measure ye mete, it shall be measured unto you" are not merely expressions of religious enthusiasm: they are scientific truths.

Unfortunately the majority of people recognize and apply only one aspect of the law of giving and receiving — the receiving. They are only too willing to take, to acquire and to hold, but very reluctant to give a fair equivalent for that which they receive and most unwilling to render service without expectation of reward. From this one-sided application of the law of compensation in social life arises much of the injustice, cruelty and suffering which partakes of the nature of hell on this earth. The keynote of the higher life is that of unselfish, loving service. Our present day social, commercial and political customs and usages are largely dictated by selfishness and greed. These tend to breed poverty and privation on the one hand, and luxury on the other. They are causes of constant strife between capital and labour and of great wars. In commercial pursuits too the interests of seller and buyer are often hostile. Only too often is there enmity between servant and master, with hatred on one side, arrogance, contempt and lack of consideration on the other.

Fortunately, the relationship between physician and nurse on the one hand and the patient on the other is often more harmonious and congenial. No matter how selfish and inconsiderate a person may be, he usually shows the best side to those from whom he expects the healing of his ailments. The best and most successful physicians and nurses are those who are able to establish between themselves and their patients a sympathetic understanding and on this basis mutual faith and confidence. Thus the practice of healing brings out the best and finest qualities of human nature. Every institution for the healing of the sick should be a centre of spiritual power and there is no better way of generating and concentrating healing power than by meetings and lectures in which the principles of true healing are discussed and demonstrated. The intellectual, magnetic and spiritual atmosphere of a centre conducted for healing in the right spirit is a powerful aid to the treatment of difficult chronic and so-called incurable cases. Nervous, mental and psychical ailments are especially influenced and benefited by the operation of higher and finer forces. To surround people suffering from various forms of abnormal psychism and obsession with these vitalizing, harmonizing and protecting influences is the most effective part of the treatment. It is on this basis only that I have been able to explain to myself and to others the rapid cures of such cases which could not possibly result from physical treatment alone. This seems to be confirmed by the fact that in psychical cases as a rule we are not able to obtain satisfactory results in the ordinary home surroundings.

The weakness in chronic disease and the inability of the organism to arouse itself to acute activity is caused by a deficiency of vital energy. The beneficial effect of magnetic treatment is not so much due to the transmission of vital force from operator to patient as to the arousing and stimulating of the latent positive electromagnetic and vitochemical energies of the sufferer — in the polarizing of his magnetic forces. The positive magnetism of the operator stirs up and intensifies the inactive vital energies in the body of the patient, very much as a piece of iron is magnetized by rubbing it with a magnet. The magnet does not impart its own magnetism to the piece of iron, but the active electromagnetic energy in the magnet arouses the latent vibratory activity in the iron. This is proved by the fact that the magnetized iron retains its power so long as it is used for magnetizing other substances and that its magnetic qualities will diminish and disappear entirely with disuse. A healthy person, animated by lofty ideals and the earnest desire to allay pain and suffering, is constantly radiating healing power whether he is aware of it or not. Use of this power for the healing of the sick cannot deplete and weaken the physician; on the contrary, the more he gives of these higher and finer energies, the more he receives from the inexhaustible storehouse of life and healing power. However, the work of the healer will generally gain in effectiveness in direct proportion to the conscious and concentrated effort he makes to benefit his patients.

The electromagnetic energies of the organism can be controlled by the will and either concentrated in or sent away from any part of the body just as the circulation of the blood can be controlled. The latter I saw done by a hypnotist who made the blood flow into and out of the arms and hands of one of his subjects by the power of his will. While this was accomplished by means of a destructive process, it taught a most valuable lesson regarding the power of the will to control the physical conditions and vital energies. I have frequently noticed in my own manipulative work how much the conscious and concentrated effort of the will has to do with the effectiveness of treatment. Often when I have given the usual massage or neurotherapy treatment and the patient still complained of pain in a certain locality of the body, I would lay my hands on the affected area and concentrate my will upon dissolving the congestion in that particular part and upon harmonizing its discordant vibrations. Very shortly, usually within a few minutes, the congestion would be relieved

259

and the pain lessened. You can try this for yourself. Next time you have a headache, recline comfortably in a chair or on a couch, relax completely and then will the blood to flow away from the brain in order to relieve the congestion and the attendant pain. Many of our patients have learned to treat themselves or members of their family in this way. It is obvious that magnetic treatment will not permanently remove pain if the latter be due to irritation caused by a luxated bone, by some foreign body or by local accumulation of morbid matter and poisons in any part or organ. In all such cases the local cause of the irritation must be removed before the pain can subside or disappear.

Mesmer, a French physician, was the first to experiment scientifically with human magnetism and to use it for healing purposes. From him this method was called Mesmerism. Unfortunately the term is also used to designate hypnotism and has thus contributed to the confusion as to the true nature and meaning of these greatly differing practices. Mesmer made his discoveries towards the end of the eighteenth century. About the middle of the nineteenth century, Baron von Reichenbach, a German scientist, took up the work where Mesmer had left it and brought actual proof of the existence of the electromagnetic energies and their manifestation in the aura. He conducted his experiments in a dark chamber impervious to light rays from without. Psychically sensitive persons, after remaining in the dark chamber for a short time, were able to perceive the aura more or less distinctly in the form of light or bluish vapour emanating from living objects placed before them. Clairvoyant psychics, or "sensitives" as he called them, were able to distinguish various colours of the aura.

Von Reichenbach was one of the greatest chemists of his or any other age. He was the first to prepare paraffin and some of the analin dyes from coal tar. The latter part of his life he devoted almost entirely to the study of the electromagnetic fluids emanating from living bodies. He called this emanation Od-Kraft, after Odin, the highest deity of Scandinavian mythology. He wrote a number of valuable treatises on this subject. The title of one booklet is "Who is Sensitive and Who is not?" In this he gives many rules and methods for determining the degree of psychic sensitivity of a person. I ascribe this sensitivity to a high degree of refinement of the sensory organs of the physical body or to the functioning of the sensory organs of the spiritual body. Matter on the physical plane is perceived by the sensory organs of the physical body only, while spiritual matter and its emanations of light, colour, sound, etc. are perceived by the sensory organs of the spiritual body only.

The following experiments will make the purely physical emanations of the aura visible to ordinary sight: In a room dark enough to leave the hands just visible, alternately approach and separate the finger tips. If a person is in good, healthy physical condition streaks of bluish light or vapour will appear between the finger tips. The bluish streams can be stretched out and moved in various directions like rubber bands. If you wish to see the aura emanating from the body, prepare a room containing one window in the following manner: On the wall opposite the window hang a curtain of dull, black cloth. The window should have a shade which can be raised or lowered as may be required. Cover the lower part of the window with some fabric impervious to light and in front of the black curtain place a person nude to the waist. The observers stand in front of and with their backs turned to the window. The transition between daylight and darkness is the best time of day for this experiment. The inflow of light into the dark chamber is regulated by pulling the window shade down to a narrow slit so as to admit just enough light to leave the room in semi-darkness. When the condition of light, or rather of darkness, in the room is perfectly adjusted, the observers, with their backs to the window and their gaze fixed upon the subject, will soon see around the nude body a bluish light or vapour. The emanation will be more or less strong and distinct according to the positive or negative condition of the subject. The healthier and stronger physically, intellectually and morally the person, the more voluminous and distinct will be his aura. The bluish vapour, visible to the physical eye, represents the purely physical emanation of the subject. The higher and finer intellectual, emotional and moral emanations are visible only to clairvoyant sight. I found that about eight or nine persons in ten were capable of seeing the physical aura when the conditions were right. To spiritual sight the physical emanation appears, as before explained, red — the colour of blood. I have elsewhere explained that the aura disappears entirely during sound sleep and reappears with the awakening of consciousness, with the beginning of physical and mental activity; and that during the hours of sleep the body acts as a storage battery for the accumulation of vital energy. When this is exhausted in the daily work the tired feeling makes its appearance and there is a desire for rest and sleep. Sleep is the great restorer of vital energy.

Vital energy is active not only through the laying on of hands, or magnetic passes, but also through the eyes, the sound of the voice and, most of all, through the breath. The principle rule to be observed by the physician when administering magnetic treatment is to place himself in such a position to the subject that opposite parts of their bodies come into juxtaposition, that is the right hand must touch or pass over the left side of the patient, and vice versa. Magnetic passes must proceed from the head downwards over the body, the hands returning in a sweeping outward, circular movement so as not to counteract the downward passes. If you should treat a person from behind or while he is lying on his stomach your hands must be crossed and passed over the body in that way from the head downward in order to cover the opposite poles in the body of the patient.(1)

Magnetic treatment can usefully be used in the treatment of poor circulation in the extremities. The patient should lie on a couch or bed with shoes and stockings removed; lay your hands flat against the soles of his feet or grip his feet firmly around the ankles. Slight friction will aid reaction. While thus applying your magnetic current, will the vital fluids to flow into the extremities and to warm them with the glow of life. I have cured in this manner many cases of chronic cold feet and always advise our nurses and operators to apply this natural treatment in place of the hot water bottle, which brings about a cold reaction and in the long run makes the circulation more inactive.

When giving the magnetic passes in a sitting position the subject should remain in a comfortable, relaxed and receptive condition. The more receptive and sensitive the subject, the more distinctly he will feel the magnetic vibrations like a mild current from an electric battery. A simple experiment to test the existence and strength of the magnetic emanations of a person, is the following: The subject stretches out his hands horizontally while the operator approaches them from below, his finger tips approaching each other and turned upwards. As he slightly moves the finger tips in close proximity to the palms of the subject the latter will feel the magnetic vibrations, according to his degree of sensitiveness, as a slight breath of air or as a more or less powerful electric current. The degree of sensation will vary according to the negativity or sensitivity of the subject and the positivity of the operator.

One of the best ways of administering magnetic treatment is through magnetized water. Water may be charged with positive or negative magnetism as required by the character of the ailment. Positive magnetism has a relaxing effect. Positive magnetism, therefore, would be in

---

(1)
It appears that different sides and different parts of the body have a different polarity and when the hands are used to convey energy, as in magnetic treatment, this must be taken into consideration if the best results are to be obtained. In this connection mention should be made of the work and ideas of the late Mr. L. E. Eeman. He maintained (1) that relaxation and conservation of energy could be promoted by the clasping or crossing of the hands and feet, thus completing a circuit, and (2) that the polarity of left-handed people is generally different from and opposite to that of right-handed people. Mr. Eeman used these ideas to develop techniques for the treatment of patients. He also made experiments in group therapy by joining up patients in circuit or in parallel like electric batteries. In all cases he was careful to bear in mind the difference in polarity of any left-handed people.

order for the treatment of chronic diarrhoea, while negative magnetism is most effective for the treatment of constipation. In order to charge water or any other fluid positively the left hand is placed under the vessel, while the right hand with fingers pointing downwards and in close proximity to the fluid makes circular passes. If a substance is to be magnetized negatively, the process would be reversed, that is the fingers of the left hand must do the charging. In like manner fabrics and other substances may be charged magnetically.

In every family a person possessed of good, healthy magnetism should train for giving this valuable method of treatment. It will be found very helpful in many forms of acute and chronic disease. I have been asked the question whether there is not danger of suppressing crises by the administration of magnetic treatment. There is no danger in this respect because the right kind of magnetic treatment arouses and stimulates the vital energies, and as healing crises are manifestations of increased vital activity magnetic treatment will help to produce them and to increase their constructive activity.

Sympathy healing is a form of treatment practised among the country population of northern Europe. It is an occult science handed down from father or mother to son or daughter in certain families known for their probity and piety. While I was studying Nature Cure in Europe my attention was repeatedly called to the seemingly mysterious and miraculous results obtained by these healers. This led me to investigate their methods and after convincing one of these healers of my sincerity of purpose, he confided to me the secrets of his art. Their remedies consist in prayers, charms and similes. Some plant or object which in some way resembles the disease is given to the person. In this connection it is interesting to remember that Jesus many times made use of material similes when performing works of healing, as when he told the leper to bathe in the River Jordan; when he rubbed the eyes of the blind man with spittle. The mystical remedies become efficient only when administered with faith, will and sympathy. The healer must have absolute faith that he can heal with the aid of the higher powers and he must have the positive will to heal and sympathy with the sufferings of the one he is trying to benefit. The work of healing must be done in silence, without reward and without vain boasting. While going and coming on an errand of mercy the healer does not utter a word unless it be of prayer. He does not accept any material reward for his services nor does he ever speak of his cures. To break any of these sacred obligations would be sacrilegious and would in his opinion bring about the loss of his power. I have plenty of proof that their methods are sometimes strangely successful but at other times they fail equally mysteriously.

The villagers of northern Europe to a large extent depend upon these occult healers for treatment and undoubtedly in most cases with more lasting results than under orthodox treatment. These primitive methods date back to the time when the Germanic matron, the Druid or tribal priest combined in their ministrations the holy offices of physician, prophet and priest. This shows that mental and spiritual methods of healing did not originate with leaders of modern mental healing cults. One cannot help but observe how infinitely more unselfish, pure and spiritual are the methods of these simple country folk than the commercialized, self-advertising practices of certain modern mental healers. If simony or trading in the gifts of the Holy Spirit and in the power of the Holy Ghost was branded as a sin and a crime by the disciples of Jesus, why is it "Christian" science now? The specious arguments of our modern healers as to "the necessity of making a living" and "the labourer is worthy of his hire" are effectively contradicted by the unselfish ministrations of the sympathy healers.

CHAPTER XXXV

THE LEGITIMATE SCOPE AND NATURAL LIMITATIONS OF MENTAL AND METAPHYSICAL HEALING

During the last generation people have perceived more or less clearly the fallacies of old school medicine and surgery. They have grown more and more suspicious of orthodox theories and practices. From allopathic "overdoing" the pendulum has swung to the other extreme of metaphysical nihilism, to the "underdoing" of mental and metaphysical systems of treating human ailments. Some of these systems and cults have met with success and wide popularity, and this is looked upon by their followers as a proof that all the claims and teachings which they make are based upon absolute truth. However, a thorough understanding of the fundamental laws of cure, as I have explained them in this volume, will reveal in how far their teachings and their practices are based upon truth and in how far they are inspired by erroneous assumptions.(1)

For many generations people have been educated in the belief that almost every acute disease will end fatally unless the patient is drugged or operated on. When they find to their surprise that the metaphysical formulas or prayers of a mental healer or scientist will cure the baby's measles or the father's smallpox just as well and possibly better than the pills and potions of the doctor, they are firmly convinced that a miracle has been performed and they become blind believers in and fanatical followers of their new idols. They simply exchange one superstition for another; the belief in the efficacy of drugs and surgical operations for the belief in the wonder working power of a metaphysical formula, a self-appointed saviour, or a reason-stultifying and will-benumbing cult. They have not been taught that every acute disease is the result of a healing effort of nature and therefore fail to see that it is vital force, "the physician

(1)
    Lindlahr's use of the word "metaphysical" would appear somewhat unusual and not to have anything much to do with the Science of Metaphysics as generally understood. He seems to mean by "Metaphysical Healing" any system based on the idea that disease can and should be overcome, not by treatment of the physical body but by thinking it away or making a change in one's mental attitude towards it. He regards Christian Science as the outstanding example of this.

within", that under favourable circumstances cures measles and smallpox as easily as it repairs the broken blade of grass or heals the wounded animal of the forest.

Faith in this vital healing force is good, but what the healer and the Scientist fail to recognize when they say: "Have unlimited faith and all will be well" is that faith needs to be accompanied by works. Though we cannot heal and give life we can in many ways assist the healer within. We can teach nature's laws, we can remove obstructions and we can make the conditions within and around the patient more favourable for the action of nature's healing forces. Obedience to laws is the secret of health and this in turn depends primarily on self-control. The rational thing to do is not to deny the existence and reality of evil and disease and to expect the laws of nature to be strained and twisted to save us from the natural consequences of the violation of those laws, but rather to learn the lessons which the evils are capable of teaching us.

As in medicine, so also in metaphysical healing, men judge by superficial results, not by the real underlying causes. The usual answer to any criticism of Christian Science or kindred methods of cure is: "See the results. Nobody can deny their wonderful cures." Let us see whether there really is anything very wonderful or supernatural about these cures or whether they can be very simply explained. In another chapter we explain the difference between functional and organic disease and show how in diseases of the functional type the life force or healing force, which always endeavours to establish normal conditions and the perfect type, may work unaided up to the reconstructive healing crises and through these eliminate the morbid encumbrances from the system and reestablish normal structure and function. It is in cases like these that metaphysicians attain their best results simply because nature helps herself. On the other hand, in cases of the true organic type, where the vitality is low and the destruction of vital parts and organs has progressed to a considerable extent, the system is no longer able to rouse itself to self-help. In such cases faith alone is not sufficient to obtain results. It must be backed and assisted by all the natural methods of treatment at our command.

In our critical examination of old school methods we found that by far the greater part of all chronic ailments is due to drugging and to surgery. People commence doctoring for little troubles which are aggravated by every dose of medicine and every surgical operation until they end in big troubles. Is it marvellous that such patients improve and that many are cured when they are weaned from drugs and the knife? Metaphysical healers unconsciously do their best and most beneficial work because they induce their followers not to suppress acute diseases and healing crises by drugs and surgical operations, thus allowing them to run their natural course in harmony with the fundamental law of Nature Cure; namely that every acute disease is the result of a cleansing and healing effort of nature. People will refrain from the suppressive drug treatment under the influence of metaphysical teachings which appeal to the miracle loving element in their natures, when they cannot be convinced by common sense Nature Cure reasoning. Thus metaphysicians assist nature indirectly by non-interference and directly by soothing fear and worry, by instilling faith, hope and confidence. Frequently they also aid nature by prohibiting the use of tobacco, alcohol and pork, and otherwise regulating the life and habits of their followers.

Let us consider the problem from another point of view. Let us assume, for argument's sake, that the average person passes in the course of a lifetime through a dozen different diseases. He recovers from eleven of these no matter what the treatment. It is only the twelfth to which he succumbs. Yet whosoever happened to treat the first eleven diseases claims to have cured them and, perhaps, to have saved the patient's life when, very often, the recovery was in spite of the treatment and not because of it. These explanations account for the seemingly miraculous results of metaphysical healing. If healers and Scientists were to explain their cures by the laws and principles of Nature Cure philosophy, mystery and miracle would be taken out of their business.

To believe that God or Nature will overcome the natural effects of our ignorance, laziness and viciousness by wonders, signs and metaphysics, or to deny the existence of sickness, sin and suffering, must lead inevitably to intellectual and moral stagnation and degeneration. I am a thorough and consistent optimist and enthusiast for new ideas, but I do not overlook the fact that in this, as in everything else, there lurks the danger of over-doing and exaggeration. The danger of the revulsion from old time pessimism to modern optimism lies in the fact that the "higher thought" enthusiast may cut from under his own feet the solid ground of reality; that he may become a dreamer instead of a thinker and a doer; and that he may mistake selfish, emotional sentimentalism for practical charity and altruism. This unhealthy "all-is-good, there-is-no-evil" emotionalism leads only too often to weakening of personal effort, a deadening of the sense of individual responsibility and thereby to mental and moral atrophy; for any of our voluntary functions, capacities and powers which we fail to exercise will in time become benumbed and paralysed. Un-prejudiced observers who come in close contact with metaphysicians cannot help perceiving the pernicious effect of their subtle sophistries on reason and character.

A chronic invalid who had been under the treatment of a faith healer for several years exclaimed when we gave her our various instructions for dieting, bathing, breathing exercises, etc: "How glad I am that you give me something to do. I fear I have been imposing too long on the goodness of the Lord, expecting Him to do my work for me." Often afterwards when recovering from life-long ailments, she expressed her happiness and contentment in that she herself was doing something which in her opinion was rational and helpful because it assisted nature's healing efforts. We firmly believe in the influence of mind over matter, in the fact that vibrations of the physical plane by continuity create corresponding vibrations on the mental and psychical planes and vice versa. We know that, in accordance with this law, anything which affects the mind or the moral life of a person affects also his physical condition; but instead of hypnotising the minds of our patients by unreasonable dogmas and formulae, we strengthen and harmonize their mental vibrations by appealing to reason, by teaching and explaining natural laws instead of obscuring and denying them. The more intelligent the patient, the more amenable he will be to such normal suggestions based on scientific truth and on the dictates of reason and common sense. While nonresistance to nature's healing efforts is better than suppression by drugs or the knife, there is something still more helpful and rational than the mere negative attitude toward disease on the physical plane assumed by metaphysical cults. That "something" is intelligent cooperation with nature's cleansing and healing efforts.

Where the old school fails by sins of commission the faith schools fail by sins of omission. Daily many patients are sacrificed through fanatical inactivity when their lives might be saved by the wet pack or cold sponge bath, by the internal bath, rational diet, judicious fasting, scientific manipulation, or other simple yet powerful natural remedies. To permit a patient to perish in a burning fever, depending solely upon the efficacy of prayers, formulae and a self-induced mental attitude, when wet packs and cold sponging would in a few minutes reduce the temperature below the danger point, is manslaughter even though it be done in the name of religion.

Incidents like the following are common in our practice: A little girl in the neighbourhood of our institution contracted diphtheria. The mother, an ardent Christian Scientist, called in several healers of her cult, but the child grew worse day by day until the false membranes in the throat began to choke her to death. A boarder in the house, who was a follower of Nature Cure, finally induced the mother to call upon us for advice by threatening to notify the City Health Department. Within an hour after the application of the whole-body packs and the cold ablutions, the blood was sufficiently drawn away from the local congestion in the throat into the surface of the body so that the child breathed easily and freely and from then on made a splendid recovery. In another case a man had been suffering from sciatic rheumatism for fifteen years. He had swallowed poisonous drugs to no avail. For several years he had been under Mental Science treatment but the suffering had grown more intense. When he applied to us for help we found that the right hip bone (the innominate) had slipped upward and backward. A few manipulative treatments replaced the bone where it belonged and the "sciatic rheumatism" was cured. In this case, the combined "concentration" and prayers of all the metaphysical healers on earth would not have succeeded in replacing the luxated bone, which required the strength of a trained manipulator. Mechanical lesions of that kind (and there are many of them) require mechanical treatment.

Another factor which makes converts to metaphysical healing cults by the hundreds is the "get-rich-quick" instinct in human nature, the desire to get "something for nothing" or for as little as possible. Herein lies the seductive pull of old time drugging and of modern metaphysics. "It does not matter how you live, when you get into trouble, a bottle of medicine or a metaphysical formula will make it all right." Our forefathers were too pessimistic; "higher thought" enthusiasts are often too optimistic. While the former poisoned their lives and paralyzed their God-given faculties and powers by dismal dread of hell's fire and damnation, our modern healers and Scientists have drifted to the other extreme. They tell us there is no sin, no pain, no suffering. If that be true, there is also no action and reaction and there is no need for self-control, self-help or personal effort. The ideal of the faith healer is really the ideal of the animal. The animal trusts implicitly, it has absolute faith. Guided by instinct, God or Nature, it follows the promptings of its appetites and passions without worrying about right or wrong. It acts today as it did ten thousand years ago. In man, reason has taken the place of instinct. We must think and manage for ourselves. We are free and responsible moral agents. If we deny this, we deny the very foundations of equity, justice and right. It behoves us to use the talents which God has given us, to study the laws of our being and to comply with them to the best of our ability so that enlightened reason may take the place of animal instinct and guide us to physical, mental and moral perfection.

CHAPTER XXXVI

THE DIFFERENCE BETWEEN FUNCTIONAL AND ORGANIC DISEASE

Much confusion concerning the curability of chronic diseases by the various methods of treatment arises through failure to understand the difference between functional and organic chronic disease. For instance there is a close resemblance between pseudo and true locomotor ataxia. Often it is difficult to distinguish functional lung trouble from the organic type of the disease. In our practice, several cases of mental derangement which had been diagnosed as "true paresis" proved to be of the functional type and under natural treatment recovered rapidly. Functional diseases may present a very serious appearance, may be labelled with awe inspiring Greek or Latin names and yet readily yield to natural methods of living and treatment.

In diseases of an organic nature, however, right living and self-treatment are usually not sufficient to insure satisfactory results. In such cases all forms of active and passive treatment must be applied and even then it is frequently difficult and sometimes impossible to produce a cure.

Chronic diseases of a functional nature develop when an otherwise healthy organism becomes saturated and clogged with food and drug poisons to such an extent that these encumbrances interfere with the free circulation of the blood and nerve currents and with the normal functions of the cells, organs and tissues of the body. Such cases resemble a watch which is losing time because its works are filled with dust. All that such a waste encumbered watch or body needs, in order to restore normal functions, is a good cleaning. Natural diet, fasting, systematic exercise, deep breathing, cold bathing and the right mental attitude are usually sufficient to accomplish this physical house cleaning and to restore perfect health. Functional disorders yield readily to the various forms of metaphysical treatment. Remove such patients from the weakening and destructive effects of poisonous drugs and surgical operations, supplant fear and worry by courage and faith, and the results often seem miraculous to those who do not understand the power of the purifying and stimulating influence of natural living and the right mental attitude.

In diseases of the organic type, however, good results are not so easily achieved. A body affected by organic disease resembles a watch whose mechanism has been injured and partly destroyed by rust and corrosive acids. If such be the case, cleaning and oiling alone will not be sufficient to put the timepiece in good working order. The watchmaker has to replace the damaged parts. That is easy enough in the case of the watch but it is not so easily done in the human body. Besides, in many instances the corroding acids are the very medicines which were given to cure the disease, and the injury or destruction of vital parts and organs is only too often the direct or indirect result of surgical operations. The watchmaker may remove those parts of the watch which are suffering from "organic" trouble and replace them by new ones. This the surgeon cannot do. He can extirpate but he cannot replace. Operative treatment leaves the organism forever after in a mutilated condition and often prevents or seriously interferes with nature's cleansing and healing crises.

It is often claimed by metaphysical healers that they can cure organic diseases as easily and as quickly as functional ailments. If they better understood the difference between functional and organic disorders as explained in the foregoing pages, they would not make such deceptive and extravagant claims. They would then realize the natural limitations of metaphysical healing. When waste matter, ptomaines or poisonous alkaloids and acids produced in the body as a result of wrong diet and other violations of nature's laws have brought about destruction and corrosion in vital parts and organs — when dislocations and subluxations of bony structures or new growths and accumulations in the forms of tumours, stones or gravel obstruct the blood vessels and nerve currents, shut off the supply of vital fluids, and thus cause malnutrition and gradual decay of the tissues — when in addition to this the organism has been poisoned or mutilated by drugs and surgical operations, then its purification and repair become a tedious and difficult task. Not only must the mechanism of the body be cleansed and freed from obstructive and destructive materials, but the injured parts must be repaired, morbid growths and abnormal formations dissolved and eliminated, and lesions in the bony structures corrected by manipulative treatment. In organic diseases the vitality is usually so low and destruction so great that the organism cannot arouse itself to self-help. Even the cessation of suppressive treatment and the stimulating influence of mental and metaphysical therapeutics are not sufficient to bring about the reconstructive healing crises. This can only be accomplished by the combined influences of all the natural methods of living and treatment.

It is in cases like these that metaphysical healing and hygienic living find their limitation. Such organic defects require systematic treatment by all the methods, active and passive, which the best Nature Cure sanitariums can furnish. It may be slow and laborious work to obtain satisfactory results and if the vitality be too low or the destruction of vital parts and organs have too far advanced, even the best and most complete combination of natural methods of treatment may fail to produce a cure. However, this can only be determined by a fair trial of natural methods. The forces of nature are ever ready to react to persistent, systematic effort in the right direction and when there is enough vitality to keep alive there is likely to be enough to purify and reconstruct the organism and in time to bring about improvement and cure. This explains why, in the organic types of disease, metaphysical methods of treatment alone are insufficient. At least one half of the patients who come to the Nature Cure Physician have faithfully tried these methods without avail, but the failures are easily excused by "lack of faith", "wrong mental attitude", or "something wrong with the patient or his surroundings".

In our experience, too, with patients who had formerly tried metaphysical methods of healing faithfully but without results, we sometimes come face to face with a curious and amusing phase of human nature. As our patients improve under the natural regimen and treatment they gradually return to their "first love" and ascribe the good effects of natural treatment to a better understanding of Science. As health and strength return they say: "Formerly I did not know how to apply Science, but now I know and that is why I am growing better"! I suppose this form of self-deception is due to the fact that people feel flattered by the idea that Providence has taken a special interest in their case and cured them by miraculous intervention, or that the cure has been effected by a mysterious metaphysical principle. It is so much more interesting to be cured by some occult principle than by simple diet and cold water. Undoubtedly it is this mystery-loving element in human nature that makes metaphysical healing so much more popular than common-sense Nature Cure.

Not long ago Professor Munsterberg investigated the claims made by Christian Scientists that they were "constantly curing diseases of the organic type". He reported his findings in a series of articles in McClure's Magazine (1908) stating that he enquired personally into one hundred cases said to have been cured by Christian Science and found that ninety-two of them had been of the functional type, while eight were claimed to have been organic but that in no instance could this be proved beyond doubt.

CHAPTER XXXVII

THE TWOFOLD ATTITUDE OF MIND AND SOUL

The following is an extract from a letter sent to me in response to one of my articles in the Nature Cure Magazine. "Sometimes you say we must rely on our own personal efforts and at other times you teach dependence upon a higher power. This to me is contradictory and confusing. I cannot understand how, consistently, we can do both at the same time. Which is right? Is it best to rely upon our own power and our personal efforts or upon the 'Higher Power'?"

There is nothing contradictory or incompatible in the teachings of Nature Cure philosophy concerning the physical and metaphysical methods of treating human ailments. Both the independent and dependent attitudes of mind and soul are good and true and may be entertained at the same time. It is necessary for us to rely on our own personal efforts in carrying out the dictates of reason and of common sense. But this need not prevent us from praying for and confidently expecting a larger inflow of vital power and intuitional discernment from the source of all intelligence and power in the innermost parts of our being. This twofold attitude of mind and soul is justified not only by reason and intuition, but also by the anatomical structure of the human organism and its physiological and psychological faculties, capacities and powers. The activities of the human organism are governed by two different systems of nerves, the autonomic or sympathetic and the cerebrospinal or sensory-motor. The sympathetic nervous system is the conveyor of vital force to the organs and cells of the body. Just what this vital force is and where it originates we do not know. It is the manifestation of that which we term God, Nature, Life, the Higher Power or the Divine Within.

Heart action, the circulation of the blood, respiration, digestion, assimilation of food, elimination and all other involuntary activities and functions of the human organism are controlled by means of the sympathetic nervous system. The nature of the controlling force itself is not known to us. We do know that it is supremely powerful, intelligent and benevolent. The more we study the anatomy, physiology and psychology of the human organism, the more we wonder at its marvellous complexity

273

and ingenuity of structure and function. Every moment there are enacted in our bodies innumerable mechanical, chemical and psychological miracles. Who or what performs these miracles? We do not know. Yet every moment of our lives depends upon the infinite care and wisdom of this unknown intelligence and power. Why, then, should we not trust the one so faithful? Why should we not ask aid from one so powerful? Why not seek enlightenment from one who is so wise and so benevolent?

However, not all of the human entity is dependent upon a controlling power, nor are all its functions involuntary. Within the house prepared by the Divine Intelligence there dwells a sovereign in his own right and by his own might. He is endowed with freedom of desire, of choice and of action. He creates in his brain the nerve centres which control the voluntary activities of the body and from these brain centres he sends his commands through the fibres of the motor nerves to the voluntary muscles and makes them do his bidding, some he commands to walk, others to laugh, to eat, to speak, etc. This independent principle in man we call the ego, the individual intelligence. It imagines, desires, reasons, plans and works out, by the power of free will and independent choice, its own salvation or destruction, physically, mentally, morally and spiritually. By means of the motor nervous system this thinker and doer directs and controls from the headquarters in the brain all the voluntary functions, capacities and powers of the human organism. This part of the human entity can evolve and progress only through its own conscious and voluntary personal efforts.

In this Man differs from the animal creation. The animal is able to take care of itself shortly after birth. It inherits, fully developed, those brain centres for the control of the bodily functions which the new born human must develop slowly and laboriously through patient and persistent effort in the course of many years. Of voluntary capacities and powers the new born infant possesses little more than the simplest unicellular animalcule, about all it can do is to scent and swallow food. Its cerebral hemispheres are as yet blank slates to be inscribed gradually by its conscious and voluntary exertions. Before it can think, reason, speak, walk or do anything else it must first develop in its brain special centres for each and every one of these voluntary faculties and functions. Through these persistent personal efforts, reason, will and self-control are gradually evolved and developed; while the animal, being hereditarily endowed with the functions and faculties necessary for the maintenance of life, has no occasion for the development of the higher faculties and powers and therefore remains an irresponsible automaton which cannot be held accountable for its actions.

To recapitulate: Freedom of choice and of action distinguish the human from the animal. In the animal kingdom, reasoning power and freedom of action move in the narrow limits of heredity and instinct, while man through his own personal efforts is capable of unlimited development physically, mentally, morally and spiritually, both here and hereafter.([1]) We say physically advisedly, for in the spiritual realms in the life after death the physical (spiritual material) body also is capable of deterioration or of even greater refinement and beautification. Through the right use of his voluntary faculties, capacities and powers Man is enabled to become the master of himself and of his destiny.

Thus we find that the human organism consists of two distinct parts or departments, the one acting independently of the ego and deriving its motive force from an unknown source and the other under the conscious and voluntary control of the ego. The twofold nature of the human entity justifies the twofold attitude of mind and soul — on the one hand the prayerful and faithful dependence upon that mysterious power which flows into us and controls us through the sympathetic nervous system and on the other hand the conscious and voluntary dominion over the various faculties, capacities and powers with which nature has endowed us. It is our privilege and our duty to maintain both attitudes, the dependent as well as the independent. The desire and the will to plan, to choose and to perform are ours, but for the power to execute we are dependent upon a higher source.

([1])
It can be argued that reasoning power does exist in a rudimentary form in some animals and that it can be trained and developed. This is particularly so in animals which have been specially bred, domesticated or trained by man for his purpose.

CHAPTER XXXVIII

THE SYMPHONY OF LIFE

Human life appears to me as a great orchestra in which we are the players. The great composition to be performed is the "Symphony of Life", its infinitude of dissonances and melodies blending into one colossal tone picture of harmony and grandeur. We players must study the laws of music and the score of the great symphony and we must practise diligently and persistently until we can play our parts unerringly in harmony with the concepts of the Great Composer. At the same time we must learn to keep our instrument, the body, in the best possible condition; for even the greatest artist, endowed with a profound knowledge of the laws of music and possessed of the most perfect technique, cannot produce musical and harmonious sounds from an instrument with strings relaxed or over tense, or with its body filled with rubbish. The artist must learn that the instrument, its material, its construction and its care are just as much subject to law as are the harmonies of the score.

In the final analysis, everything is vibration acting in and on the universal ethers which are held to be the primordial substance. Possibly the ethers themselves are modes of vibration. That which is constructive is harmonious vibration. That which is destructive is inharmonious vibration. Against this it may be urged that devolution has its harmonies as well as evolution, that every symphony is made up of dissonances as well as of harmonies. To this I answer, "Unadulterated harmony may, solely from lack of change, become monotonous; but discords alone never create harmony, health or happiness".

As the artist seeks vibratory harmony between his instrument and the harmonics of the universe of sound, so the health seeker must endeavour to establish vibratory unison between the material elements of his body and nature's harmonics of health in the physical universe. The atoms and molecules in the wood and strings of the violin, as well as the sound produced from them, are modes of motion or vibration. In order to bring forth musical and harmonious notes, the vibratory conditions of the physical elements of the violin must be in harmonious vibratory relationship with nature's harmonics in the universe of sound. The elements and forces composing the human body are also vibratory in their nature. They also must be kept in a certain well balanced chemical combination, mechanical adjustment and physical refinement, if they are to vibrate in unison with nature's harmonics in the physical universe and thus produce the harmonies of health and strength and beauty. If our instrument is out of tune or if we ignorantly or wilfully insist on playing in our own way regardless of the score, we create discords not only for ourselves but also for our fellow artists in the great orchestra of life. Sin, disease, suffering and evil are but discords produced by the ignorance, indifference or malice of the players. Therefore we cannot attribute the discords of life to the Great Composer. They are of our own making and will last as long as we refuse to learn our parts and to play them in tune with the Great Score. For in this way only can we ever hope to master the art and science of right living and enjoy the harmonies of peace, self-content and happiness.

CHAPTER XXXIX

THE THREEFOLD CONSTITUTION OF MAN

The following diagram and accompanying explanations will serve to illustrate the Three Planes of Being, the corresponding Threefold Constitution of Man, and their analogy to the artist and his instrument.

Planes of Being	Threefold Constitution of Man	Analogy
Moral or Psychic	Soul	Music, Laws of Harmony
Mental	Mind	Player
Material	Bodies (Physical and Spiritual)	Violin

Man lives and functions on three distinct planes of being: the physical and spiritual material, the mental and the soul (psychical or moral) planes. He may be diseased upon any one or more of these planes. The true physician must look for causes of disease and for methods of treatment upon all three planes of being. The purely materialistic physician concentrates all his study and effort upon the physical material plane of being. To him mental, spiritual, psychical and moral phenomena are merely "chemical and physiological actions and reactions of brain and nerve substance". He has nothing but contempt and derision for the man who believes in or knows of a spiritual body or a soul. He is like an artist who says: "My violin is all there is to music. The musician's art consists in keeping his instrument in good condition. Technique and the laws of harmony are matters of imagination and of superstitious belief". On the other hand, mental healers, Christian Scientists and faith healers concentrate all their efforts upon either the mental or the soul plane, frequently making no distinction between the two. In the treatment of disease they ignore the conditions and needs of the physical body and some of them even deny its existence. These metaphysicians are like the artist who devotes all his time and energy to the study and practice of technique, counterpoint and harmony, neglecting his instrument and taking no heed whether its mechanism is out of order or its interior filled with rubbish. His knowledge of the laws of harmonics and his execution may be ever so perfect; but with his instrument out of tune he will produce discord instead of harmony.

The true artist realises that Mind, the player, must study Soul, the harmonics; and that the mind must also have its instrument, the Body, in perfect condition in order to interpret perfectly and artistically the harmonies of the "Symphony of Life". Likewise the Nature Cure physician will look for causes of disease and for means of cure upon the material, mental and psychical planes of being. Thus will higher civilization and greater knowledge lead back to the natural simplicity of primitive races, where physician and priest are one. After all, physical health is the best possible basis for the attainment of mental, moral and spiritual health. All building begins with the foundation. We do not first suspend the steeple in the air and then build the church under it. So also the building of the temple of human character should begin by laying the foundation in physical health.

We have known people who have attained high moral and spiritual development and then suffered utter shipwreck physically, mentally and in every other way, because ignorantly they had violated the laws of their physical natures. There are others who believe that the possession of occult knowledge and the achievement of mastership confer absolute control over nature's forces and phenomena on the physical plane. These people believe that a man is not a master if he does not miraculously heal all manner of disease and raise the dead. If such things were possible, they would overthrow the laws of cause and effect and of compensation. They would abolish the basic principles of morality and constructive spirituality. If it is possible in one case to heal disease and to overcome death through the fiat of the will of a master, then it should be possible in all cases. If so, then we can ignore the existence of nature's laws, indulge our appetites and passions to the fullest extent and when the natural results of our transgressions overtake us, we can go to the healer or master and have our diseases "instantly and painlessly" removed, like a bad tooth. I say this with all due reverence for and faith in the efficacy of true prayer, and with full knowledge of the healing power of therapeutic faith; but I do not believe that God, or nature, or a master, or metaphysical formulae can or will make good in a miraculous way for the inevitable results of our transgressions of the natural laws that govern our being. If such miraculous healing were possible and of common occurrence, what occasion would there be for the exercise of reason, will and self-control? What would become of the scientific basis of morality and constructive spirituality?

All this leads us to the following conclusions: If there is in operation a constructive principle of nature on the ethical, moral and spiritual planes of being with which we must align ourselves and to which we must conform our conscious and voluntary activities in order to achieve individual completion and happiness, then this constructive principle must be in operation also in our physical bodies and in their correlated physical, mental and emotional activities. If the constructive principle is active in the physical as well as in the moral and spiritual realms, then the harmonic relationship of the physical to the constructive law of its being must constitute the morality of the physical; and from this it follows that the achievement of health on the physical plane is as much under our conscious and voluntary control as the working out of our individual salvation on the higher planes of life.[1]

To recapitulate: First, our well being on all planes and in all relationships of life depend upon the existence, recognition and practical application of the great fundamental laws and principles just explained. Second: Physical health as well as moral health is of our own making. We are personally responsible not only for our own physical and mental health, but we are also morally responsible for the hereditary tendencies of our offspring toward health or disease. Third: The attainment of physical health through compliance with nature's laws is just as much our duty as is our ethical, moral and psychical development.

That which we call God, Nature, the Creator or the Universal Intelligence is the great central cause of all things, and the vibratory activities produced by or proceeding from this central or primary cause continue through all spheres of life, as the light waves of the sun, moon and fixed stars penetrate through the intervening spheres of life to our plane of earth. Therefore all powers, forces, laws and principles which manifest on our plane proceed and continue from the innermost Divine to the outermost external plane in physical nature. This explains the continuity,

[1]
It must nevertheless be admitted that spiritual healings and so-called miraculous cures do occur sometimes without the patient actually knowing that he is being treated, without his having any deep faith and without his making or knowing how to make any great change in his way of life by following any special regimen or routine of bodily treatment. The explanation of this would appear to be that miracles do occur but that they are not miracles in the sense of being suspensions or overridings of natural laws or principles. They are, rather, a sign that the body can be healed by having brought to bear upon it energies or forces which do exist but which are outside the physical as we now understand it. There are evidences that these forces are particularly strong in certain places (e.g. Lourdes) and that there are healers of all religions and of none, who have a special power of manipulating them.

stability and correspondence on all planes of being of that which we call "Natural Law". In other words, "Natural Law is the established harmonic relationship of effects and phenomena to their causes, and of all particular causes to the one great primary cause of all things."

CHAPTER XL

MENTAL THERAPEUTICS

The new psychology and the science of mental and spiritual healing teach that the lower principles in man stand or should stand under the dominion of the higher. The physical body with its material elements is dominated and guided by the mind. The mind is inspired through the inner consciousness which is an attribute of the soul. The soul of man is in communion with the over-soul which is the source of all life and all intelligence animating the universe. Wherever this natural order is reversed there is discord and disease. Too many people think and act as though the physical body were all in all, as though it were the only thing worth caring for and thinking about. They exaggerate the importance of the physical and become its abject slaves. The physical body is the lowest and least intelligent of the different principles making up the human entity. Yet people allow their minds and their souls to become dominated and terrified by the sensations of the physical body. When the servants in the house control and terrify the master, when the master becomes their slave and they can do with him as they please, there can be no order and harmony in that house. We must expect the same results when the lower principles in man lord it over the higher. When physical weakness, illness and pain fill the mind with fear and dismay, reason becomes clouded, the will atrophied and self-control is lost.

Every thought and every emotion has its direct effect upon the physical constituents of the body. The mental and emotional vibrations become physical vibrations and structures. Discord in the mind is translated into disease in the body, while the harmonies of hope, faith, cheerfulness, happiness, love and altruism create in the organism the corresponding health vibrations. Have you ever noticed how the written or printed notes of a tone piece or the perforations on the paper music roll of an automatic player are arranged in symmetrical and geometrical figures and groups? Dry sand strewn on the top of a piano on which harmonious tone combinations are produced shows a tendency to arrange itself in symmetrical patterns. In this you have a visual illustration of the translation of harmonious sound vibrations, which express "the harmonics of the soul's emotions", into correspondingly harmonious arrangements and configurations in the physical material of the paper roll. A jumble of discords of sound, if reproduced on a music roll, would present a chaotic jumble of perforations. Thus the purely mental and emotional is translated into its corresponding discords or harmonies in the physical. As the perforations on the paper music roll arrange themselves either symmetrically or without symmetry and order, in strict accordance with the harmonies or discords of the composition, so the atoms, molecules and cells in the physical group themselves in normal or abnormal structures of health or of disease in exact correspondence with the harmonious or the discordant vibrations conveyed to them from the mental and emotional planes.

Another illustration: Two violins, as they leave the shop of the maker are exactly alike in material, structure and quality of tone. One of the two instruments is constantly used by beginners and persons incapable of producing pure notes. The other passes into the hands of an artist who understands how to use the instrument to the best advantage and draws from it only musical tones that are true in pitch and quality. After a few years compare the two violins again. You will find that the one used by the tyros in music has deteriorated in its musical qualities, while the one in the hands of the artist has greatly improved in quality and purity of tone. What is the reason? The atoms and molecules in the wood of the two instruments have grouped themselves according to the discords or the harmonies that have been produced from them. If this rearrangement of atoms is possible in 'dead" wood, how much easier must be this adjustment of atoms, molecules and cells to discordant or harmonious vibratory influence in the living, plastic and fluidic human organism?

What harmony is to music, hope, faith, cheerfulness, happiness, sympathy, love and altruism are to the vibratory conditions of the human entity. These emotions are in alignment with the constructive principle in nature. They harmonize the physical vibrations, relax the tissues and open them wide to the inflow of the life force. Swedenborg truly says: "The warmth of life is the heat of the divine love permeating and animating the universe". The more we possess of hope, faith, love and kindred emotions, the more we open ourselves to the inflow of the vital energies. The good natured, cheerful, sympathetic person is more alive than the crabbed, morose, selfish individual. It has been proved over and over again by everyday experience that mental and emotional conditions positively affect the chemical composition of the tissues and secretions of the body. The destructive emotions of fear, worry, anger, jealousy, revengefulness, envy, etc., actually poison the fluids and tissues of the body. The bite of an angry man may cause blood poisoning, and prove as fatal as the bite of a mad dog. Sudden fear, anger or any other destructive emotion in the nursing mother may cause illness or even death of the infant. In psychological laboratories it has been found by scientifically conducted experiments that under the influence of destructive mental and emotional conditions, the secretions and excretions of the body show an increase of morbid and poisonous elements. Selfishness, fear and worry contract and congeal the blood vessels, the nerve fibres and the other channels through which life forces are conveyed to different parts of the physical body. The flow of the life currents is impeded and diminished. Such are the actual physiological effects of fear, anxiety and egotism on the physical organism. A man under the influence of great fear and one exposed to freezing present the same outward appearance. In both cases death may result through the congealing of the tissues and the shutting out of the life currents. The person afflicted with the worry habit may not die suddenly like one overcome by great and sudden fear. Nevertheless, fear and worry vibrations constantly maintained will surely obstruct and diminish the inflow of life force, lower the vitality and therewith the resistance to the encroachment of influences inimical to the health of the organism.

The cells of the body are negative, or at least they should be negative to the positive mind. The relationship of the mind to the cell should be like that of hypnotist to subject. If the mind could not exert such absolute control over the cells and cell groups, it would be impossible for us to walk, talk, write, dodge danger, etc. with almost automatic ease. The cells are not able to reason upon the truth or untruth of the suggestions conveyed to them from the mind. They accept its promptings unqualifiedly and act accordingly. Thus, if the mind constantly thinks of, say, the stomach as being in a badly diseased condition, unable to do its work properly, the mental images of weakness and disease with their accompanying fear vibrations are telegraphed over the efferent nerves to the cells of the stomach, and these become more and more weakened and diseased through the destructive vibrations sent to them from the mind. I often advise my patients to procure a book on anatomy and physiology and to study and keep constantly before their mind's eye the normal structure and functions of a healthy stomach or liver or whatever organ may be involved in any particular case.

The foregoing explains why affirmations of health are justifiable in face of disease. The health conditions must first be established in the mind before they can be conveyed to and impressed upon the cells. The well-being of the human body as a whole depends upon the health of the billions of minute cells which compose it. These cells are so small that they have to be magnified several hundred times under a powerful microscope before we can see them. Yet they are independent living beings which grow, assimilate food, work and die like the big cell, Man. These little cells are congregated in communities which form the organs and tissues of the body and in these communities they carry on the complicated activities of citizens living in a large city. Some are carriers, bringing food materials to the tissues and organs or conveying waste and morbid matter to the excretory channels of the body. Other cells manufacture chemical substances such as sugar, fats, ferments, etc. for the production of which complicated factories are required. The marvellous work performed by these minute organisms, as well as observations made in the dissecting room and under the microscope, strongly indicate that these cells are endowed with some sort of individual intelligence. They do their work without our aid or conscious volition. Nevertheless, they are greatly influenced by the varying conditions of the mind. While their activities seem to be controlled through the sympathetic nervous system, they stand in direct telegraphic communication with "headquarters" in the brain and every impulse of the mind is conveyed to them. If there be dismay and confusion in the mind, this condition is telegraphically conveyed over the nerve trunks and filaments to every cell in the body, and as a result these little workers become panic-stricken and incapable of rightly performing their manifold duties.

The cell system of the body resembles a vast army. The mind is the general at the head of it. The cells are the soldiers, divided into groups for special work. Much of the work of the army is carried on through well established departments, as the commissariat, hospital service, scouts and pickets, etc. Though the life and the activities of the army are so well regulated that they seem automatic, nevertheless much depends upon the commander. The vital processes of the human organism, digestion, assimilation, elimination, respiration, circulation of the blood, etc., are going on without our volition whether we be awake or asleep. These involuntary activities are impelled by the sympathetic nervous system, while the voluntary functions of the body are controlled through the motor nervous system. This division, however, is not a sharp one, the two departments frequently overlapping one another. The sympathetic nervous system resembles the commissarial department of the army which attends to the material welfare of the soldiers, while the motor nervous system, with headquarters in the brain, corresponds to the commander with his executive staff, the nerve centres in the spinal cord and other parts of the body being the subordinate officers in the field. While the physical wellbeing of the army depends upon the almost automatic work of its various departments, its mind and soul is the man commanding it. He determines the spirit, the energy and the efficiency of the vast organization. If the commander-in-chief lacks insight, force and determination, the discipline of the army will be lax and its efficiency greatly impaired. If he be a craven, without faith in himself and in the cause he represents, his doubt and indecision will communicate themselves to the whole army, resulting in discouragement and defeat. The most successful commanders have been those who were possessed of absolute confidence in themselves and in the efficiency of their army, who in the face of grave danger and discouraging situations pressed on to the predetermined goal with dogged courage and resolution. Determination and pertinacity of this kind create the magnetic power which imparts itself to every individual soldier in the army and makes him a willing subject, even unto death, to the will of his commander.

When pestilence was invading Napoleon's army, that great general entered the hospitals where the victims of the plague were lying, took them by the hand and conversed with them. He did this to overcome the fear in the hearts of his soldiers and thus to protect them against the dread disease. He said: "A man whose will can conquer the world, can conquer the plague". To my mind, this was one of the greatest deeds of the Corsican. At a time when "New Thought" was practically unknown, the genius of this man had grasped its principles and was making them factors in his apparent success. "Apparent" because, while we admire his genius we deplore the ends to which he applied his wonderful powers. At times when the battle seemed lost, Napoleon would go to the front where the danger was greatest, and by the mere sight of him the hard pressed soldiers under his command were inspired to superhuman effort and final victory. As long as the glamour of invincibility surrounded him Napoleon was invincible, because he infused into his soldiers faith and courage which nothing could withstand. But when the cunning of the Russian broke his power and decimated his ranks on the icebound steppes, the hypnotic spell was broken also. Friends and enemies alike recognized that, after all, he was but a man, subject to chance and circumstance. From that time on he was vulnerable and suffered defeat after defeat.

The power of the mind over the physical body and its involuntary functions (those controlled through the sympathetic system) may be illustrated by the demonstrated facts of hypnotism. Through the exertion of his own imagination and his willpower, the hypnotist can so dominate the brain and through the brain the physical body of his subject, as to influence not only the sensory functions but also heart action and respiration. By the power of his will the hypnotist is able to retard or accelerate pulse and respiration and even to subdue the heart beat so that it becomes hardly perceptible. If it is possible thus to control by the power of will the vital functions in the body of another person, it must be possible also to control these functions in our own bodies. Many Hindoo fakirs and yogi have developed this power of the mind over the physical body to a marvellous extent. Here lies the true domain of mental therapeutics. We can learn to dominate and regulate the vital activities and the life currents in our bodies so that they will do their work intelligently and serenely even under the stress of illness or danger. We can by the power of will direct the vital currents to those parts and organs which need them most, and we can relieve congested areas by equalizing the circulation, by drawing therefrom the surplus of blood and nerve currents and distributing the vital fluids over other parts of the body. We must be careful, however, to use our higher powers in conformity with nature's intent; that is, we must not endeavour to suppress nature's cleaning and healing efforts. It is possible to do this by the power of will as well as by ice bags and drugs. Mentally and emotionally as well as physically we must work with nature, not against her. When we understand the fundamental laws of disease and cure we cannot well do otherwise.

CHAPTER XLI

HOW SHALL WE PRAY?

Shall we say, "Father, give me this", "Father, do for me that", or "Behold I am perfect. Imperfection, sin and suffering are only errors of mortal mind"? Or shall we pray: "Father, give me Thy strength that I may live in harmony with Thy law, for thus only will all good come to me"? The first of these alternatives is to beg, the second to steal, the third to earn by honest effort. Our fathers who prayed in the first way did not understand the great law of compensation which demands that we give an equivalent for everything we receive. Every living thing in some way or other gives an equivalent for its existence. With man the fulfillment of the law of service and of compensation becomes conscious and voluntary and his self-respect refuses to take without giving. Those who pray according to the second alternative which affirms that imperfection, sin and suffering are errors of mortal mind are to be found among certain metaphysical healers and their disciples. To assume the possession of goodness and perfection without an earnest effort to develop and to deserve these qualities is to steal the glory of the Perfect One. The assumption of present perfection precludes the necessity of striving and labouring for its attainment. If I am already all goodness, all love, all wisdom and all power, what remains for me to strive for? Herein lies the danger of metaphysical idealism. While it may dispel pessimism, fear and anxiety, it inevitably weakens the will power and the capacity for self-help and personal effort. The ideal of the metaphysician is the ideal of the animal. The animal does not worry about right and wrong, nor, with few exceptions, does it make provision for the future. Its care and forethought extend only to the next meal. But this perfect, ideal, passive trust in nature's bounty causes the animal to remain animal and prevents its rising above the narrow limitations of habit and instinct. The inherent faculties, capacities and powers of the human soul can be developed only by effort and use. The savage, living in the most favoured regions of the earth, depending for his sustenance in perfect faith and trust on nature's bounty, has remained savage. Through ages he has risen but little above the level of the beasts that perish. The great law of use ordains that those faculties and powers which we do not develop remain in abeyance and those which we possess weaken and atrophy if we fail to exercise them.

This is the same law which the Master, Jesus, emphasized in many of his parables and sayings. "For whosoever hath, to him shall be given, and he shall have more abundance; but whosoever hath not, from him shall be taken away even that he hath". What does this mean? Those who have the desire and the will to work out their own salvation, acquire greater knowledge and power in exact proportion to their well directed efforts; but those who have neither the desire nor the will to help themselves, lose their natural endowments and the possibilities and opportunities which these would have conferred upon them. The anatomy and physiology of the human brain reveal the fact that for every voluntary faculty, capacity and power of the body, mind and soul which we wish to develop, we have to create new centres in the brain. In this respect nature gives no more and no less than we deserve and work for. If we try to cheat by usurping the perfection and the power which we have not honestly earned and developed, then some time, somewhere, we shall have to balance the account.

After all, the only true prayer is personal effort and self-help. This does not mean that we should not invoke the help of the higher powers, of those who have gone before us, of the Great Friends and Invisible Helpers and of the Great Father, the giver of all life, all wisdom and all power. We should pray for strength to do our work, not to have it done for us. The wise parent will not do for the child the home tasks assigned to him at school. Neither will the powers on high or the Great Friends perform our allotted tasks for us. This life is a school for personal effort. If it were not so, life would be meaningless. From the cradle to the grave, our days are one continuous effort to learn, to acquire, to overcome difficulties. Only in this way can we develop our latent faculties, capacities and powers. These cannot be developed by having our tasks done for us, nor by assuming that we already know and possess everything. The athlete must do his own training. No one else can do it for him. Therefore the assumption of superiority over his opponent will not develop his suppleness of body and strength of muscle. To be sure, faith and courage are essential to victory, but they must be backed by careful and persistent training. Vainglorious boasting alone will not win the contest. So in the battle of life, the more faith we have in God, in the Great Friends and in our own powers, the wider do we open ourselves to the inflow of wisdom and strength from all that is good and true and powerful in the universe. But through persistent and well directed effort alone can we control the powers and fashion the materials which nature has so lavishly bestowed upon us.

The creative will, actuated by desire and enlightened by reason, brings order and harmony out of chaotic forces and materials. And yet certain metaphysicians tell us that we ourselves must do nothing to overcome weakness, sin and suffering; that we must depend entirely upon the efficiency of metaphysical formulae; that the deity and the powers of nature are jealous of our personal efforts; that we must not try to help ourselves lest we forfeit their good will. Is it not blasphemous to assume that God would blame us and withold his aid because we dared to use faculties, capacities and powers with which he has endowed us? Yet this is the teaching of a popular healing cult. Its members are forbidden, on penalty of expulsion, to use in the treatment of human ailments the most innocent natural remedies. The giving of an enema or the common sense regulation of diet are regarded as sufficient to nullify the power of their metaphysical formulae and to prevent the working of nature's healing forces.

One of our patients who had been under such treatment until she was in a dying condition told us afterwards that her bowels often did not move for a week and when she complained to her "healer" about this condition and asked permission to take an enema he answered: "Pay no attention. The Lord is taking care of that in some other way". This "healer" had been a prominent allopathic physician who, like so many others ignorant of nature's simple laws, had swung from one extreme to the other, from allopathic overdoing to metaphysical underdoing. In this instance the Lord "took care" of the patient's bowels until she was down with a severe attack of appendicitis and peritonitis. Amid all the extremes, Nature Cure points the common sense middle way. Basing its teachings and its practices on a clear understanding of the laws of health, disease and cure, it refrains from suppressing acute diseases with poisonous drugs or the knife, knowing that they are in reality nature's cleansing and healing efforts. Neither does it sit idly by and expect the Lord or metaphysical formula to do our work and to make good for our violations of nature's laws. Understanding the Law, Nature Cure believes in cooperating with it; in giving the Lord a helping hand. It teaches that "God helps him who helps himself", that He will not become angry and refuse His help if His children use rightly the reason, the will power and the self-control with which he has endowed them so that they may achieve their own salvation.

We claim that Nature Cure is in truth a grand and true prayer. It teaches the law on all planes of being — the physical, the mental, the moral and the spiritual; and it insists that the only way to attain perfect health of body, mind and soul is to comply with the law to the best of our ability. When we do that we place ourselves in alignment with the constructive principle in nature, and in exact proportion to our intelligent and voluntary cooperation with the laws of our being, all good will come to us. Therefore we pray: "Father, give me Thy strength that I may live in harmony with Thy law, for thus only will all good come to me."

CHAPTER XLII

SCIENTIFIC RELAXATION AND NORMAL SUGGESTION

Under the strain of workaday hurry and worry, your nerve vibrations are apt to become more and more intense and excited. They run away with you until, as the saying goes, you are "flying all to pieces". A good illustration of this condition of the nervous system may be found in a team of horses shying at some object in the path. The driver, panic stricken, drops the reins, the frightened horses take the bit between their teeth and dash headlong down the road, until their master regains control, checks the animals in their maddened course and compels them to resume their ordinary pace. So the highstrung, oversensitive individual must gain control over his nervous system and must subdue his runaway mental and emotional activities into restful harmonious vibrations. This is done by insuring sufficient rest and sleep under the right conditions and by practising scientific relaxation at all times.

The nervous person gets easily excited. Comparatively little things will cause an outbreak of intense irritation or emotional hyper-activity. Usually, the victim of unbalanced nerves is of the high-strung, sensitive type, naturally inclining to more rapid vibrations on all planes, capable of greater achievement than the solid, heavy, slow-vibrating person who "doesn't know that he has any nerves", but also is in greater danger of mental and emotional overstrain and physical depletion as a result of the excessive and uncontrolled expenditure of life force and nervous energy. Watch your nervous friend while performing some trivial task, picking up something from the floor or putting a book in its accustomed place. The fitful, jerky movements betray the inner impatience and irritability. Worry, hurry and flurry do not hasten the task in hand; they only retard it. They cause neglect and bungling, which require more time to straighten out than deliberate and patient work in the first place. Watch him, too, while he is resting or sleeping. Instead of "letting go" of the body his muscles are drawn and tense. The body is screwed up into all sorts of awkward positions and acrobatic distortions. He nervously clutches the arm chair, or strenuously clings to the bed, as though these aids to rest and comfort were trying to escape from under him. The sleep is fitful and disturbed, as are the physical and mental vibrations. To the sensitive the aura is visible, indicating continuous expenditure of nervous force. This interferes with the accumulation of vital energy in the millions of tiny storage batteries in the brain, the spinal cord and the sympathetic ganglia, with the result that during sleep not sufficient reserve force is stored for the work of the following day. Such an one expends as much vitality while sleeping as another who has learnt the art of restful relaxation expends while working. No wonder he feels all fagged out in the morning — as tired as when he went to bed.

At first glance the idea of relaxation while working may seem paradoxical. However, experience proves that it is not only possible but absolutely necessary that we perform our work in a relaxed and serene condition of body and mind. The most strenuous physical or mental labour will then not cause as much exhaustion as light work done in a state of nervous tension, irritability, fretfulness or worry. Relaxation while working necessitates plan and system. Most nervous breakdowns result not so much from overwork as from the vitality wasted through lack of orderly procedure. Therefore, take some time to plan and arrange your work and form the habit of doing certain things that have to be done every day as nearly as possible in the same way (making sure that it is the right way) and at the same time of the day. Orderly system will soon become habitual and result in saving much valuable time and energy. Always cultivate a serene and cheerful attitude of mind and soul, taking whatever comes as "part of the day's work", doing your best under the circumstances but absolutely refusing to worry and fret about anything. Do not "cross a bridge before you get to it" and do not waste time regretting something which cannot be undone.

It is important also to obtain relaxation while sitting. Sit upright in a comfortable chair without strain or tension, spine and head erect, the legs forming right angles with the thighs (the chair should be neither too high nor too low), feet resting firmly upon the floor, toes pointing slightly outward, the forearms resting lightly upon the legs with the hands upon the knees. This must be accomplished without effort, for effort means tension. Now dismiss all thoughts of hurry, care, worry or fear and dwell upon such thoughts as the following: "I am now completely relaxed in body and mind. I am receptive to nature's harmonious and invigorating vibrations — they dispel the discordant and destructive vibrations of hurry, worry, fear and anger. New life, new health, new strength are entering into me with every breath, pervading my whole being." Repeat these thoughts mentally, or if it helps you say them aloud several times quietly and forcefully, impressing them deeply upon your inner consciousness. After practising relaxation in this manner, lie down for a few minutes' rest if circumstances permit, or practise rhythmical breathing. Then return to your work and endeavour to maintain a calm, trustful, controlled attitude of mind. If you are inclined to be irritable, suspicious, jealous, fault-finding, envious, etc. dwell on the following thought pictures: "I am now fully relaxed, at rest and at peace. The world is an echo. If I send forth irritable, suspicious, hateful thought vibrations, the like will return to me from other minds. I shall think such thoughts no longer. God is love, love is harmony, happiness, heaven. The more I send forth love, the more I am like God; the more of love will God and men return to me; the more I shall realize true happiness, true health, true strength, and true success."

Relaxation before going to sleep is, perhaps, the most important of all. When ready to go to sleep lie flat on your back so that as nearly as possible every part of the spine touches the bed, extend the arms along the sides of the body, hands turned upward, palms open, every muscle relaxed.(1) Dismiss all thought of work, annoyance or anxiety. Say to yourself: "I am now going to sleep soundly and peacefully. I am master of my body, my mind and my soul. Nothing evil shall disturb me. At . . . a.m., neither earlier nor later, I shall awaken rested and refreshed, strong in body and mind. I shall meet tomorrow's tasks and duties promptly and serenely." Simple as this formula may seem, it has helped cure many a case of persistent insomnia and nervous prostration. Having thus set your "mental alarm clock", with a few times practice you will be able to wake up, without being called, at the appointed time and to demonstrate to yourself the power of your mind over your body. The quality of your sleep and its effect upon your system depend on the character of the mental and psychic vibrations carried into it. If you harbour thoughts of passion, worry or fear, these destructive thought vibrations will disturb your slumbers and you will awake in the morning weak and tired. If, however, you repeat mentally a formula like the above, suggesting harmonious, constructive thoughts, until you lose consciousness, you will carry into your slumbers vibrations of rest, health and strength, producing corresponding effects upon the physical organism. After a perfectly relaxed condition of body and mind has been attained, it is not necessary to remain lying on the back. Any position of the body may then be assumed which seems most restful. My patients frequently ask what

---

(1)
    Mention has been made above of Mr. L. E. Eeman, a recent exponent of the art of relaxation, who maintained that the crossing of the feet and the linking of the hands over the region of the solar plexus were a help to conserving energy and promoting relaxation. Also it would appear to be more conducive to relaxation to keep the backs of the hands turned forwards in the position of pronation at all times when they are not in use.

position of the body is best during sleep. It is not good to lie continuously in any one position. This tends to cause unsymmetrical development of the body and to affect unfavourably the functions of various organs. It is best to change occasionally from one position to another, as bodily comfort seems to indicate and require. Many people fret and worry if sleep does not come as quickly as desired. They picture to themselves in darkest colours the dire results of wakefulness. Such a state of mind makes sleep impossible. If persisted in, it will inevitably lead to chronic insomnia. Instead of indulging in hurtful worry, say to yourself: "I do not care whether I sleep or not. Though I do not sleep I am lying here perfectly relaxed, at rest and at peace. I am strengthened and rested by remaining in a state of peaceful relaxation." However, the "I do not care" must be actually meant and felt, must not be merely a mechanical repetition of words. Nothing is more conducive to sleep, even under the most trying circumstances, than such an "I-don't-care" attitude of mind. Try it and the chances are that just because you do not care you will fall fast asleep.

CHAPTER XLIII

MAN'S DEMANDS ARE GOD'S COMMANDS

Our critics say: "If Nature Cure is all that you claim for it, why is it not more generally accepted by the medical profession and the public?" The greatest drawback to the spreading of the Nature Cure idea is the necessity of self-control which it imposes. If our cures of so-called incurable diseases could be made without asking the patients to change their habits of living, without the demand for effort on their own part, Nature Cure sanitariums could not be built fast enough in this country. No matter how marvellous the results of the natural methods, when investigators learn that the treatment necessitates the control of indiscriminate appetite and self-indulgence and the persistent practice of "natural" living and all that this involves, they exclaim: "The natural regimen may be all right, but who can live up to it? You are asking the impossible. You are looking for a perfection which does not exist. Your directions call for an amount of will power and self-control which nobody possesses." Fortunately, however, this is not true. Human nature is good enough to comply with nature's laws. Furthermore, the natural ways must be the most pleasant in the end or nature is a fraud and a cheat. True enjoyment of life and happiness are impossible without perfect physical, mental and moral health, and these depend upon natural living and natural treatment of human ailments.

If I were asked the question: "What do you consider the greatest benefit to be derived from the Nature Cure regimen?" I should answer: "The strengthening of will-power and self-control." This is the very purpose of life. Upon it depends all further achievement. Self-control is the "master's key" to all higher development on the mental, moral and spiritual planes of being; but before we can exercise it on the higher planes, we must have learned to apply it on the lower plane in the management and control of our physical appetites and habits. When we have learned to control these, "higher development" will come easily.

A good method for strengthening the will power is auto-suggestion. The most opportune moments in the twenty four hours of the day for practising this "mental magic" are those before dropping to sleep. At

296

this time there is the least disturbance and interference from outside influences, the mind is most passive and susceptible to suggestion, and impressions made under these favourable conditions upon the "phonograph records" of the subconscious mind are the most lasting and the most powerful to control physical, mental and moral activities. When thoroughly relaxed, at rest and at peace, say to yourself: "Whatever duties confront me tomorrow I shall execute them promptly without wavering or hesitation. I shall not give in to this bad habit which has been controlling me. I shall do only that which reason and conscience approve."

In order to be more specific and systematic and to obtain results more surely and quickly, concentrate upon one weakness at a time. When that has been overcome, take up another, until in this way you have attained perfect control over your thoughts, feelings and actions. Suppose you have acquired the habit of remaining in bed and dozing after your mental alarm clock has given its signal to arise, and you dread the effort of going through your morning exercises and ablutions. Then, the night before impress upon the subconscious mind deeply and firmly the following suggestions: "Tomorrow morning on awakening I shall jump out of bed without hesitation and go through my morning exercises with zest and vigour." Or, suppose you are subject to the fear and worry habit, say to yourself: "Tomorrow or any time thereafter when depressing, gloomy thoughts threaten to control me, I shall overcome them with thoughts of hope and faith and with absolute confidence in the divine power of the will within me to overcome and achieve." Or, when in need of strengthening guidance, "Almighty Love, Creative Love, purify, strengthen, enlighten me." In this manner you may give the subconscious mind suggestions and impressions for overcoming bad habits and for establishing and strengthening good habits.

If a serious problem is confronting you and you are unable to solve it to your satisfaction, think upon it just before you are dropping off to sleep and confidently demand that the right solution come to you during the hours of rest. The inner consciousness is always awake. It is the watchman who awakens you at the appointed time in the morning. It will work upon your problem while you sleep. There is a real justification for the popular phrase: "Before I decide the matter I'll sleep on it." In the practise of mental magic of this kind, as in everything else, success depends upon patience and perseverance. It would be entirely useless to go through these mental drills occasionally and in a desultory fashion; but if persisted in faithfully and intelligently, they will prove truly magical in their effects upon the development of will-power and self-control, and on these depend the mastery of conditions within and without, the conquest of fate and destiny.

Constructive Affirmations or Prayers which can be of use

Desire and will are the open doors to heaven and hell.

I am spirit: I rejoice in an abundance of life, health, strength, wisdom and divine love.

I am Thy child created in Thy likeness. Help me to know the power that Thou hast given me.

I radiate Faith, Power, Goodness and Love.

I am thankful because Faith has taken the place of fear, and knowledge the place of ignorance and superstition. All good will come to me as I obey the laws of my being.

I am Harmony: I radiate Health and Happiness.

Thou art my physician: Thou renewest my body with the waters of Life, of Health and of Strength.

I am made whole through the renewing of my mind.

My soul draws to itself the vitality and healing currents of nature.

I am now living in harmony with the Law, and the Law will make me whole.

"The Kingdom of Heaven is within you."

The Divine Energy within me harmonizes and puts in order the material elements of my body.

Only as I live above the attraction and discord of mortal things and fill my mind with immortal truth do I realize the peace and perfection of divine being.

All good comes to me because I am learning to live in harmony with the laws of my being.

Infinite Love and Faith fill my mind and thrill my body with Healing Life.

My mind now rests from all material activity. I am at peace in the health and strength-giving life of the Spirit.

My flesh is alive with the Life, Strength and Intelligence of the Healing Spirit.

My doubts and fears are dissolved and dissipated. I rest in confidence and peace in Thy unchanging law.

My faith makes me whole.

The Divine Will within me rises victorious over disease and death. I am the Master of my fate.

My soul is radiant with Divine Peace. Every cell in my body is vibrant with Divine Harmony and Power.

I will be what I will to be.

I now vibrate in unison with all that is good and true and perfect on the Higher Planes of Being.

My mind my kingdom is: my will the King.

The more I live in harmony with things spiritual the more I am freed from the bondage of things physical.

Health is the natural state of man. Do not allow any thought opposed to this to dominate your mind. Say with positive assurance, "The Peace and Harmony of Divine Mind makes me perpetually whole."

I am one with God, I am one with the Great Life Principle, I am one with Eternal Vitality — I am almighty Energy.

With every breath I absorb Infinite Omnipotent Life.

Faith and Will are the Master Keys which unlock to us the treasures of the Universe.

The more I give the more I receive from the Infinite and Everlasting Storehouse of riches and power.

Mighty Spirit: In Thy strength I am strong; in Thy healing atmosphere I am realizing health; from Thy vital spirit flows the vigour that my body needs.

I am the centre for the concentration and radiation of spiritual power; as I give so I receive.

Fear destroys. Through Faith I am quickened into Life.

"Talk Faith: The world is better off without your uttered ignorance and morbid doubt. If you have Faith in God or man or self, say so; if not, push back upon the shelf of silence all your thoughts till Faith shall come; no one will grieve because your lips are dumb."

(Ella Wheeler Wilcox)

"Resist not evil, but overcome evil with good."

"Faith opens wide the flood gates of life."

He who thinks he can, develops within himself the power that can.

Nature is full of music, as it exists through the laws of harmony. Man only is discordant and out of tune.

"He that believeth on Me, the works that I do he shall do also. And greater works shall he do."

"Where two or three are gathered together in My name, there am I in the midst of them."

Impatient demand drives things away. Calm demand brings all good things in time.

As man learns to rule his Universe within he learns to master the Universe without.

"Father, give me of Thy strength and Thy wisdom that I may comply with Thy law in all things. Thus only can I come into the possession of the divine heritage which Thou hast prepared for me from the beginning."

The active principle in my will is the force which creates and governs the Universe.

"Be still, my soul, and know that peace is thine; Be steadfast, heart, and know that strength divine belongs to thee; Cease from thy turmoil, mind, and thou the everlasting rest shall find."

Only as I give the best that is within me can I receive the best that is without me.

Suffering is often the greatest blessing to humanity. It compels us to search out and remove its cause and thus we learn the beauties of eternal law.

A vivid imagination, a positive faith and a powerful will are the workers of mental magic.

Each man his prison makes. You are not bound but as you bind yourself. Within deliverance must be sought.

The way of peace is the way of power. It brings us repose without lethargy, activity without effort, love without anxiety, and joy without reaction.

> "Our lives are songs, God writes the words,
> And we set them to music at leisure,
> And the song is sad or the song is glad
> As we choose to fashion the measure."

We attract to ourselves whatever influences we choose.

The greatest force in the universe is the power of many minds united in purpose, faith and will. The higher and better the motive, the greater the power.

"As a man thinketh in his heart so is he."

The only death imaginable is stagnation.

I am today what my past thoughts and emotions have made me.

I am a free-born citizen of this boundless Universe. Nothing can bind, hold me or limit me but my own opinions and my own actions.

Almighty Love, creative Love, purify, strengthen, enlighten me.

> "God of the granite and the rose,
> Soul of the sparrow and the bee —
> The mighty tide of being flows
> Through every creature, Lord, from Thee.
> It leaps to life in bird and flowers,
> Through every grade of being runs,
> Till from creation's radiant towers
> Its glories flame in stars and suns.
> Know that like bird and grass and flower,
> The life within thee is divine;

Nor time, nor space, nor human power,
The God within thee can confine.
God of the granite and the rose,
Soul of the sparrow and the bee —
The mighty tide of being flows
From every creature back to Thee;
Thus round and round the circle runs —
A mighty sea without a shore —
While men and angels, stars and suns,
Unite to praise Thee evermore."

APPENDIX I

EPIDEMICS

Epidemics and the communicability of disease do undoubtedly present problems and difficulties of explanation to those who believe that they are not merely a matter of chance or of "bad luck". Daniel Mackinnon, the disciple and pupil of Henry Lindlahr, in his book "The Conquest of Pain" has added to what Lindlahr has to say on the subject. According to him the Law of Resonance is one of the universal laws to which the body is subject and its action is capable of explaining to a great extent the phenomena of epidemics and the communicability of disease.

He says: 'This Law of Resonance, also known as the Law of Sympathetic Vibration or the Law of Similars has been defined by writers on the subject of Physics as follows: "A system free to execute vibrations of a definite period is capable of selecting and absorbing from the surrounding medium energy in the form of vibrations of the same period as those which it can execute." This in fact means that the natural vibratory period, and the resulting energy emanations, of a specific chemical unit of toxic material in a human body will attract to itself similar vibratory emanations which are radiating from an adjacent body. This disturbance will be in proportion to the quantity of the toxic material acted upon. To develop this idea in relation to epidemic disease it can be suggested that there would seem to be two somewhat distinct types of epidemic disease. (1) A type resulting from actual poisonous matter, or other sufficiently irritating material contained in air, water, food, etc. Illustrations of this type are to be found in influenza, which, according to these ideas, results from the presence of a poisonous gas in the air, present in sufficient quantity to be inimical to the human body; in typhoid, resulting from the end-products of protein putrefaction in water and milk particularly, and sometimes from the eating of decaying fish or from fish which has not been properly cleaned; and, in hay fever, from the effects of certain vegetable matter, not necessarily poisonous, floating in the air, and on being inhaled, acting upon certain poisonous substances present in the bodies of those who are susceptible to hay fever. (2) A type transferable from one individual to another by reason of energy emanations. Measles, mumps, chicken-pox, small-pox, scarlet fever, whooping cough, and diphtheria are typical instances of this variety.

Epidemic diseases, which will come to be explained not so much as a result of bacteriological investigation as of the work of accomplished chemists and physicists, can be understood only as the basic laws underlying them are understood. In connection with the Law of Resonance we can, by the use of two pianos tuned to the same pitch, demonstrate three different types of physical phenomena.

(a) As a result of striking any string on one piano, the identical string on the other piano will commence to vibrate, and, consequently, the original sound is augmented or amplified, and it is heard as a louder note.

(b) If one string on one piano is struck repeatedly, and with sufficient force, the corresponding string on the other instrument can be broken.

(c) If, for example, the middle C string is removed from one of the pianos, then none of the other eighty odd strings which remain on the instrument will respond perfectly to the note of the middle C sounded on the other instrument.

These phenomena are in harmony with the principle involved in the Law of Resonance, and they can be demonstrated in many different ways, with materials ranging from liquids to solids of the most dense types.

If the Law of Resonance is a fundamental, natural, universal law affecting all physical organizations, then it must of necessity affect the human body. Consequently, it should be entirely possible to reproduce and demonstrate the above piano-string phenomena in human bodies. It is suggested that they can be so demonstrated, and that they constitute the basis for a reasonable theory and explanation of problems of epidemics and immunity. To make this clearer, let us take an example. Five children are at play together, and one of them happens to be in the incubation stage of measles; his temperature is going up slowly, his eyes and nose are running, and he is beginning to cough. What brought this measles condition into existence? In the foregoing pages it has been suggested that measles result from certain toxic material carried into the body of the yet unborn child by the blood of the mother. This toxic material is a specific, definitely formed chemical organization which may be called X toxaemia. It is a self-existing, physical organization, made up of chemical elements, and, as such, it can exist only by taking energy into its body, and, in turn, radiating energy off. The nature of the wave lengths of energy radiating off from any substance determines the basic or individual nature of that substance. The only thing which can be changed with regard to the energy given off by a particular substance is the intensity or speed with which it leaves that substance; its natural wave-length cannot be changed. Let us then consider the X toxaemia suggested above as being present in the body of the child developing the case of measles. The total amount of energy at work in the body of this child is sufficient to resent the presence of this toxic material, and, because the child is at an age where natural processes of elimination are most likely to take place, this will result in an augmentation and concentration of energy first of all in the heat-controlling centre of the brain, located in the medulla; this will be followed by an increase of heart action, and a consequent increase in the movement of blood in the body generally. Resulting from these factors, there will be a corresponding increase of activity of certain internal organs, especially the liver and spleen, and, in proportion as these large organs become congested with blood, so will the temperature rise. When it rises to a certain point, it will bring about combustion or oxidation of the X toxaemia, and as this proceeds, whatever energy is released by it will leave its point of origin with great speed and with considerable force behind it. In other words, a maximum of force is behind the wave-lengths of energy released from the burning toxic material. This energy, travelling at great speed, radiates from the body of the sickened child. In the case of the children at play together, these energy vibrations penetrate the bodies of all the children in proportion to proximity. Let us say that two more of these five playing children have the same X toxaemia in their bodies, but in an inactive or latent condition. The toxaemia in this instance will be like the middle C of the piano which constantly radiates off a minimum of energy until a stronger stream of energy of the same pitch is released somewhere near to it; when this happens, the energy out-put of the string will be increased from a minimum to a maximum flow. As the increased vibrations from the body of the sickened child pass through the bodies of all the children present, it finds a responsive chord only in the two children containing the same toxaemia. The final result of this is that there will be three children affected with measles. The two other children of the five who are minus the X toxaemia are in the same condition as the piano with the middle C string removed. There is nothing in the shape of X toxaemia in their bodies which can be acted upon by such radiations emanating from another body, consequently they are immune to measles. Thus we can arrive at a reasonable explanation of why some people contract certain acute diseases while others are not affected by contact with them. It must, however, be remembered that susceptibility is affected also by factors such as Periodicity and Vitality. There are, for instance, periods and times at which congenital and other toxaemias tend to be cleaned out of the bodies of children and young persons and these will be times of great susceptibility. Vitality also is an important factor in determining

304

whether or not a person can respond to energy vibrations. For various reasons vitality may be lowered to such an extent that an acute reaction cannot be produced.'

I have quoted this extract because it seems to provide a useful contribution to the study of epidemics and immunity. The idea that a better understanding of these things can be brought about by the work of physicists and biochemists rather than by that of bacteriologists and virologists seems very revolutionary in these days, but if we accept the view that bacteria are a secondary manifestation of disease rather than its cause, it is a very reasonable one. Whatever else the physical body may be it is a physico-chemical organization and as such must be subject to physical and chemical laws. The chemical state of the body and its tissues must be one of the most important factors by which its health is conditioned and its susceptibility to disease is determined. The chemical state of the body in turn depends to a great extent on what is breathed into it through the lungs and what is put into it in the form of food and drink. It may well be that the science of Epidemiology has been hindered rather than helped by the germ theory of disease, at least in its present form. To say that a certain micro-organism causes a certain disease tends to raise more questions than it answers, for one is driven to ask what causes the micro-organisms to appear and what gives them their virulence. Moreover, the idea that every infection and epidemic is caused by a specific micro-organism leads to an endless search for new forms and strains of bacteria and viruses and for methods of killing them when found; whereas the answers to many important questions of epidemiology are little sought for and remain obscure. For instance, we know that many diseases are endemic and flare up into epidemics in places where hygiene and living conditions are poor, but the details and mechanism of why and how this is so are little understood. We know, too, that there is some connection between pestilence and war which has been noticed from the earliest times but which has never been much elucidated. We know from our history books that the most destructive epidemics have sometimes spread over large areas and that they sometimes do so still, especially in primitive countries. Such epidemics would seem often to wax and spread for a time and then wane and disappear for no very obvious reasons, and not always to be greatly influenced by the methods of prevention or treatment which are being employed. Another subject which seems to call for more investigation is the cause of the seasonal, periodic and climatic or cosmic factors which undoubtedly exercise an influence on the appearance and course of certain diseases and epidemics. Finally, the assumption that when disease is communicated it happens as the result of micro-organisms passing from person to person would not seem to be proven, though it may sometimes be possible artificially to convey disease from one person to another in this way. Though it is conceivable that with very close contact air-borne organisms could be conveyed from one person to another, the evidence is strong against "pathogenic" organisms remaining alive or virulent in the air for any length of time. The idea that the communicability of disease is usually due to the operation of the Law of Resonance is, surely, at least as plausible as the explanation that it is due to infection by germs.

APPENDIX II

SPECIFIC IMMUNITY AND PROPHYLAXIS

Lindlahr affirmed that the kind of vaccination and immunization procedures which are used in orthodox medical circles are a perversion, distortion or misapplication of homoeopathic principles and methods. Mackinnon has explained this somewhat more fully in one of his letters to the editor. He says: 'The School of Natural Therapeutics is not entirely antagonistic to the use of morbidific material in the treatment of disease. Its principle cause of disagreement with the advocates of serum therapy is with their practice, and not so much with the principle involved. Somewhere about the year 1500 Paracelsus used and advocated the idea of Isopathy — that is the theory that a disease may be cured by administering one or more of its own products. Paracelsus proved the worth of his ideas by curing almost every case of cholera that he had to deal with when his colleagues were utterly helpless. Homoeopathy has made a special study of this particular idea of therapeutics, and homoeopathic physicians of the older school were uniformly successful in protecting their patients, and their patients' children by the administration of potentized products of disease. These were administered orally, and not hypodermically, and that is a very significant difference. Some of the materials used for this purpose are as follows: Diphtherinum, made from the actual membranous material that is peculiar to diphtheria; Variolinum, made from the actual exudate of small-pox pustules; Medorrhinum, made from the actual gonorrheal discharge, and so on. These peculiar remedies are known to homoeopathic physicians as Nosodes. These nosodes are used only in very high potencies, running from, say, the Mth up to the 5CMth. If you understand how this business of potentizing is done, you will readily appreciate the fact that if a few powders of the CMth potency are given to a child or to an adult, it would clearly be impossible for it to do very much in the way of harm. The homoeopathic physician of the older school was intent upon amplifying the energy of his medicines, so that the energy that was released in the bodies of his patients would act as a sounding keynote that would aggravate every symptom in the body to such an extent that it would result in the neut-

ralization of the disease particles or entities within the body. The homoeopathic physician is dealing with energy only. In serology, the practitioner
is using gross amounts of material that, in themselves, are highly dangerous
to the human body, to say nothing of the fact that these materials are
injected hypodermically into the body, which is not a natural way of
putting anything into such a highly complicated machine.'

There is no doubt that as far as medication is concerned the homoeopathic treatment of acute infectious diseases once these have developed
is highly successful, but homoeopaths have always contended that their
remedies can also be used to give protection and confer immunity in
advance. If this is so it is highly important that it should be more widely
realized and publicised. The anti-vaccinationists would find their task very
much easier if they could be in a position to point to an alternative by
which the protection which the various vaccines and serums are designed
to afford can be harmlessly provided in another way. In this connection
it may be noted that there does appear to be some tendency among
modern orthodox immunologists, without perhaps understanding what
they are doing, to move somewhat in the direction of homoeopathy,
both in respect of dosage or attenuation and method of administration
(per mouth), and perhaps in other ways too. If this is so it would be a
great advantage if this movement could become more rapid and more
conscious.

It should be noted, however, that it is the Nature Cure contention that
the fever and bacterial action which takes place in acute diseases are
constructive and useful and in some cases are the only means by which
pathogenic substance in the body can be broken down and eliminated.
If this is so, it would seem doubtful whether it is desirable to try to produce
an absolute immunity to all infectious diseases, even if it is possible to
do so. It would appear that the protection which one would hope to
afford by a nosode or other homoeopathic remedy would be relative
rather than absolute and that it would work by causing the body to
make a favourable reaction to an infection rather than to be unaffected
by it. The ultimate aim of Nature Cure as set forth by Lindlahr is to
produce a condition of health so perfect that immunity will naturally
arise. Meanwhile the aim must be to combat disease conditions by
methods which are eliminative rather than suppressive and homoeopathy
is one of these methods. In the process of treatment of this kind crises
will inevitably arise and, if rightly dealt with, will be helpful and beneficial,
but the wise physician will work to bring about improvements by lysis
rather than by crisis so far as this is possible.

APPENDIX III

PARASITISM

If we accept the biochemical or Nature Cure theory of acute disease it necessitates a complete change in generally accepted views of the relation of micro-organisms to disease and an abandonment of the belief in the parasitic character of most disease processes. But if the bacteria which are found in most forms of acute disease are in fact scavengers rather than parasites, it still appears that parasitism is a common natural phenomenon which provides an explanation for a number of diseases. Infestations of lice, worms and flukes and such diseases as scabies have the appearance of being genuinely parasitic and similar in character to certain parasitic diseases met with in animals and plants. However, though parasitism does exist there is much evidence that it is rarer in its pure form than is supposed and that it is much less destructive, meaningless and one-sided than it appears to be. Healthy animals in the wild state would not usually seem to be infested with parasites to any great extent, though they may tend to become so when they grow old or ill. In man it has been found possible by homoeopaths and Nature Cure practitioners to treat parasitic diseases successfully without making any direct attempt to destroy the parasite. In other words it has been found that the presence and activity of the parasite are dependent on the condition of the host. Lindlahr gives many instances of cases in which the activity of the parasites was clearly a benefit to the host and in which the parasites disappeared as mysteriously as they had come when their work had been done. It has also been found that plants grown on impoverished soil or soil manured and cultivated in an unnatural way are very prone to "parasitic" disease, but that plants grown on scientifically prepared soil are almost or entirely free from it. Sir Albert Howard, the pioneer of organic agriculture, writes as follows:— "The evidence in favour of the view that disease resistance in plants and animals depends on soil fertility is also considerable ... Insects and fungi are not the real cause of plant diseases, and only attack unsuitable varieties of crops which are imperfectly grown. Their true role in agriculture is that of censors for pointing out the crops which are imperfectly nourished. Disease resistance seems to be the natural reward of healthy and well-nourished protoplasm ... In regard to animal diseases my experience in India was very similar. For twenty-one years I was able to study the reaction of well fed animals to the epidemic diseases such as rinderpest, foot and mouth disease, septicaemia, and so forth, which frequently devastated the countryside. None of my animals was segregated; none was inoculated; they frequently came in contact with diseased stock. No case of infectious disease occurred. The reward of well-nourished protoplasm was a very high degree of disease resistance which might even be described as immunity." Though there is still much to be discovered before the phenomena of parasitism can be fully understood and explained, it is safe to contend that parasitism, like everything else in nature, has a purpose and a meaning and that parasites are playing a definite part in the general scheme of things. It will also be found that even when dealing with "parasitic" diseases it is generally best to treat the patient rather than the disease, and that the parasite will disappear when the conditions which make its activity possible cease to exist. It may be noted that much interest is now being shown in biological methods for the control of pests in order to avoid the use of poisonous substances which contaminate air, soil, water and crops. It is also being recognized that both in the animal and the vegetable world affinities and symbioses exist which are of benefit to both of the parties concerned.

APPENDIX IV

SOIL AND SEED

by Lady Eve Balfour

(formerly Organizing Secretary of the Soil Association)

If nutrition is a cycle — a flow of vitalized materials from the soil and back to the soil again — then it must be studied as a whole and any specialised study of the part must be recognised as a study of the part. Its relation to all other parts must never be lost sight of. Given that our major contention is correct, we may in fact be led seriously astray if we attempt to diagnose cause and effect, in any manifestation of living organisms, without taking into consideration their relationship to this wider whole. It is therefore of great practical importance to discover if this cycle is purely hypothetical, or if it exists in fact.

I have recently come across strong supporting evidence for its existence in a summarised report, by Dr. F. M. Pottinger, of a feeding experiment on cats, printed in the American Journal of Orthodontics and Oral Surgery, Volume 32, No. 8, August, 1946. The experiment extended over 10 years and involved 900 animals.

The main purpose was a comparison between cooked and raw food, though there were various sub-divisions using different combinations, such for instance as groups of cats fed on raw meat with pasteurised milk, and others on cooked meat with raw milk. The animals who received an all-raw food diet, both milk and meat, remained healthy and bred normal healthy litters from generation to generation, while all those of which cooked food formed the major portion of the diet, whether this were meat or milk, became progressively degenerate through succeeding generations. For example 25% of abortions occurred in the first generation and 70% in the second. The animals also fell prey to a varied range of diseases, all listed in the report, and in many cases by the third generation the kittens had become so degenerate that they failed to survive for six months. A further experiment with different kinds of milk produced the same result. The raw milk fed cats remained healthy and bred normally from generation to generation, while all those fed on other forms of milk suffered from increasing degrees of sickness, degeneration and skeletal malformation in this order — pasteurised milk, evaporated milk, and sweetened condensed milk. In later experiments cats whose general metabolism had been deranged by the cooked food were returned to a raw food diet. Complete regeneration, where it was not too late to achieve this, took four generations. This is a striking parallel to the experience of organic cultivators with plants.

Now here is the part of these experiments which particularly concerns farmers and gardeners. "After we performed these experiments," says the report, "the pens in which all these animals were housed lay fallow for several months. Weeds sprang up in each pen. The fact that the weeds grew so luxuriantly in the pen which housed the raw meat and raw milk fed animals, as compared with those which grew in the other pens, led us to perform another experiment.

This experiment consisted of planting two kinds of beans in each pen, and the report contains a photograph showing these beans growing in four pens previously occupied by cats fed on the four milk diets mentioned above, namely raw milk, pasteurised milk, evaporated milk, and sweetened condensed milk. The growth of the crops followed exactly the same pattern as the health of the cats, and was in the same order, vigorous healthy beans in the raw milk pen, less good in the pasteurised, very poor in the evaporated and practically no growth at all in the sweetened condensed milk pen.

The report ends with this extremely significant statement: "The principles of growth and development are easily altered by heat and oxidation, which kill living cells at every stage of the life process from the soil, through the plant and through the animal. Change is not only shown in the immediate generation but as a germ plasm *which manifests itself in subsequent generations of plants and animals.*

The important point about these experiments is not the evidence that heat kills living cells, we knew that already, but that devitalised food, fed to an animal, could start a train of malnutrition that continued to manifest its effects right round the cycle, for when the food was devitalised, not only did the cats which fed on it become devitalised, but the soil to which their excreta was returned was able to produce only devitalised plants. Vital living food on the other hand produced vital healthy cats whose excreta in its turn produced vital soil capable of producing vigorous healthy plants. From this fact it seems to me that we must draw the conclusion that plants can only reach their maximum vitality when grown in fully vitalised soil, and that soil can only reach its maximum vitality when it is fed with the waste products of fully vitalised

312

plants and animals, for one thing is very certain, we cannot create vitality in a laboratory.

Is it surprising then that we set up a vicious circle when we first feed our soil on the lifeless product of the factory; then subject the weakened plants that result to every kind of life destroying poison powder and spray; then feed them to our livestock — often further devitalised by heat processing — and finally partake ourselves of food derived from such plants and animals, usually still further devitalised by various methods of sterilization or processing?

It is against this destructive vicious circle that the ever growing numbers of organic cultivators are in revolt. They endeavour to substitute for it an ever mounting spiral of increased fertility by seeking to operate the nutrition cycle in the opposite and creative direction, fostering the living principle in all its phases. This is why they lay such stress on growing their own seed, or buying it only from other organic cultivators. It is why, too, they endeavour as far as possible to feed their livestock and themselves on their own produce, for they know that soil, seed and animals, and their waste products all go together and that maximum health and vitality, with the disease resistance that goes with it, cannot be built up in one generation, or from good seed alone.

Many examples exist to confirm the truth of this. Here are two. In a letter to "Mother Earth" the journal of the Soil Association, (Spring 1949), Mrs. Mann writes: "I cultivate on compost lines, but also attempt to go a stage further and use the Steiner Bio-Dynamic methods. As one result, we have succeeded in producing, by five years' effort, tomato seed which retains disease resistance even if planted among other tomato plants attacked by red spider, mildew, etc. I have also received already excellent reports from growers concerning stamina, quality and quantity of crop. I think the main point of interest here is that the quality of our seed was developed without selection or hybridization, and thus resulted from environmental influences alone; and these were transmitted through the seed, not necessarily as a result of treatment given to the plants it produced. I had reports from people who had used neither compost, nor any organics for that matter. They had houses that were riddled with tomato diseases — and my seed produced healthy plants. This rather confirms my view that a healthy plant has active selective capacity, which our methods of cultivation and selection tend to suppress."

This shows that stamina, built up through the integration of living soil and seed for several generations, can overcome adverse environmental conditions, at any rate for one generation.

My next example illustrates the same rule in the opposite sense. On the Soil Association stand at the Royal Show in 1949 we had several growing plots. One of them was barley. The bed was divided into three, the two outside plots were both composted and the centre plot received nothing. Half the bed was sown with barley grown for five generations on the organic section of the Haughley Research Farms, and the other half with barley of the same original stock, but grown for five generations on the chemical section of the farm. The line of demarkation between these two lots of seed came in the middle of the untreated plot.

The bed was deturfed on April 8th and the barley sown on April 9th. Acute drought conditions set in immediately afterwards and a serious wireworm attack followed. When I saw the bed in May I was doubtful if there would be a crop at all by July, but at my next visit at the end of June, this is what I saw:—

At the half-way division, clear through the middle of the untreated part of the bed, one could see, to a line, where the compost-grown seed stopped and the chemically-grown seed started. Not only was the former taller and generally more robust, but it had, in large measure, thrown off the wireworm attack — whereas the chemically-grown seed had succumbed to an extent of over 50% of the plants, even on the composted plot. By the time the Royal Show opened, the contrast was even more marked.

Here once again were seed and soil operating together in the previous life history of the plant. Well composted soil could not, by itself, in one generation, enable the crop, raised for five generations on devitalised soil, to withstand the wireworm attack, while the crop from the same original seed, raised for five generations on a vital soil did so, even on the untreated plot.

One of our visitors to the Royal Show, after seeing this demonstration, told me the following story: There were two fields near together; one had been treated organically for some time and the other chemically. The crop on the chemically treated field suffered very badly from a wireworm attack. A count was taken and the wireworm on this field were found to be 2,000,000 to the acre. A count was then also taken in the neighbouring organically treated field, where no signs of wireworm damage was visible. Here the count was no less than 5,000,000 to the acre!

It is thus not the presence of the pest or disease organism that matters, so much as the vitality of soil, plant and animal.

We have thought too long in terms of destruction as the only remedy for the ills that beset us. Kill, burn or poison, is the advice we get, more often than not, if we seek it in official circles. It is the advice of despair. Let us try for a change the constructive approach, and endeavour to build vitality and natural resistance through the operation of the nutrition cycle. It will get us further.

APPENDIX V

The following is an extract from a communication by Dr. John B. Fraser to the Canada Lancet, June 1916 (vol. 49, no. 10, p. 447), with regard to certain experiments carried out by him:

The reasons for questioning the germ theory are mainly three, viz.:

1. The divergent views of bacteriologists as to which germ caused the disease.

2. The stronger claim of the bio-chemic theory.

3. The absence of germs at the onset of disease (as the following sample cases show).

    a. A man crossing a river broke through the ice, was rescued, later became ill, and the doctor fearing pneumonia, tested for pneumo-cocci — there were none present; when the pneumonia developed they appeared.

    b. After an oyster supper some men had cramps and diarrhoea, followed by typhoid fever — no Eberth bacilli were present in the first stools but were present later.

    c. Hurrying, a girl arrived at her shop sweating; as the shop was cold, she became very chilly, next day complained of a sore throat, but no Klebs-Loffler bacilli were found; later, when a diphtheritic patch appeared, the bacilli were present.

Here in each case the bacilli followed the onset of the disease. Believing that the above germs were the result and not the cause of the diseases, tests of the germs of diphtheria, typhoid and pneumonia were made.

The first test was whether the Klebs-Loffler bacilli would cause diph-theria, and about 50,000 were swallowed without any result; later 100,000, 500,000 and a million and more were swallowed, and in no case did they cause any ill effect.

The second series of tests was to decide whether the Eberth bacillus would cause typhoid, but each test was negative; even when millions were swallowed. The third series of tests showed that one could swallow a million (and over) pneumo-cocci without causing pneumonia, or any disturbance.

The investigations covered about two years, and forty-five (45) different tests were made giving an average of fifteen tests each.

I personally tested each germ (culture) before allowing the others to do so; and six persons (3 male, 3 female) knowingly took part in the tests and in no case did any symptom of the disease follow.

The germs were swallowed in each case, and were given in milk, water, bread, cheese, meat, head-cheese, fish and apples — also tested on the tongue.

Most of the cultures were grown by myself — some from stock tubes furnished by Parke, Davis & Co., and one tube furnished by the Toronto Board of Health through one of their bacteriologists.

As the tests were carefully made, they prove that there is not the danger from germs that bacteriologists claim; they also may stimulate other Canadians to undertake further experimental work, for the actual test on man decides the truth of the theory.

REFERENCE INDEX

ABSCESSES—product of inflammation, 58; in appendicitis, 92; treatment, 92.
ACID—uric acid diseases, 171, 208; cell waste acid, table, 207; neutralized, 208; composition of, 210; Dr. Haig on uric acid diseases, 209; uric acid, how precipitated, 211; results of precipitation, 212; effect of stimulants, 212-213; treatment of acid diseases, 214; role in body, 215; acidity during healing crisis, 217; acidity of urine, 217.
ACTION AND REACTION—acute reactions, 20; law of, 44; of drugs, 155-157; of water, air, 157; in homoeopathic treatment, 181; 184.
ACUTE DISEASE—definition of, 9, 19.
ADENOIDS—eliminating organs, 60; removal of, 117-119.
ADHESIONS—curable by natural treatment, 123.
AFFIRMATIONS—positive, 284; constructive, 298.
AFTER EFFECTS—of drug or ice treated typhoid, 77; of surgical operations, 83; of wrongly treated appendicitis, 94; of vaccination, 98-100, 113-114; of vaccines, serums, shown in eye, 102; of vaccination, a case, 103-104; of vaccination, epilepsy, a case, 104-105; of vaccination, diphtheria, 106; anterior poliomyelitis from vaccination, 107-108; of diphtheria antitoxin, 111-112; of diphtheria do not occur under natural treatment, 113; of removal of tonsils, 118-119; of curetment of womb, 122; of womb operations, 125-126; of extirpation of wen, 136; of suppression of eruptions, 135; of laxatives, 155, 156; harmful after effects of manipulative suppression of fever, 251.
AIR BATHS AND LIGHT—in chronic diseases, 157.
ALCOHOL—stimulates by paralysis, 223-226; effect on mind, 226; effects of, 227.
ALKALOIDS—poisonous, 60; of putrefaction, 137; diagram 207.
ALLOPATHY—inconsistency of theory and practice, 42, 165; use of poisons, 43; mistakes effect for cause, 44; treatments suppressive, 45; treatment of venereal disease, 51; interpretation of inflammation, 55; has adopted natural treatment for typhoid, 78, 169; conception and handling of appendicitis, 85; treatment of diphtheria, 111; treatment of tonsilitis 117; treatment of leucorrhoea, 122; treatment of prolapsus, 124; treatment of climacteric, 127-128; confirmation of our theories as to the cause of chronic diseases, 134; chronic means incurable, 141; treatment makes and keeps the chronic, 141; lays more stress on diagnosis than treatment, 142; treats symptoms as disease, 145; defence of drugs, 155; use of digitalis, 156; forced to adopt natural methods, 168; Dr. Osler on Medicine, 168-169; legitimate scope of medicine, 170; inorganic minerals and poisons harmful, 174; action of allopathic dose of belladonna, 180; view of high blood pressure, 217.
ANAESTHETICS—encourage indiscriminate operations, 80; beneficial and destructive effects of, 80; has inflicted more wounds than has healed, 80.
ANIMAL—unreliability of experiments on, 70; dogs cured of cancer, 135; kingdom, what controlled by, 201; instinct, 201; elements in, 205; difference between man and animal, 274.
ANTERIOR POLIOMYELITIS—caused by vaccination, 107.
ANTHRAX—67, 70.
ANTISEPTICS—confirmation of our theories from the battlefields of Europe, 13; use in leucorrhoea and birth control, 122;
ANTITOXINS—natural and allopathic, 57; diphtheria, effects of, 111; for prevention, 112; effects shown in eye, 113.

317

APPENDICITIS—allopathic description and treatment, 85; foreign bodies in appendix, 86; true cause of, 89; prevention of, 90; treatment of acute, 91; abscesses, 92; case of, 93; after effects, 94.
APPENDIX—foreign bodies in, 86; uses of, 87; a case, removal, 94.
ARTERIOSCLEROSIS—after effect of mercury, 52; from excess of salts, 206; from excess of pathogen, 209, 213; curable by natural treatment, 217.
ATOMS—composition of, 13; vibration, 24; positive and negative, 197.
AURA—pale in nervous temperaments, 191; cause of, visible only during waking hours, 256; colours of, 256; experiments to make visible, 260.

BACTERIA—not cause of disease, 9; originate from microzymes, 10, 65, 68, 36; thrive in diseased organisms only, 37; secondary cause of disease, 11, 39; found in healthy bodies, 38; inability of to create disease, 39; why epidemics, 38; immunity by right living, 39; test by Dr. Rodermund in smallpox, 39; action of serum and antitoxins, 41; arrest of, 57; development of microzymes into, 61; Pasteur's theory of, 66; morbid soil necessary to growth, 69; not cause but effect of disease, 69; diphtheria bacteria how developed, 106.
BÉCHAMP—theory of microzymes, 9-14, 62; discovery of microzymes, 66; "The Blood", organic matter, 172,200.
BELLADONNA—homoeopathic use, 181.
BIRTH CONTROL—means and results, 122.
BITES—snake and insect, 40.
BLOOD—normal and abnormal composition, 31; pathogenic obstruction, 62; proportion of white and red corpuscles, 64; contamination by vaccines, 101; root of cancer in, 135; "The Blood" quotation from, 172; what chemical composition depends on, 188; precipitation of uric acid into, 211; high blood pressure produced, 211; composition of, 215; cause and cure of high blood pressure, 217; high blood pressure curable by natural treatment, 217; charged with positive mineral elements, 254; flow controlled by will-power, 259.
BRAIN—effect on of operations on genital organs, 126; effects of stimulants on, 226; construction of, 227; most powerful electro-magnetic battery in the body, 255.
BRANDT, DR.—on water treatment of typhoid fever, 169.
BREAD—white constipating, 89; whole grain action of, 90.
BRIGHTS DISEASE—how caused, 210.
BROMIDES—benumb and paralyze brain and nerve centres, 48.

CALCULI—must be dissolved by rendering blood alkaline, 193; from accumulation of pathogen, 206,209.
CANCER—Dr. Senn on, 50; psora cause of, 135; as result of wen removal, 136; experiments of Dr. Ross, 136; relation of meat eating to, 138; experiments on mice, 133; radium and X-ray for, 133.
CARBON—compounds, 200.
CATARRH—of genital organs, 122.
CAECUM—description, use, 87.
CELLS—origin of microzymes, 10; composed of microzymes: 13; permanent cells of adult present in procreative cell, 13; life requirements of, 28; health and disease resident in, 30; germinal, 35; nutrition of, 61; elimination from, 62; not structural unit of life, development and division, microzymes of, 67; health of, 69; in chronic disease, 146; needs of, 147; interference with activity of cells creates disease, 148; dose for, 182; cell nutrition, composition, waste, diagram, 206; are negative, 254; cell system, 255; cell protoplasm is hydrogen plus negative substances, 254, see Microzymes.
CHEMICAL—processes of health and disease, 205; chemical substances disease producing, 206; chemical composition of tissues affected by mental and emotional conditions, 254.
CHILD—creation and rearing in accord with natural law, 17; disease heredity, 35; hereditary taints shown in the eye, 35; diseases, 49; prenatal influences, 232; need of sex instruction, 233.
CHIROPRACTIC—definition of, 238; school of adheres to allopathic idea of acute disease, 250; theory of fevers, 250; harmful effects of chiropractic suppression of

318

fever and other crises, 251.

CHRISTIAN SCIENCE—in appendicitis, 92-93; argument of, 218; faith without works is dangerous, 267; a case, 268; limitations of, 271; dangers of, 288; see also Metaphysical Healing.

CHRONIC DISEASE—definition of, 19; cause of, 50; confirmation of Nature Cure theories of origin, 134; time to cure, 139; must pull the roots, 140; should chronic be left to fate, 141; natural treatment only hope of chronic, 141; treatment of, 145; caused by suppression of acute disease, 146; relation of cell life to, 146-149; why meat has bad effect, 149; cold water and manipulative treatment for, 149; air and light baths, exercise, right mental attitude, 150; healing crises, 154; do we fail, 158; law of crises dominates cure of, 159; healing crises periodicity, 160; law of sevens in, 164; why many not cured, 166; causes of uric acid disease, 171; many caused by drugs, 177; importance of natural diet, 177,188; fasting in, 192; why healing crises necessary in, 208; acid diseases, 208; why metaphysical healers cannot cure, 266, 272.

CINCHONISM—see Quinine.

CIVILISATION—Senn on diseases of, 50; artificiality of, cause of, 50.

CLEANLINESS—health is, 148.

CLIMACTERIC—Change of Life, see Women's Ailments.

CLOTHING—unhygienic, 124.

COFFEE—effect on uric acid condition, 212; paralysing effect on nervous system, 224; effects of stimulation, 225; effect on mind, 226.

COLD—catching a, 73; cause of, 74; cure of, 74.

COLLEMIA—60, 212.

COMPRESSES—see Packs.

CONGESTION—see Inflammation.

CONSTITUTION—three-fold constitution of man, 278-281; diagram of, 278.

CONSTRUCTIVE—principle in nature, 18; natural treatment in conformity with, 20; thoughts, 283; affirmations, 298.

CONTAGION—safety from if in good condition, 39; explained, 69.

CORPUSCLES—white, see Leucocytes; electric, 199.

CRISES—healing, definition of, 20; disease, 20; lice, 49; childhood diseases, 49; elimination of drugs, 53; healing crises as eruptions in natural treatment of cancer, 135; healing crises essential to cure of chronic disease, 140, 153; healing and disease crises described, 152; healing crises properly conducted not fatal, 154; law of crises, 158; Swedenborg on crises of soul, 158; periodicity of, 160; Friday periods, 162; should not fear healing crises, 162; the law of sevens in febrile diseases, 164; in chronic diseases, 164; character and approach of healing crises shown in eye, 165; former symptoms appear in healing crises, 165; how many, 166; healing crises often accompanied by depression, 167; homoeopathy and the law of crises, 181; fasting in, 190; time for fasting, 194; why necessary in morbid conditions, 208; acidity during, 216-217; called by chiropractors "retracing", 245; effect of treatment of crises, 250-251.

CURE—definition of, 20; general application, 42; unity of, 55; in metaphysical healing, 266.

CURETMENT—of womb destructive, not curative, 122.

DAIRY—products, composition of milk close to red arterial blood, 188.

DANDRUFF—caused by elimination of systemic poisons through scalp, 48.

DEANE, DR. TENISON—"Crime of Vaccination", 113.

DESTRUCTIVE PRINCIPLE—definition of, 18; disease conforms to, 25;

DIAGNOSIS—from the eye see Iridiagnosis and prognosis, 142; Allopathy lays more stress on diagnosis than treatment, 142; cure more important than diagnosis in Nature Cure, 142; our method more thorough, 143; from eye of great interest and importance, 144.

DIARRHOEA—effect of suppression by opiates, 48.

DIETETICS—function of natural, 31; wrong diet cause of appendicitis, 89; white bread constipating, 89; action of whole grain bread, 90; use of salt, 176; importance of natural diet, 177; natural diet based on the composition of milk, 188; allopathic mistakes in, 188; necessity for vegetarian diet, 189; negative vegetarian diet, 192; positive and negative foods, 199; meat not necessary for animal magnetism, 202;

FEAR—and the germ theory, 37.
FERMENTATION—life a succession of, 23; cause of, 67.
FEVER—see Inflammation; chiropractic theory of, 250; harmful effects of suppression by manipulative treatment, 252.
FOOD—see Dietetics; and food and drink in themselves cannot convey life-force, 220-222; see Life-Force.
FRUITS—seed-bearing fruit not cause of appendicitis, preventive of, 90; juice as drink in diphtheria case, 115; are neutralizing and eliminating, 189, 193; juice in fasting, 194; are acid reducing, 216.
FUNCTIONAL—disease, 242, 270; see Disease.

GASTRITIS—acute, treatment of by neurotherapy, 249.
GENITAL ORGANS—curetment of, 122; extirpation, case of gonorrheal infection, 123; prolapsus and displacement of, 124; inflammation of cured by natural treatment, 124; prolapsus may prevent conception, 124; results of operations in later pregnancies, 126; cutting in the brain, 126.
GERMS—originate from microzymes, 10, 64-65; see Bacteria.
GLANDS—function of spleen and lymphatic, 60; engorgement of, 62; effect of massage on, 64; effect of removal of thyroid and spleen, 81; of Lieberkuhn, 88; tonsils, use, removal, etc., 117.
GONORRHOEA—see Veneral Disease.

HABITS—how to overcome bad habits and acquire good ones, 296-297.
HAHNEMANN—134, 183.
HAIG, DR.—on uric acid poisoning, 209.
HARDENING OF ARTERIES—see Arteriosclerosis.
HARMONICS—relation with life, 18; established harmonic relations, 25; of health, 32; 278-281.
HEADACHE POWDERS—paralyze brain, results of use, 45.
HEALING CRISES—see Crises.
HEALTH—definition of, 19, 25; positive, 29, 199, 205; resident in cell, 30; relation of thought to, 71.
HAEMORRHOIDS—chronic after-effects of suppression, 146.
HEREDITY—new light on, 13; and acquired disease taints, 29; disease tendencies, 35; in cancer, 134, 137; of abnormal sexuality, 232.
HIGH BLOOD PRESSURE—see Blood.
HIPPOCRATES—42; on law of Periodicity in Crises, 160; quotation from Encyclopaedia Britannica, 160.
HISTORY—of Nature Cure, 15.
HOMOEOPATHY—medicines, 174, 180; how prepared, how act, 180; belladonna, 180; high potency dose, 182; and law of crises, 184; economics of, 185; complement of Natural Therapeutics, 185.
HOOF AND MOUTH DISEASE—news item, 100; government agent on, 102; natural treatment of, 103.
HUMAN BODY—a unit, 82; elements in, 205; body great electric battery, 254.
HUME E. DOUGLAS—"Life's Primal Architects", 10; quotations, 70.
HYDROTHERAPY—effects in acute disease, 116; fear of cold water, 139; why we use cold water, 139; how cold water acts in chronic disease, 149, 156.
HYPNOTIC—control by fasting, 191; difference between hypnotic process and magnetic treatment, 253.
HYPNOTISM AND OBSESSION—228; destructive, 253.

ICE—suppression by, 75; after effects of ice treated typhoid, 77.
IMMUNITY—natural, 36, 38; antitoxin for, 111.
INDIGESTION—resulting from wrong treatment of typhoid, 77.
INFECTION—see Contagion.
INFLAMMATION—suppressed by serums, antitoxins, 41; constructive tendencies of, 55; orthodox interpretation of, 55; Nature Cure interpretation of, 59; diagram, 57; Powell's Theory, 59; old theory reversed, 61; suppression of first two stages, 72; suppression of third stage, 75; suppression of fourth and fifth stages, 77; of genital organs cured by natural treatment, 123; is eliminative, 55; luxations of bony separate structures may be caused by, 249.

321

INHIBITORY NERVOUS SYSTEM—224; paralysed by stimulants, 224.
INTESTINES—action of, 87; danger spot in, 88; case of operation on, 94; effect of suppression of haemorrhoids, 145; effect of laxatives, 155.
INORGANIC MINERALS AND POISONS—175; salt, 175, difficult to eliminate, 176.
INSANITY—from operation on genital organs, 126; during climacteric, 126.
INSOMNIA—suppressed by sedatives, 45; cure by relaxation, 293-294.
IODISM—secondary cause of disease, 29.
IRIDIAGNOSIS—proofs by, 53; typhoid or lymphatic rosary, 77; results of vaccines traced by, 102; after effects of vaccination, a case, 103; showing epilepsy after vaccination, a case, 104; signs of vaccination, 105; effects of antotixin in eye, 112; itch spots (psoric), 134; not depended on alone but of great importance, 144; proves poisons accumulate in the system, 170, 175, 176.
IRIS—see Iridiagnosis.
ITCH—see Psora.

KIDNEYS—salts eliminated through are neutralised acids, 206.
KOCH—postulates contradicted, 67.

LAHMANN—experiments in re sweating, 157.
LAW OF ACTION AND REACTION—see Action and Reaction.
LAW OF COMPENSATION—basic law of universe, 257; see Action and Reaction.
LAW OF DUAL EFFECT—see Action and Reaction.
LAW OF SEVENS—see Periodicity.
LEUCOCYTES—11; allopathic explanation of, 56; Powell's theory of, 60-62; explanation of granular and nucleated appearance and amoeboid motion, 63; decrease of, 64; standard of, 65.
LEUCORRHOEA—cause of, 122; allopathic treatment of, 122.
LICE—see Parasites.
LIFE—conceptions of, 23; elements, 199; vitamins, 203; positive mineral elements carriers of life elements in lower kingdom, 203; force 209, 221; symphony of, 276; force in human organism transmuted into electromagnetism and vito-chemical energy, 283; see also Vital Force.
LUETIC DISEASES—see Venereal Diseases.
LUXATIONS—see Spinal Manipulation.
LYMPH—abnormal composition of, 28, 31; nodes condense pathogen, 61.
LYMPHATIC—glands, functions of, 60; swelling in tuberculosis, 62; signs in iris, 77.

MAGIC—modus operandi of white and black, 184.
MAGNETIC—treatment, how administered, 253, 261; difference between magnetic treatment and hypnotism, 253; magnetic healer does not attempt to control will-power, 253; treatment does not deplete power of operator, 257; operator must have faith, will and sympathy, 257; history of magnetic healing, 260; treatment for poor circulation, 262; experiment to test strength of magnetic emanations, 262; magnetised water, 262; sympathy healing, 263.
MAGNETISM—what is it, 198; in re life force, 209; effects in massage, 252.
MALASSIMILATION—resulting from wrong treatment of typhoid, 77.
MALNUTRITION—resulting from wrong treatment of typhoid, 77.
MALIGNANT—see Cancer and Tumours.
MANIPULATIVE TREATMENT—internal, Thure Brandt, 125; in chronic disease, 150; see Spinal Manipulation and Massage.
MARRIAGE—Relations, 232.
MASSAGE—action of, 64; Thure Brandt, 125; internal stimulation secured by, 250; effects of, 252; electromagnetic effects of, 252; more positive the operator the more positive the effects, 252.
MASTURBATION—see Onanism.
MATTER—and vital force, 23-24; influence of mind over, 32.
MacEWAN, DR.—opposes removal of appendix, 87.
MEAT—sale of vaccine calves for meat, 102; composition of meat and effects of eating, 189; effect on uric acid condition, 212-213.
MEDICINES—are they in conformity with natural treatment, 21; Osler on, 168;

Nature Cure regarding, 170; Tissue Remedies, 172; medicinal remedies, 173; homoeopathic, 174; minerals and poisons used by allopathy, 174; stimulating effects of, 226.

MENSTRUATION—see Women's Ailments.

MENTAL—states, influence of, 32; importance of mental state in cure of chronic disease, 150; therapeutics cannot correct bony lesions, 248; healing not modern, 264; healing, 265, 282; healing, limitations of, 271; three-fold constitution of man, 278; conditions affect composition of tissues and secretions, 283; also see Emotions.

MERCURY—secondary cause of disease, results of, 51,52,53; how it acts, 45.

METAPHYSICAL HEALING—21, 218; nihilism, 265; healing from within, 265; self control the whole law, 266; cures, 266; faith without works dangerous, 267; a case, 268; ideal of the faith healer is the ideal of the animal, 269; limitations, 271; dangers of, 288.

METCHNIKOFF—theory of bacteria, 59; contemporary of Béchamp, 66.

METHODS OF TREATMENT—see Treatment.

MICROORGANISM—see Bacteria.

MICROZYMES—explanation of heredity, 35, 62; develop into bacteria in morbid soil, 61; discovery of, 66; create wild cells, 137; necessary to produce live, organised foods, 172; digestive ferments produced by, 173; size of dose for, 182; development into bacteria, 208.

MILK—standard for natural dietetics, 188.

MILK SCURF—see Eruptions.

MIND—errors of mortal, 26; effects of stimulants on, 226; and soul, 273; the player, 279; two-fold attitude of the mind and soul, 273; see Mental.

MINERALS—substances must be in live organised form, 171; vegetable extracts, how prepared, 172; difference between organic and live organised, 172; inorganic, 174; use of salt, 175; difficult elimination of inorganic minerals, 175; structure of, 200; positive mineral elements carriers of life elements to lower kingdom, 203.

MOUTH BREATHING—cure of, 118-119.

MORAL REGENERATION—Swedenborg, 158.

MORBID MATTER—bacteria product of, 9; accumulation of interferes with cell drainage and nutrition, 28; soil for bacteria, 36; see Microzymes; accumulation of from meat eating, 189; product of cell and food metabolism, 208-212.

NAPRAPATHY—definition of, 238; school adheres to allopathic idea of acute disease, 250.

NATURAL DIETETICS—see Dietetics.

NATURAL LAW—violation of, cause of disease, compliance necessary to overcome, 26;

NATURAL THERAPEUTICS—definition of includes Nature Cure, see Announcement; value of spinal manipulation from viewpoint of, 248; each method of treatment supplemented by all others, 249; see Nature Cure.

NATURE—return to, 29; not a poor healer, reliable, 166; orderly and intelligent in repair, 166; law of polarity or sex in, 198; four kingdoms of, 199.

NATURE CURE—history of, 15; definition of, 18; included in Natural Therapeutics, see Announcement; of venereal diseases, 51; of inflammation, 57; of suppressed pneumonia, 75; treatment of typhoid adopted by allopathy, results of, 78, 169; operations obviated by, 82; viewpoint of appendicitis, 85; in Germany and America, 114; of tonsilitis, 119; of gonorrhoea, 123; of disorders of genital organs, 123; during climacteric, 127; of cancer, 135; nature cures cancer, a case, 135-136; Natural Therapeutics only system that combines all that is good in healing, 140, 222; why achieves results, only hope of chronic, 141; diagnosis not important, 142; diagnosis most thorough, 142; helps nature remove disease, 145; treatment of chronic diseases, 149-151; do we ever fail, 158; correctness of methods proved by crises, 165-166; allopathy adopting methods of, 168; position regarding medicines, 170; treatment, foods and remedies, vegetable extracts, 172; use of homoeopathic remedies, 174, 180; importance of natural diet, 177; homoeopathy, complement of, 185; how it works, 290; why not more generally accepted, 296.

NEGATIVE—disease is, 29,197, 205; electrons, 198; what is negative, 199; food, 199; quality of sex, 203; producing diet, 205; cell waste negative, 206-207.

NERVOUS SYSTEM—223; motor, inhibitory, sympathetic, 223-224; inhibitory paralysed by stimulants, 224; manipulative stimulation of, 250; action of, 285.
NERVOUSNESS—from operations, 126.
NEUROPATHY—definition of, 238.
NEUROTHERAPY—in chronic diseases, 150; definition of, 239; aims at results other than correction of lesions, 249; treatment in acute gastritis, 249.

OBSESSION—see Hypnotism.
ONANISM (MASTURBATION)—cause of, 231; effects of meat eating, 233; effects of, 234; how to regenerate, 235; parents should warn children, 236.
OPERATIONS—see Surgery.
OPSONINS—11, 66, 57.
ORGANIC—difference between organic and live organised, 172, 200; difference between organic disease and functional, 270-272; disease—see Disease.
ORGANISED—live organised form of mineral salts, 171, 200; difference between organised and organic forms, 172, 200.
OSLER, Sir WILLIAM—on medicine, 168-170.
OSMOSIS—62.
OSTEOPATHY—definition of, 237; school adheres to allopathic idea of acute diseases, 250.

PACKS—in appendicitis, 91; in smallpox, 108.
PARALYSIS—of brain by bromides, 48; caused by diphtheria antitoxin, 111-112; by suppression of haemorrhoids, 146; stimulation caused by, 223.
PARASITES—head lice, 48; suppression, crises, 49; suppression of, 134; removing head lice, 135.
PASTEUR—9, 11; germ theory, 66-71.
PATHOGENIC—bacteria product of pathogenic conditions, 9; Powell's theory verified by records of our patients, 12,64; obstruction starts inflammation which develops microzymes into bacteria, 12; theory of inflammation, 59.
PATHOGEN—lymph nodes condense, 60; producing diet, 205-206.
PERIODICITY—the law of sevens, 160; taught by Hippocrates, 160-161; Pythagoras on matter, 161; Friday periods, superstitions relating to, 161; should not fear crises periods, 162; law of sevens applied to individual life, 162; law of sevens in febrile diseases, 164; in chronic diseases, 164; Nature Cure methods proved by crises, 165-166.
PERITONITIS—natural treatment, 92.
PERSPIRATION—see Sweating.
PHAGOCYTES—Powell's theory of, 11; allopathic explanation, 56; theory of inflammation, 59; see Leucocytes.
PHAGOCYTOSIS—Powell's theory of, 11; allopathic theory, 56; facts opposed to, 62; see Leucocytes.
PNEUMONIA—suppression by ice, 75; natural treatment, 76.
POLARITY—29; health is satisfied polarity, 33; law of, 198; of substance, and life elements, 199; sexual, 203; mental and emotional, 203; psychical, 203.
POSITIVE—health is, 29, 197, 205; what is, 199; food, 199; mineral elements, carriers of life elements in lower kingdom, 203; quality of sex, 203; the more positive the masseur the better effects of massage, 252; affirmations, 284.
POTENCY—high potency doses of drugs, 180; are they effective, 182.
POWELL, DR. THOMAS—pathogenic theory, 11; theory of inflammation, 59; earlier statement in Nature Cure literature, 59; on leucocytes, 63.
PRAYER—must be backed by right living, 280; how shall we pray, 288; right way to pray, 289.
PREGNANCY—effects of intercourse during, 231.
PRIESSNITZ—founder of Nature Cure, 15.
PROTOPLASM—cell, 206-208.
PSORA—soil for parasites, 49; internal cause of cancer, 134; suppression of, sign in eye, 134; eruptions in natural treatment of cancer, 136.
PSYCHISM—abnormal induced by fasting, 191, 192; psychic polarity, 203.
PTOMAINES—60.
PURGING—artificial, first and permanent effects, 155, 156.

PUS—composition of, 56.
PYTHAGORAS—theory of numbers, 24; taught law of crises, 160; on composition of matter, 198; "primordial substance" of Pythagoras, 199.

QUININE—symptoms and elimination of, 53; allopathic effect of, 185.

RADIUM—in cancer, 133.
REACTION—see Action.
REASON—benumbed by stimulants, 224; benumbed by hypnotism, 228; has taken the place of instinct, 269.
RELAXATION—by neurotherapy treatment, 250; scientific, 292; while working, 293; before sleeping, 294.
RHEUMATISM—fasting in, 192; caused by morbid deposits, 206, 211; effect of coffee and meat on, 212; arthritic stage, 213.
RODERMUND DR.—experiment with smallpox exudate, 39.
ROSS DR. H. C.—experiments in cell proliferation, 136-137.

SALT—use of, 175.
SALTS—neutralised acids, too much formed, 205; diagram, 207; role in body, 215.
SALVARSAN (606)—iodides, etc., effect of in venereal disease, 52.
SCHEUSSLER—"Tissue Remedies", 172.
SCROFULA—a secondary cause of disease, 29.
SCURVY OR SCORBUT—cause of, cure, 176; on German raider, cause of, 218.
SEDATIVES—dual action on brain and nervous system, 45.
SELF-CONTROL—the master key, 26; effect of fasting on, 195; benumbed by hypnotism, 228; the whole law of healing, 266; strengthening of, 296.
SENN, DR. NICHOLAS—on cancer, 50.
SEPTIMAL LAW—see Periodicity.
SEQUELAE—see After Effects.
SERUMS—suppressive, 57; see also Vaccines.
SEX—law of, 198; sexual polarity, 203; indulgence not necessary to health, 232; need of sex instruction before marriage, 232; marriage relation, 232; effect of meat eating, 233; need of sex instruction for child, 233.
SKIN—Elimination of neutralised acids through, 206.
SMALLPOX—experiment by Dr. Rodermund, 39; natural immunity, 99; beneficial effects of under natural treatment, 108; case in author's family, 108; see also Vaccination.
SOUL—life element, 200; twofold attitude of mind and soul, 273; soul the harmonics, 279; powers of developed by use, 288; spiritual love highest vibratory activity of, 257.
SPINAL MANIPULATION—history of, 237; osteopathy, 237; chiropractic, 238; naprapathy, 238; spondylotherapy, 238; neurotherapy, 239; anatomy of spine, 239; mechanics of the skeleton, 240; spinal lesions and their causes, 241; nature and effects of lesions, 242; detection of lesions, 244; structural analysis, 244; corrections of lesions, 244; value of curative gymnastics in restoring normal curves, 246; relation of neurotherapy to other methods of healing, 246; cannot make good for an unbalanced diet, 248; luxations may be caused by inflammatory conditions, 249; chiropractic theory of fevers, 250; harmful effects of suppression by, 251; properly applied is helpful in acute disease, 251.
SPIRITUAL—life element, 200; life active in body after death in physical body, 209; institution for healing should be centre for spiritual power, 258.
SPLEEN—see Glands.
SPONDYLOTHERAPY—definition of, 238; see also Spinal Manipulation.
STIMULANTS—effect on nervous system, 224, 226; effect on mind, 228.
ST. VITUS DANCE—caused by removal of tonsils and adenoids, 119.
SUPPRESSION—of inflammation by serums, 41; conventional treatment of acute diseases is suppression, 47; of diarrhoea, venereal diseases, etc., 48; of children's diseases, 49; the cause of chronic diseases, 50, 145; cases of, 51; of inflammation, 57; results of, during first stages of inflammation, 72; results of, during third stage of inflammation, 75; by ice, 75; of last stages of inflammation, 77; after effects of drug or ice treated typhoid, 77; of diphtheria, 112-113; by surgical treatment of tonsilitis and adenoids, 117-119; of colds, etc,. result in catarrhal

condition of genital organs, 121-122; of psora, cause of cancer, 134; of haemorrhoids causes paralysis, 146; of fever, by chiropractic, harmful effects of, 251.

SURGERY—promiscuous surgery not constructive, 21; suppressive, 47; length of life after operation, 47; results of use of anaesthetics, 80; when indicated, 80; extirpation not cure, 80-81; removal of thyroid and spleen, 81; effect of major operation, 82; Zone Therapy in relation to, 83; after effects not immediately manifest, 83; on genital organs, 83; warning against operations by surgeon, 87; dangers of operation in appendicitis, 92; removal of haemorrhoids and appendix, a case, 94; removal of tonsils and adenoids, effects of, 117-119; curetment of womb, 122; treatment of prolapsus of genital organs, 124; results of womb operation in later pregnancy, 126; effects of on brain, 126; in cancer not cure, 133.

SWEATING—Dr. Lahman, experiments, artificial, natural, 157.

SWEDENBORG, EMMANUEL—quotation, 158.

SYCOTIC ERUPTIONS—see Eruptions.

SYMPHONY—of life, 276.

SYPHILIS—see Venereal.

TAINTS—disease, hereditary, 35; see also Disease.

TEA—why injurious, 213; see also Disease.

THURE BRANDT MASSAGE—125.

THYROID GLAND—See Glands.

"TISSUE REMEDIES"—see Schuessler, inorganic, 172.

TONSILITIS—surgical treatment of, effect, 117-119; prevention and cure, 119.

TONSILS—eliminating organs, 60; removal of, 117; use of, 117-118; effects of removal, 118.

TREATMENT—constructive and destructive, 20, 21; unity of, 29, 55; natural methods, 29; allopathic treatment of appendicitis, 85; natural treatment of appendicitis, 90-91; natural treatment of hoof and mouth disease, 102-103; natural treatment of smallpox, 108; surgical treatment of tonsils and adenoids, 117; natural treatment of tonsilitis, 119; natural treatment of woman's ailments, 125; natural treatment in chronic diseases, 149-151; natural treatment of acid diseases, 214; neurotherapy treatment of acute gastritis, 249.

TUBERCULOSIS—62.

TUMOURS—caused by curetting, 123; caused by pessaries, 125; Dr. Ross's experiments, 137.

TYPHOID FEVER—after effects when drug or ice treated, 77; rosary, 77; allopathy adopted natural methods of treatment, results of, 78; fasting in, 194.

UNIT—human body, a, 82.

UNITY OF CURE—see Treatment.

UNITY OF DISEASE—see Disease.

URIC ACID—see Acid.

URINE—acidity of, 217.

VACCINATION—discovery of, 96; does it exterminate smallpox? does it protect? 97; after effects, 97; effect on mammary glands, 98; produces acute and chronic disease, 99; after effects, a case, 103; epilepsy caused by, a case, 104; signs in eye, 105-106; diphtheria caused by, 106; anterior poliomyelitis caused by, 107; cause of diphtheria, 113.

VACCINES—what they contain, 100; responsible for hoof and mouth outbreak, 100; manufacture of, 101; calves producing vaccine sold for meat, 102; results of shown in eye, 102; government agent on hoof and mouth disease, 102.

VEDIC TEACHING—71.

VEGETABLE—extracts, how prepared and administered, 172; negative vegetable diet, 192; kingdom, 200; diet and animal magnetism, 202.

VEGETARIAN DIET—see Dietetics.

VENEREAL DISEASES—gonorrhoeal discharges and syphilitic ulcers suppressed, 48; effects of suppression of, 51; cured by natural methods, 51; from vaccination, 98, 100; case of gonorrhoeal infection, 123.

VIBRATION—and life, 24; in health and disease, 33; four ranges of vibration control kingdoms of nature, 199; mechanical electrical vibration too coarse for human bodies and treatment of disease, 255; vibratory quality of aura constitutes repulsion or attraction, 256; spiritual love highest vibratory activity of the soul, 257; of magnetic healer must be harmonious, 257; constructive, destructive, 276; emotional, 282.

VIOLATION OF NATURE'S LAWS—see Natural Law.

VITAL FORCE—definition, 23; economy of, 29, 209; not derived from food and drink, when vital force leaves body at death, production of vital energy ceases, 255.

VITALITY—lowered, 28, 29, 220; to increase, 222; reserve, 223; storing of during sleep, 224.

VITAMINS—meaning of, 203.

VITOCHEMICAL—life element, 200, 202; vitochemical energy from life force, 254.

WATER—treatment, see Hydrotherapy.

WHITE BLOOD CORPUSCLES—see Leucocytes and Phagocytes.

WILL POWER—benumbed by stimulants, 224; benumbed by hypnotism, 228; strengthening, 296; can control electromagnetic energies and blood flow, 286.

WOMAN'S AILMENTS—primitive woman exempt from, abnormal menstruation result of, 121; leucorrhoea caused by, 122; birth control, 122; curetment of womb, 122; extirpation of organs not cure, natural treatment can cure, 123; case of gonnorrhoeal infection, 123-124; prolapsus and displacement of genital organs, 124; unhygenic clothing, 124-125; pessaries, 125; natural treatment, 125; result of womb operation in later pregnancy, 125-126; climacteric, cause of disturbances accompanying, 126; menses, 127; climacteric under allopathic treatment, 128.

WOMB—see Genital Organs.

XANTHINS—what are they, 60.

X-RAY—in cancer, 137.

YEAST GERM—experiment of Béchamp, 10, 57. See also Germ.

ZONE THERAPY—relation to surgery, 83.